eHEALTH APPLICATIONS

eHealth Applications: Promising Strategies for Behavior Change provides an overview of technological applications in contemporary health communication research, exploring the history and current uses of eHealth applications in disease prevention and management. This volume focuses on the use of these technology-based interventions for public health promotion and explores the rapid growth of an innovative interdisciplinary field.

The chapters in this work discuss key eHealth applications by presenting research examining a variety of technology-based applications. Editors Seth M. Noar and Nancy Grant Harrington summarize the latest in eHealth research, including a range of computer, Internet, and mobile applications, and offer observations and reflections on this growing area, such as dissemination of programs and future directions for the study of interactive health communication and eHealth.

Providing a timely and comprehensive review of current tools for health communication, *eHealth Applications* is a must-read for scholars, students, and researchers in health communication, public health, and health education.

Dr. Seth M. Noar is an Associate Professor in the School of Journalism and Mass Communication and a Member of the Lineberger Comprehensive Cancer Center at the University of North Carolina at Chapel Hill. His research addresses health behavior theories and message design, mass media campaigns, eHealth applications, and methodological topics, including meta-analysis and evaluation.

Dr. Nancy Grant Harrington is a Professor in the Department of Communication and Associate Dean for Research in the College of Communications and Information Studies at the University of Kentucky. Her research focuses on persuasive message design in a health behavior change context, particularly as it relates to risk behavior prevention/health promotion and interactive health communication using computer technology.

ROUTLEDGE COMMUNICATION SERIES

Jennings Bryant/Dolf Zillmann, Series Editors

eHEALTH APPLICATIONS

Promising Strategies for
Behavior Change

Edited by Seth M. Noar and
Nancy Grant Harrington

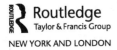

Routledge
Taylor & Francis Group

NEW YORK AND LONDON

First published 2012
by Routledge
711 Third Avenue, New York, NY 10017

Simultaneously published in the UK
by Routledge
2 Park Square, Milton Park, Abingdon, Oxon OX14 4RN

Routledge is an imprint of the Taylor & Francis Group, an informa business

© 2012 Taylor & Francis

The right of Seth M. Noar and Nancy Grant Harrington to be identified as the author of the editorial material, and of the authors for their individual chapters, has been asserted in accordance with sections 77 and 78 of the Copyright, Designs and Patents Act 1988.

Library of Congress Cataloging in Publication Data

eHealth applications : promising strategies for health behavior change / edited by Seth M. Noar and Nancy Grant Harrington.
  p. ; cm. — (Routledge communication series)
Developed from a pre-conference at the 2010 Kentucky Conference on Health Communication.
Includes bibliographical references.
I. Noar, Seth M. II. Harrington, Nancy Grant. III. Kentucky Conference on Health Communication (2010 : Lexington, Ky.) IV. Series: Routledge communication series.
[DNLM: 1. Health Communication—methods—Congresses. 2. Health Promotion—methods—Congresses. 3. Cellular Phone—Congresses. 4. Internet—Congresses. 5. Medical Informatics—methods—Congresses. 6. Video Games—Congresses. WA 590]
610.285—dc23   2011041240

ISBN: 978-0-415-88817-2
ISBN: 978-0-415-88818-9
ISBN: 978-0-203-14909-6

Typeset in Bembo
by Apex CoVantage, LLC

To Eva—for your spark, your sweetness, your silliness, and
most of all . . . your love. And to Elisa . . . for everything
SMN

To Troy—for your constant support, patience, and love
NGH

We dedicate this volume to Marci Campbell, who spent her
career tirelessly developing innovative eHealth applications
and making them accessible to those most in need
SMN, NGH

CONTENTS

FOREWORD

Allow me to outline a brief history of eHealth research:

- *Frustration* with the status quo.
- *Prediction* that computers were going to play an increasing role in our lives.
- *Research* using eHealth approaches.
- *Dissemination* into health care, employer, school, and government sectors.

Yes, *frustration* was an early motive for eHealth, stemming from a growing awareness that other approaches to population-based behavior change were largely ineffective (e.g., mass media), had very low potential to reach large populations (e.g., individual or group therapy programs), or were costly (e.g., telephonic coaching). This triad—efficacy, reach, and low cost—has always been essential to population-based behavior change initiatives; it's also what makes these efforts so vexing. By the late 1990s, the historic period of the Internet's emergence, eHealth seemed to offer a solution to this Rubik's Cube.

It didn't take a rocket scientist to *predict* that computers were going to play an increasing role in our lives. It's only recently, however, that most researchers and practitioners in our field have paid much attention to the emergence of interactive communications technologies, digital biometric devices, and computerized health records. As a result, the research community failed to keep up with the real world. Filling the void through the early 2000s were Wild West snake oil salesmen with online pamphlet racks and crude search engines. The paucity of research attention kept the bar for the quality of eHealth programs very low while also minimizing the potential value of these programs.

Much has changed since the early 2000s. This book by Seth Noar and Nancy Harrington provides evidence that we responded to the unprecedented changes in health and communications technologies with a significant, if not vast, amount of relevant *research* in this emerging field. *eHealth Applications: Promising Strategies for Behavior Change* not only tells us where we stand today but provides direction for our future.

In the real world, the snake oil salesmen are going away. Practitioners from health care organizations, employers, schools, and government are increasingly aware of, and demanding, an evidence base for eHealth products. Expectations for efficacy, reach, and low cost from eHealth programs are becoming more realistic, and there is a growing understanding of the challenges that require resolution. Also important, the research community is recognizing the potential contributions of commercial efforts, particularly from the current superhighways of new media such as Facebook and Google.

Noar and Harrington have assembled all the right pieces of the eHealth puzzle. An early chapter presents a detailed history of the eHealth field. To minimize the repetition of old mistakes, understanding this history is essential, although it's often unknown to new researchers and practitioners in the field. This book also contains entire chapters focusing on elements fundamental to eHealth, including interactivity, tailoring, gaming, social media, and avatars. Other chapters focus on the communications technology of eHealth, including the Internet, mobile devices, and interactive voice response (IVR). A number of chapters provide an understanding of how these eHealth elements and technologies may be applied to specific public health problems, including chronic illness, sexually transmitted disease, cigarette smoking, weight management, and many other problems.

Finally, this book also addresses the *dissemination* of eHealth. While dissemination is perhaps not as sexy as other chapter topics, allow me to put this as subtly as I can: Chances are good that your new killer health app will fail. It won't fail because the app wasn't killer, it will fail because you didn't bother to read the chapters related to policy and dissemination. The authors of these chapters recognize and clearly discuss the issues involved in adoption, implementation, and maintenance of innovative technologies. Dude, dudette (female version of "dude"—check Wikipedia), read these chapters.

The eHealth research and practice communities aim to help individuals make better decisions about their health and then to help these individuals act on their decisions through lasting behavior change. This book represents a milestone in this endeavor, demonstrating that the eHealth bar is now higher, with an expectation for more engaging, innovative products; more published evidence; more useful theory; greater assurance of privacy; and better dissemination to those in greatest need.

It's exciting to watch highly talented researchers and practitioners move this field forward. The unprecedented rate of change in the eHealth field and the ages of its innovators often have me feeling that if I can't get out of the road, I should lend a hand.

I'm here to lend a hand. I hope you are as well.

Victor J. Strecher
Professor and Director of Innovation and Social Entrepreneurship,
University of Michigan School of Public Health

ACKNOWLEDGMENTS

We would like to thank the Kentucky Conference on Health Communication (KCHC) Planning Committee for letting us run with this idea for the KCHC 2010 preconference. We thank the Department of Communication at the University of Kentucky for sponsoring KCHC, and we especially thank Phil Palmgreen for his support of this project. We also thank UNC's Lineberger Comprehensive Cancer Center for their support. We acknowledge the excellent contributions of the chapter authors and their responsiveness to our suggestions. Special thanks go to Amber Williams and Nick Iannarino for their very careful editorial work on the chapters and index and Leticia Mazon for help with the index. Finally, we thank Linda Bathgate for her wonderful support and encouragement throughout the entire project.

PREFACE

The world is changing ever so rapidly, and perhaps the best example of this is the rapid growth and evolution of computer and media technologies. Such advances are nothing short of revolutionary in many areas, with examples including the changing nature of the news industry, the ways in which we shop for goods and services, and the ways in which we communicate with one another. Moreover, it seems difficult to remember a time when terms like "Facebook," "YouTube," and "iPhone" were not a part of our common lexicon, even though each of these was developed well within the past decade.

For those of us interested in health communication, new technologies provide a wealth of opportunities for innovative health promotion and disease prevention efforts. Whereas traditional health communication efforts have tended to be interpersonal (e.g., face-to-face counseling) or mediated by traditional media (e.g., print, radio, television), technologies such as the Internet and mobile devices are opening up new doors for innovative health communication efforts. Indeed, there is much excitement surrounding these developments—and for a number of reasons. Compared to more traditional health promotion approaches, these newer technologies may be capable of delivering health content that is more (1) individualized, interactive, and multimedia capable; (2) convenient, accessible, appealing, low cost, and disseminable; and (3) standardized, flexible, and automated (Fotheringham, Owies, Leslie, & Owen, 2000; Robinson, Patrick, Eng, & Gustafson, 1998; Strecher, 2007). For these reasons, such technological applications are increasingly being developed, implemented, and evaluated, with reviews of this literature showing much promise (Fjeldsoe, Marshall, & Miller, 2009; Murray, Burns, See, Lai, & Nazareth, 2005; Noar, Black, & Pierce, 2009; Portnoy, Scott-Sheldon, Johnson, & Carey, 2008).

Recognizing these important changes in the technology and media land-scape, and in particular the implications for health communication, we organized a technology-focused preconference for the 2010 Kentucky Conference on Health Communication (KCHC). The focus of this preconference was specifically on the application of innovative technology to behavior change interventions. Several top speakers were brought in to present on technology application in areas such as Internet-based interventions, mobile programs, health video games, and virtual agents. In addition, a number of local speakers from the faculty of the Department of Communication at the University of Kentucky, who were conducting related work, also spoke. At the end of the day, a roundtable discussion and dialogue with the audience ensued regarding the application of technology for health communication and behavior change.

The current volume was borne out of the preconference. Indeed, during the process of organizing the KCHC preconference we came to realize that a volume bringing together the wealth of research on these interactive applications did not exist. While edited volumes have appeared in this general area, none has brought together a collection of work that focuses on these technologies as applied to public health promotion and health behavior change. An older edited volume focused on interactive technology and health (Street, Gold, & Manning, 1997), but this volume is largely dated now. Previous edited volumes on the Internet and health communication (Rice & Katz, 2001) have focused primarily on health information and clinical applications on the Internet. Finally, a new volume on new media and health has its major focus on clinical applications and health care (Parker & Thorson, 2009). Thus, recognizing an important gap that we believed we could help fill, we decided to undertake the task of putting together the current edited volume.

This volume is intended to be a sourcebook for the use of health communication technologies/applications for health promotion and health behavior change. One collective term used earlier on in the literature for such technologies is *interactive health communication,* which is defined as "the interaction of an individual—consumer, patient, caregiver, or professional—with or through an electronic device or communication technology to access or transmit health information or to receive guidance and support on a health-related issue" (Robinson et al., 1998). As we discuss in our opening chapter, this term has largely been replaced by *eHealth,* which is defined as "the use of emerging information and communication technology, especially the Internet, to improve or enable health and health care" (Eng, 2001, p. 1). While in some cases terminology in this field is still emerging and evolving (e.g., *mHealth* is now used to refer to mobile health), it is clear that eHealth has quickly become the term to describe this compelling and quickly growing interdisciplinary field. While the current volume is thus focused on eHealth applications, we give a great deal of attention to what was recognized early on as a key defining aspect of those applications—*interactivity.*

The current edited volume focuses on eHealth applications and includes a range of chapters covering computer, Internet, and mobile applications for promoting health behavior change. Its focus is primarily on using these technology-based interventions for public health promotion and disease prevention. The purpose of this volume is to (1) provide an overview of eHealth applications, including their history and conceptual bases; (2) feature chapters on research examining a variety of eHealth applications, including a range of computer, Internet, and mobile applications; and (3) address key issues related to practice, policy, and dissemination of eHealth programs and conclude with observations and reflections on this important and growing research terrain.

This volume is likely to be of interest to many audiences, and it has been written and edited to make it as accessible as possible for diverse audiences. Given the inter-, multi-, and trans-disciplinary nature of this area, this volume will be relevant to several disciplines, including communication, public health, psychology, nursing, medicine, education, sociology, and anthropology, among others. A host of researchers, practitioners, and students interested in and/or currently conducting work on technology and health communication will likely find the current volume of interest. Indeed, it is our hope that the book is useful to researchers and students at a variety of universities, institutes, centers, and agencies and to practitioners working in a variety of contexts, including government agencies, community agencies, health clinics, and other settings.

In terms of chapter structure, contributing authors were asked to cover several areas relevant to their eHealth application. These areas included definitions of the application along with illustrative examples, target populations to which the application has been applied, theoretical bases for the application, contexts in which the application has been applied, effects that the application has demonstrated, dissemination potential for the application, advantages of their particular eHealth application, and limitations of the application and future directions for research. This "outline" was used to ensure that chapter contributors covered what we believed to be key elements, and it also provided some structure for authors and comparability across chapters for readers. At the same time, we strove to give some flexibility to authors so that their own unique voices could be heard throughout the chapters (and so that the chapters would not feel too formulaic).

Beyond the specific eHealth application chapters, we also include chapters that provide important background and context. The volume begins with a chapter on the history of eHealth applications (Bull, this volume), followed by in-depth coverage of the concept of interactivity and its importance to health behavior change (Chung, this volume). Given the increased focus on implementation and dissemination research at the National Institutes of Health and elsewhere, we include a chapter focused on dissemination of eHealth applications (Rabin & Glasgow, this volume). Related to this, those researchers interested in moving eHealth applications from research to practice need to be attuned to the policy environment and understand how it affects such applications, so the book includes a chapter on policy issues related to eHealth applications (Baur, this volume). Finally, we end the book with a chapter that reflects on the authors' contributions; discusses key research, practice, and policy issues that cut across eHealth as an emerging field; and paves the way for future dialogue, debate, dissemination, and inquiry into eHealth applications.

Our hope is that by covering the growing research terrain in eHealth in one volume, we will contribute to a broader conversation about the utility of eHealth for health promotion and disease prevention. Ultimately, we believe that the exciting work being conducted in this area has the potential to advance the health of individuals and communities in the United States and in countries worldwide. A careful understanding of the history, applications, research trajectories, dissemination issues, and policy environment that comes from this volume will hopefully bring us closer to increasing the engagement of many populations with effective eHealth applications.

Seth M. Noar
University of North Carolina at Chapel Hill
Nancy Grant Harrington
University of Kentucky

References

Eng, T. R. (2001). *The eHealth landscape: A terrain map of emerging information and communication technologies in health and health care.* Princeton, NJ: Robert Wood Johnson Foundation.

Fjeldsoe, B. S., Marshall, A. L., & Miller, Y. D. (2009). Behavior change interventions delivered by mobile telephone short-message service. *American Journal of Preventive Medicine, 36*(2), 165–173.

Fotheringham, M. J., Owies, D., Leslie, E., & Owen, N. (2000). Interactive health communication in preventive medicine: Internet-based strategies in teaching and research. *American Journal of Preventive Medicine, 19*(2), 113–120.

Murray, E., Burns, J., See, T. S., Lai, R., & Nazareth, I. (2005). Interactive health communication applications for people with chronic disease. *Cochrane Database of Systematic Reviews, (Online)*(4), CD004274.

Noar, S. M., Black, H. G., & Pierce, L. B. (2009). Efficacy of computer technology-based HIV prevention interventions: A meta-analysis. *AIDS, 23*(1), 107–115.

Parker, J. C., & Thorson, E. (2009). *Health communication in the new media landscape.* New York: Springer Publishing Co.

Portnoy, D. B., Scott-Sheldon, L. A. J., Johnson, B. T., & Carey, M. P. (2008). Computer-delivered interventions for health promotion and behavioral risk reduction: A meta-analysis of 75 randomized controlled trials, 1988–2007. *Preventive Medicine, 47*(1), 3–16.

Rice, R. E., & Katz, J. E. (2001). *The Internet and health communication: Experiences and expectations.* Thousand Oaks, CA: Sage.

Robinson, T. N., Patrick, K., Eng, T. R., & Gustafson, D. (1998). An evidence-based approach to interactive health communication: A challenge to medicine in the information age. *Journal of the American Medical Association, 280*(14), 1264.

Strecher, V. J. (2007). Internet methods for delivering behavioral and health-related interventions (eHealth). *Annual Review of Clinical Psychology, 3,* 53–76.

Street, R. L., Gold, W. R., & Manning, T. (1997). *Health promotion and interactive technology: Theoretical applications and future directions.* Mahwah, NJ: Lawrence Erlbaum Associates.

Historical and Conceptual
Foundations

1

eHEALTH APPLICATIONS

An Introduction and Overview

Seth M. Noar and Nancy Grant Harrington

The Case for Behavior Change

The twenty-first century has begun with major health challenges both in the United States and worldwide. While for decades the advancement of medical technologies and therapies has led to extension of life and enhanced quality of life, a significant number of chronic health problems continue to ail societies because of their root behavioral causes. For example, in the United States, the five leading causes of death are heart disease, cancer, stroke (cerebrovascular disease), diabetes, and chronic obstructive pulmonary disease (Jemal, Ward, Hao, & Thun, 2005). Although genetic factors contribute to many of these diseases, several analyses indicate that human behavior also contributes significantly (Danaei et al., 2009; McGinnis & Foege, 1993; Mokdad, Marks, Stroup, & Gerberding, 2004). In fact, one analysis suggests that *half* of all annual deaths in the United States are due to preventable causes, with the largest contributing factors being smoking, poor diet, and physical inactivity (Mokdad et al., 2004). Other exacerbating factors include alcohol consumption, exposure to microbial and toxic agents, motor vehicle crashes, incidents involving firearms, unsafe sexual behaviors, and illicit use of drugs (McGinnis & Foege, 1993; Mokdad et al., 2004). A World Health Organization (WHO) report also identifies many of these same behavioral factors as significant contributors to disease worldwide (World Health Organization, 2008).

As a case in point, the spread of HIV/AIDS continues to have no medical solution, with behavioral risk reduction in relation to sexual behavior and drug use being key strategies for prevention. While biomedical strategies are becoming a significant component of future prevention efforts (Coates, Richter, & Caceres, 2008), biomedical strategies also often require behavioral change. For instance, the International AIDS Conference in Vienna in 2010 reported results of a groundbreaking research trial in which a microbicide was successful in reducing transmission of HIV/AIDS by 39%. This microbicide is a topically applied gel that contains an antiretroviral drug that prevents HIV infection from replicating in the body, allowing a person's immune system to expel the virus before it takes hold. Such news is very promising because these results, if replicated, will lead the way to a development that has eluded researchers for decades: a safer sex method that *women* can control and use. However, just because a medical product ultimately comes to market does not mean it will be widely adopted. Will people *want* to use this new product, particularly high-risk populations? If people do use the product, will they use it *correctly*? Will the fact that it is *not* 100% effective deter its use? How can this new product be promoted effectively? Finding answers to these questions will require behavioral and health communication research (De Wit, Aggleton, Myers, & Crewe, 2011).

The behavioral data and examples above suggest that even in a world with sophisticated medical technologies, effective approaches for changing health behavior are still greatly needed. Reducing smoking-related illnesses, reversing the upward trend of diseases that result from poor diet and physical inactivity, and ending the HIV/AIDS epidemic will all require persons, couples, families, groups, and communities to make behavioral changes. In order to understand how to effectively accomplish these changes, research examining a host of approaches to health communication and health behavior change is necessary.

Changing Health Behavior: A Health Communication Perspective

The study of health behavior change spans many disciplines and decades, and several recent volumes have documented the diversity of approaches taken and lessons learned (DiClemente, Crosby, & Kegler, 2009; Glanz, Rimer, & Viswanath, 2008; Hornik, 2002; Shumaker, Ockene, & Riekert, 2009). Given the important role that communication plays across so many contexts, the critical role of the *health communication* field has been increasingly recognized (Bernhardt, 2004; Freimuth & Quinn, 2004; Kreps & Maibach, 2008). *Healthy People 2010* defines *health communication* as "the art and technique of informing, influencing, and motivating individual, institutional, and public audiences about important health issues" (Healthy People 2010, 2000, p. 11). Bernhardt fused this definition with a definition of *public health* to arrive at the term *public health communication,* which is defined as "the scientific development, strategic dissemination, and critical evaluation of relevant, accurate, accessible, and understandable health information communicated to and from intended audiences to advance the health of the public" (p. 2051). These conceptual foundations all contribute to the perspective taken in the current volume: the central role of health communication in promoting healthy behavioral changes among a host of diverse audiences. Thus, a guiding question is the following: How can we develop, implement, evaluate, and disseminate health communication programs that are both efficacious and reach large proportions of the intended audience?

While the above question seems like a simple one, the answer has been elusive. Communication researchers have long noted that while interpersonal communication approaches are the most persuasive (but have the lowest reach), mass communication approaches achieve the greatest reach (but traditionally have had low efficacy) (Rimal & Adkins, 2003). Similarly, public health researchers have recognized that impact on health behaviors and conditions is not only a function of *efficacy* but also one of *reach* (Abrams et al., 1996). To date, however, developing interventions that are capable of achieving both high efficacy and broad reach has been challenging. Also, recent work has criticized the traditional *phases of research* that are followed in most behavioral research (Glasgow, Lichtenstein, & Marcus, 2003). Most notably, several observers have noted that even when efficacy trials are successful, the efficacious interventions are rarely integrated into practice (Glasgow, Vogt, & Boles, 1999; Solomon, Card, & Malow, 2006). In addition to programs that work (*efficacy*) and for which broad exposure to and engagement with the target audience is possible (*reach*), a high priority is developing programs that can be successfully disseminated into practice (*translation*). Moreover, cost-effectiveness is also a critical part of the equation when we consider what programs have a real chance of being disseminated (Hutchinson & Wheeler, 2006; Strecher, 2007).

Computer Technology and Interactivity

The emergence of computer technology, which has advanced from personal computers to the Internet to fully functional mobile computers (i.e., smartphones), has brought with it immense opportunities for health communication and health behavior change. While interactive interventions were previously the sole territory of the interpersonal domain, computer technologies introduce the opportunity for interactivity in the absence of human interaction. The term *interactivity* has been the subject of much scholarship and has been defined in myriad ways (Bucy & Tao, 2007; Kiousis, 2002; Sundar, Kalyanaraman, & Brown, 2003; also see Chung, this volume). Observers have noted that interactivity can be defined and measured from the perspective of message exchange between users, structural attributes of a technology itself, or by perceptions of the user (Bucy & Tao). Kiousis reviewed the extensive literature and arrived at the following definition:

> Interactivity can be defined as the degree to which a communication technology can create a mediated environment in which participants can communicate (one-to-one, one-to-many, and many-to-many), both synchronously and asynchronously, and participate in reciprocal message exchanges... it additionally refers to their ability to perceive the experience as a simulation of interpersonal communication. (p. 372)

Similarly, Bucy and Tao (2007) took a comprehensive approach to the literature and proposed the following integrative definition: "Interactivity is conceptualized as technological attributes of mediated environments that enable reciprocal communication or information exchange, which afford interaction between communication technology and users or between users through technology" (p. 656).

These definitions make clear that interactivity takes place using communication technology; it involves an exchange of messages and/or information; and it mimics the experience of interpersonal communication. While research demonstrates that *perceived interactivity* is important (Kiousis, 2002), this variable is perhaps more accurately conceptualized as a *mediator* of the effects of interactivity (an objectively operationalizable, effects-independent variable) on attitude/behavior change (Bucy & Tao, 2007).

The relationship between interactivity and behavior change may be a significant one. For instance, Cassell, Jackson, and Cheuvront (1998), in their analysis of the persuasion literature, argue that interactivity is a necessary condition for behavior change. In particular, they argue that conditions necessary for persuasion to take place include that communication is *transactional,* meaning that the interaction allows for give and take of both persuader and target, and *response dependent,* in which a receiver-driven (rather than source-driven) process ultimately leads to the messages being viewed as more personally relevant. In another analysis, Street and Rimal (1997) discuss the promise of interactive media for health promotion. In a comparative analysis across several media types (including print and television), only interactive media scored high on interactivity, sensory vividness, networkability, and modifiability. Such an analysis highlights the fact that "new" media offer many more opportunities for interactive engagement than more traditional media.

Moreover, while computer technologies in and of themselves have created new opportunities for health communication, perhaps the most significant "game changer" has been the Internet. From a health communication perspective, the Internet has been described as a *hybrid* communication channel with the persuasive properties of interpersonal communication and the broad reach of mass communication (Cassell et al., 1998). Scholars have described interactive health communication programs, often delivered online, as a "revolution" in health and health care (Ahern, 2007; Kreps & Neuhauser, 2010). With the Internet as a delivery system, interactive health communication programs are now capable of reaching the majority of the North American, European, and Australian populace (Strecher, 2009), with access growing with each passing day.

Interactive Health Communication and eHealth

Recognizing that interactive health communication (IHC) was becoming a major force in health promotion, the Office of Disease Prevention and Health Promotion of the U.S. Department of Health and Human Services convened a Science Panel on Interactive Communication and Health in the late 1990s. The panel, made up of a multidisciplinary group of 14 experts, was given a mandate to "clarify major medical and public health issues raised by the rapidly growing field of communication technology" (Robinson, Patrick, Eng, & Gustafson, 1998, p. 1264). The panel conducted significant conceptual work in this area, meeting nine times over more than two years. They defined IHC as "the interaction of an individual—consumer, patient, caregiver, or professional—with or through an electronic device or communication technology to access or transmit health information or to receive guidance and support on a health-related issue" (Robinson et al., 1998, p. 1264). They made a distinction between IHC and the applications that deliver IHC, defining those as "the operational software programs or modules that interface with the end user. This includes health information and support websites and clinical decision-support and risk assessment software (which may or may not be online)" (Eng, Gustafson, Henderson, Jimison, & Patrick, 1999, p. 10). The panel also developed a reporting template for IHC applications (Robinson et al., 1998) and provided guidance on evaluation of IHC applications (Eng et al., 1999). Dissemination of information from this effort was achieved via a website (http://www.scipich.org), a full report (Science Panel on Interactive Communication and Health, 1999), and a special section of the *American Journal of Preventive Medicine* (volume 16, no. 1).

While IHC represents one of the earliest and richest conceptualizations of applications in the technology and health area, several other terms have also been used, including *interactive behavior change technology* (Glasgow, Bull, Piette, & Steiner, 2004), *new media health programs* (Abroms, Schiavo, & Lefebvre, 2008), *technology-based health promotion* (Bull, 2011), and *consumer health informatics* (Houston, Chang, Brown, & Kukafka, 2001). All of these terms come from different quarters and even different disciplines, and they represent applications that overlap a great deal with one another. Our database searches (of PsycINFO, Medline, CINAHL, Communication Abstracts, and Library, Information Science, and Technology Abstracts) conducted in May 2011, however, indicate that use of some of these terms is quite infrequent (e.g., *technology-based health promotion* had no citations and *interactive behavior change technology* had just three total citations). The use of other terms has been relatively steady but is not commensurate with the growth of the field. For example, use of the terms *interactive health communication* and *consumer health informatics* has been relatively steady since the mid- to late 1990s, with 74 and 94 *total* citations through 2010, respectively (see Figure 1.1). Although the use of these particular terms has remained steady (albeit at a low level), the field itself has expanded considerably during this time period (Bull, 2011; Kreps & Neuhauser, 2010; Strecher, 2009).

In contrast to these findings, searches for *eHealth* revealed 763 total hits and explosive growth in the use of this term over time (see Figure 1.1). While the year 2000 registered only 13 citations using this term, the most recent full year searched (2010) registered 136 citations (more citations in a single year than the *totals* for either *interactive health communication* or *consumer health informatics*). Moreover, several other developments indicate that *eHealth* is becoming the key term to represent this burgeoning field. A report released by the Office of Disease Prevention and

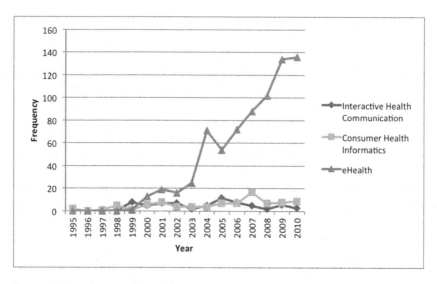

Figure 1.1 Database searches of three terms used to describe research in technology and health

Health Promotion in 2006, which essentially provided an "update" to the interactive science panel already described, replaced *interactive health communication* with the term *eHealth* (Office of Disease Prevention and Health Promotion, 2006). Also, some of the newest and most cutting-edge reviews of the field use this term (Cushing & Steele, 2010; Gerber, Olazabal, Brown, & Pablos-Mendez, 2010; Kreps & Neuhauser, 2010; Neuhauser & Kreps, 2010). Further, recent work focused on critical issues in this field, including health literacy (Bodie & Dutta, 2008), interactivity (Hawkins et al., 2010), user engagement (Lefebvre, Tada, Hilfiker, & Baur, 2010), methodological issues (Ahern, 2007), evaluation and dissemination (Curry, 2007; Glasgow, 2007; Strecher, 2007), and research agenda (Ahern, Kreslake, & Phalen, 2006; Jones et al., 2005) has all used the eHealth term. In fact, eHealth is now viewed as a field in and of itself, with much discussion regarding precisely how the term should be defined (Oh, Rizo, Enkin, & Jadad, 2005; Pagliari et al., 2005) and how such an interdisciplinary field can operate most effectively (Pagliari, 2007).

While terminology in the area of technology and health will no doubt continue to evolve (as exemplified by the even newer term *mHealth* or *mobile health* [Akter, D'Ambra, & Ray, 2011]), it seems clear at this juncture that eHealth has become *the* term that describes this rapidly growing interdisciplinary field. Definitions for eHealth (and mHealth) are presented in Table 1.1. Discussions of the eHealth field make clear that it covers a very broad set of health applications, interventions, and issues, including those impacting health information, behavior change/prevention, health self-management, online communities, decision

Table 1.1 Varying definitions for technology-based health communication programs

Term	Definition
Interactive health communication	"[T]he interaction of an individual—consumer, patient, caregiver, or professional—with or through an electronic device or communication technology to access or transmit health information or to receive guidance and support on a health-related issue" (Robinson et al., 1998, p. 1264).
Interactive health communication applications	"[T]he operational software programs or modules that interface with the end user. This includes health information and support Web sites and clinical decision-support and risk assessment software (which may or may not be online)" (Eng et al., 1999, p. 10).
Interactive behavior change technology	"[C]omputer-based tools and systems, including hardware and software, that can be used to address health behavior change" (Glasgow et al., 2004, p. 80).
New media (for health)	"[T]hose media that are based on the use of digital technologies, such as the Internet, computer games, mobile phones, and digital television" (Abroms et al., 2008, p. 3).
Consumer health informatics	"[A] subspecialty of medical informatics which studies from a patient/consumer perspective the use of electronic information and communication to improve medical outcomes and the health care decision-making process" (Houston et al., 2001, pp. 272–273).
eHealth	"[T]he use of emerging information and communication technology, especially the Internet, to improve or enable health and health care" (Eng, 2001, p. 1). "e-Health is a broad term for the heterogeneous and evolving digital resources and practices that support health and health care" (Office of Disease Prevention and Health Promotion, 2006, p. xi).
mHealth	"[T]he use of mobile communications—such as PDAs and mobile phones—for health services and information" (Akter et al., 2011).

support, disease management, and health care (Kreps & Neuhauser, 2010; Office of Disease Prevention and Health Promotion, 2006). The current volume focuses primarily on eHealth applications whose intent is to influence behavior change and, in some cases, to improve self/disease management, health information, and health care. The applications in this volume thus represent a subset of the broader literature on eHealth.

Advantages of eHealth Applications

A number of authors have written about the host of advantages of eHealth applications compared with more traditional health education and health communication approaches (Atkinson & Gold, 2002; Fotheringham, Owies, Leslie, & Owen, 2000; Neuhauser & Kreps, 2010; Rimal & Flora, 1997; Robinson et al., 1998). We summarize a number of these advantages in Table 1.2. As can be seen, such applications hold the promise of broad reach, wide appeal, convenient use, networkability, low cost, and the Internet as a delivery system. Such applications also contain several attributes thought to contribute to increased efficacy of health communication programs, including interactivity, multimedia, credible simulations, and individualized tailoring. Finally, eHealth applications hold advantages for both consumers (e.g., anonymity, convenience, low cost, increased access to information) and researchers (e.g., flexibility/modifiability, automated data collection). For these reasons, eHealth applications are increasingly being developed, applied, and evaluated (Murray, Burns, See, Lai, & Nazareth, 2005; Strecher, 2009).

Cautions Regarding eHealth Applications

While there is much excitement about eHealth applications, there is also reason to be somewhat cautious. First, while eHealth is relevant for and appealing to many populations, there may be some populations or subgroups for whom eHealth applications are not appropriate or not the best option. We need to avoid trying to make such applications fit populations that they simply may not fit, such as some segments of older populations or those with limited computer skills. Similarly, these kinds of applications may not be a fit for particular organizations or circumstances or may not be feasible in cases in which the cost of developing applications in the first place is prohibitive (Fotheringham et al., 2000). Second (and related to the first point), there are still issues related to access to the Internet. The digital divide still persists in some quarters, giving certain segments of the population an advantage when it comes to reliable and high-speed access to the Internet and thus to eHealth programs. Also, particular technologies that can deliver eHealth applications, such as smartphones, may only be accessible to those with the resources to procure such technology. Thus, we must ensure that disadvantaged populations, who are often most in need of health communication and health behavior change programs, are not left out of eHealth initiatives. Third, the ease with which eHealth applications

Table 1.2 Advantages of eHealth applications

Characteristic	Description
Anonymity	Programs can be used in an anonymous fashion, which may lead to increased reporting of sensitive behaviors and increased engagement with health communication programs
Automated data collection	Collection of data is built into the program and takes place effortlessly
Appeal	Particular applications (e.g., video games) hold appeal among certain audiences (e.g., youth), which may increase engagement in programs
Convenience/support on demand	User can interact with program whenever the need exists
Flexibility/modifiability	Ability to change and adapt program; relative ease of updating program, particularly with those programs that are online
Increased access to information	Particularly with online programs, opportunity for the user to access vast amounts of health information
Interactivity	Technological attributes of mediated environments that enable reciprocal communication or information exchange
Internet-driven delivery system	Use of the Internet as an intervention delivery system allows for broad access via desktop, laptop, tablet computers, and mobile devices
Low cost	Ability to use stand-alone programs or programs as adjuncts to other kinds of health efforts (e.g., interpersonal, mass media) can reduce costs; cost to deliver likely to be low once development is complete
Multimedia platform	Ability to use multiple forms of media, such as still images, video graphics, and sound files
Networkability	Programs online can be networked and can allow for connections with others, including other users, health educators, etc.
Simulated environment	Opportunity to role-play risky situations in a simulated environment without the possibility of harm
Tailoring potential	Ability of program to customize content to the individual, based on an assessment of the individual

can capture data, send them over a network, and deliver tailored content should give us pause. Several commercial websites (e.g., Google, Facebook) have drawn criticism for privacy concerns and questions regarding what uses of captured data are appropriate and inappropriate. Thus, there are privacy and data safety concerns that need to be carefully considered as we develop, test, and disseminate such applications. Fourth, we need to recognize that embracing eHealth means that we are moving toward a world in which health communication efforts are increasingly dependent on technology and technical support. Thus, long-term support for eHealth applications will be necessary, both because of technical difficulties that will arise and the fact that computer technology is constantly changing and thus requires frequent updates.

eHealth Applications and the Current Volume

There are a variety of ways to think about and categorize the literature on eHealth applications. We can consider that some of these applications, such as Internet-based interventions (Buller & Floyd, this volume), social media marketing (Taubenheim et al., this volume), some video games (Lieberman, this volume), and computer-tailored interventions (see chapter 8 of this volume) use the Internet for delivery and thus are "online" interventions. The remainder of applications covered in this volume, though, do not use the Internet and thus are "offline" interventions. While it is likely that offline applications will increasingly move to the Internet for delivery, there may still be contexts in the near term (e.g., doctor's office, community setting) where offline applications are entirely appropriate and useful.

Another distinction is portability. Some applications covered in this book are designed for mobile devices and thus can be accessed in more of an "on the go" fashion than others. These applications include mobile device interventions (Abroms, Padmanabhan, & Evans, this volume), text messaging interventions (Fjeldsoe, Miller, & Marshall, this volume), interactive voice response technology (Piette & Beard, this volume), and in some cases, social media interventions (Taubenheim et al., this volume). The remainder of applications covered in this book tend to be accessed on a personal computer, although with newer portable tablet computers such as the iPad, the distinction between mobile devices and personal computers may soon become somewhat blurred. Given the variety of options for eHealth application developers, what device to develop eHealth applications for is an important consideration. In making this decision, developers should consider the medium of "best fit" for their audience and for the behavior and the context in which the application will be used. Clearly, in some instances portability would be a major advantage (e.g., a mobile application in which a smoker could engage with his/her device whenever he/she gets the urge to smoke), while in others it is not necessary or could even be a hindrance (e.g., an application with a long assessment being more easily conducted on a standard computer than a mobile device).

Finally, there are applications that have more inherent entertainment value built into them, such as virtual agents (Miller et al., this volume), avatars (Fox, this volume), social media (Taubenheim et al., this volume), and video games (Lieberman, this volume). The other intervention types are likely to be more didactic and informational in nature. Again, the audience for which one is designing an application is a key consideration. When designing applications for children and adolescents, for example, entertainment value is likely to be a more important factor than when designing applications for older audiences. Still, a major advantage of many eHealth applications is appeal, and use of such applications by target audiences will be increased to the extent that the "appeal factor" can be leveraged.

While earlier in this chapter we covered a host of general advantages of eHealth applications (Table 1.2), such advantages and attributes will clearly vary from application to application. By examining the chapters in this volume, readers will become familiar with the key strengths and attributes of each type of eHealth application. In many ways, the challenge for researchers and practitioners is to advance an understanding of how we can best leverage eHealth application strengths for effective health promotion and disease prevention. Indeed, rather than simply developing applications because we can, we need a clear understanding of what applications can and should be developed in what areas in order to have the greatest possible impact on health behaviors. Indeed, over the past two decades, work by Glasgow et al. (1999, 2003) and others has made a strong statement regarding real public health impact. That is, if eHealth applications remain solely in the research domain and are not translated into practice, their ability to improve healthy behaviors and reduce the burden of major diseases such as heart disease, diabetes, cancer, and HIV/AIDS will be limited. Instead, researchers should consider not only what opportunities for intervention development exist but also how the translation, dissemination, and sustainability of interventions can be achieved. Our hope is that the current volume, with its focus not only on the research literature but also on dissemination, policy, and practice, will help lay the groundwork for the increased development, evaluation, and dissemination of eHealth applications.

References

Abrams, D. B., Orleans, C. T., Niaura, R. S., Goldstein, M. G., Prochaska, J. O., & Velicer, W. F. (1996). Integrating individual and public health perspectives for treatment of tobacco dependence under managed health care: A combined step care and matching model. *Annals of Behavioral Medicine, 18,* 290–304.

Abroms, L. C., Schiavo, R., & Lefebvre, R. C. (2008). New media cases in *Cases in Public Health Communication & Marketing:* The promise and potential. *Cases in Public Health Communication & Marketing, 2,* 3–10.

Ahern, D. K. (2007). Challenges and opportunities of eHealth research. *American Journal of Preventive Medicine, 32*(5 Suppl), S75–S82.

Ahern, D. K., Kreslake, J. M., & Phalen, J. M. (2006). What is eHealth (6): Perspectives on the evolution of eHealth research. *Journal of Medical Internet Research, 8,* e4.

Akter, S., D'Ambra, J., & Ray, P. (2011). Trustworthiness in mHealth information services: An assessment of a hierarchical model with mediating and moderating effects using partial least squares (PLS). *Journal of the American Society for Information Science & Technology, 62,* 100–116.

Atkinson, N. L., & Gold, R. S. (2002). The promise and challenge of eHealth interventions. *American Journal of Health Behavior, 26,* 494–503.

Bernhardt, J. M. (2004). Communication at the core of effective public health. *American Journal of Public Health,* 2051–2053.

Bodie, G. D., & Dutta, M. J. (2008). Understanding health literacy for strategic health marketing: eHealth literacy, health disparities, and the digital divide. *Health Marketing Quarterly, 25,* 175–203.

Bucy, E. P., & Tao, C.-C. (2007). The mediated moderation model of interactivity. *Media Psychology, 9,* 647–672.

Bull, S. (2011). *Technology-based health promotion.* Thousand Oaks, CA: Sage.

Cassell, M. M., Jackson, C., & Cheuvront, B. (1998). Health communication on the Internet: An effective channel for health behavior change? *Journal of Health Communication, 3,* 71–79.

Coates, T. J., Richter, L., & Caceres, C. (2008). Behavioural strategies to reduce HIV transmission: How to make them work better. *Lancet, 372,* 669–684.

Curry, S. J. (2007). eHealth research and healthcare delivery: Beyond intervention effectiveness. *American Journal of Preventive Medicine, 32*(5, Suppl 1), S127–S130.

Cushing, C. C., & Steele, R. G. (2010). A meta-analytic review of eHealth interventions for pediatric health promoting and maintaining behaviors. *Journal of Pediatric Psychology, 35,* 937–949.

Danaei, G., Ding, E. L., Mozaffarian, D., Taylor, B., Rehm, J., Murray, C. J., et al. (2009). The preventable causes of death in the United States: Comparative risk assessment of dietary, lifestyle, and metabolic risk factors. *Plos Medicine, 6,* e1000058–e1000058.

De Wit, J. B. F., Aggleton, P., Myers, T., & Crewe, M. (2011). The rapidly changing paradigm of HIV prevention: Time to strengthen social and behavioural approaches. *Health Education Research, 26,* 381–392.

DiClemente, R. J., Crosby, R. A., & Kegler, M. C. (2009). *Emerging theories in health promotion practice and research* (2nd ed.). San Francisco, CA: Jossey-Bass.

Eng, T. R. (2001). *The eHealth landscape: A terrain map of emerging information and communication technologies in health and health care.* Princeton, NJ: Robert Wood Johnson Foundation.

Eng, T. R., Gustafson, D. H., Henderson, J., Jimison, H., & Patrick, K. (1999). Introduction to evaluation of interactive health communication applications. Science Panel on Interactive Communication and Health. *American Journal of Preventive Medicine, 16,* 10–15.

Fotheringham, M. J., Owies, D., Leslie, E., & Owen, N. (2000). Interactive health communication in preventive medicine: Internet-based strategies in teaching and research. *American Journal of Preventive Medicine, 19,* 113–120.

Freimuth, V. S., & Quinn, S. C. (2004). The contributions of health communication to eliminating health disparities. *American Journal of Public Health, 94,* 2053–2055.

Gerber, T., Olazabal, V., Brown, K., & Pablos-Mendez, A. (2010). An agenda for action on global e-health. *Health Affairs (Project Hope), 29,* 233–236.

Glanz, K., Rimer, B. K., & Viswanath, K. (2008). *Health behavior and health education: Theory, research, and practice* (4th ed.). San Francisco, CA: Jossey-Bass.

Glasgow, R. E. (2007). eHealth evaluation and dissemination research. *American Journal of Preventive Medicine, 32*(5, Suppl 1), S119–S126.

Glasgow, R. E., Bull, S. S., Piette, J. D., & Steiner, J. F. (2004). Interactive behavior change technology: A partial solution to the competing demands of primary care. *American Journal of Preventive Medicine, 27*(2 Suppl), 80–87.

Glasgow, R. E., Lichtenstein, E., & Marcus, A. C. (2003). Why don't we see more translation of health promotion research to practice? Rethinking the efficacy-to-effectiveness transition. *American Journal of Public Health, 93,* 1261–1267.

Glasgow, R. E., Vogt, T. M., & Boles, S. M. (1999). Evaluating the public health impact of health promotion interventions: The RE-AIM framework. *American Journal of Public Health, 89,* 1322–1327.

Hawkins, R. P., Han, J.-Y., Pingree, S., Shaw, B. R., Baker, T. B., & Roberts, L. J. (2010). Interactivity and presence of three eHealth interventions. *Computers in Human Behavior, 26,* 1081–1088.

Healthy People 2010. (2000). *Healthy People 2010.* Washington, DC: U.S. Department of Health and Human Services.

Hornik, R. C. (2002). *Public health communication: Evidence for behavior change.* Mahwah, NJ: Lawrence Erlbaum Associates.

Houston, T. K., Chang, B. L., Brown, S., & Kukafka, R. (2001). Consumer health informatics: A consensus description and commentary from American Medical Informatics Association members. *AMIA Annual Symposium Proceedings, 269*–273.

Hutchinson, P., & Wheeler, J. (2006). The cost-effectiveness of health communication programs: What do we know? *Journal of Health Communication, 11,* 7–45.

Jemal, A., Ward, E., Hao, Y., & Thun, M. (2005). Trends in the leading causes of death in the United States, 1970–2002. *Journal of the American Medical Association, 294,* 1255–1259.

Jones, R., Rogers, R., Roberts, J., Callaghan, L., Lindsey, L., Campbell, J., et al. (2005). What is eHealth (5): A research agenda for eHealth through stakeholder consultation and policy context review. *Journal of Medical Internet Research, 7,* e54–e54.

Kiousis, S. (2002). Interactivity: A concept explication. *New Media & Society, 4,* 355–383.

Kreps, G. L., & Maibach, E. W. (2008). Transdisciplinary science: The nexus between communication and public health. *Journal of Communication, 58*(4), 732–748.

Kreps, G. L., & Neuhauser, L. (2010). New directions in eHealth communication: Opportunities and challenges. *Patient Education & Counseling, 78,* 329–336.

Lefebvre, R. C., Tada, Y., Hilfiker, S. W., & Baur, C. (2010). The assessment of user engagement with eHealth content: The eHealth Engagement Scale. *Journal of Computer-Mediated Communication, 15,* 666–681.

McGinnis, J. M., & Foege, W. H. (1993). Actual causes of death in the United States. *Journal of the American Medical Association, 270,* 2207–2212.

Mokdad, A. H., Marks, J. S., Stroup, D. F., & Gerberding, J. L. (2004). Actual causes of death in the United States, 2000. *Journal of the American Medical Association, 291,* 1238–1245.

Murray, E., Burns, J., See, T. S., Lai, R., & Nazareth, I. (2005). Interactive health communication applications for people with chronic disease. *Cochrane Database of Systematic Reviews* (4), CD004274.

Neuhauser, L., & Kreps, G. L. (2010). eHealth communication and behavior change: Promise and performance. *Social Semiotics, 20,* 9–27.

Office of Disease Prevention and Health Promotion. (2006). *Expanding the reach of consumer e-health tools.* Washington, DC: U.S. Department of Health and Human Services.

Oh, H., Rizo, C., Enkin, M., & Jadad, A. (2005). What is eHealth (3): A systematic review of published definitions. *Journal of Medical Internet Research, 7,* e1–e1.

Pagliari, C. (2007). Design and evaluation in eHealth: Challenges and implications for an interdisciplinary field. *Journal of Medical Internet Research, 9,* e15–e15.

Pagliari, C., Sloan, D., Gregor, P., Sullivan, F., Detmer, D., Kahan, J. P., et al. (2005). What is eHealth (4): A scoping exercise to map the field. *Journal of Medical Internet Research, 7,* e9–e9.

Rimal, R. N., & Adkins, A. D. (2003). Using computers to narrowcast health messages: The role of audience segmentation, targeting, and tailoring in health promotion. In T. L. Thompson, A. M. Dorsey, K. I. Miller, & R. Parrott (Eds.), *Handbook of health communication* (pp. 497–515). Mahwah, NJ: Lawrence Erlbaum Associates.

Rimal, R. N., & Flora, J. A. (1997). Interactive technology attributes in health promotion: Practical and theoretical issues. In R. L. Street Jr., W. R. Gold, & T. R. Manning (Eds.), *Health promotion and interactive technology: Theoretical applications and future directions* (pp. 19–38). Mahwah, NJ: Lawrence Erlbaum Associates.

Robinson, T. N., Patrick, K., Eng, T. R., & Gustafson, D. (1998). An evidence-based approach to interactive health communication: A challenge to medicine in the information age. *Journal of the American Medical Association, 280,* 1264.

Science Panel on Interactive Communication and Health. (1999). *Wired for health and wellbeing: The emergence of interactive health communication.* Washington, DC: U.S. Department of Health and Human Services.

Shumaker, S. A., Ockene, J. K., & Riekert, K. A. (2009). *The handbook of health behavior change* (3rd ed.). New York: Springer Publishing Co.

Solomon, J., Card, J. J., & Malow, R. M. (2006). Adapting efficacious interventions: Advancing translational research in HIV prevention. *Evaluation & the Health Professions, 29,* 162–194.

Strecher, V. J. (2007). Internet methods for delivering behavioral and health-related interventions (eHealth). *Annual Review of Clinical Psychology, 3,* 53–76.

Strecher, V. J. (2009). Interactive health communications for cancer prevention and control. In S. M. Miller, D. J. Bowen, R. T. Croyle, & J. H. Rowland (Eds.), *Handbook of cancer control and behavioral science: A resource for researchers, practitioners, and policymakers* (pp. 547–558). Washington, DC: American Psychological Association.

Street, R. L., & Rimal, R. N. (1997). Health promotion and interactive technology: A conceptual foundation. In R. L. Street, W. R. Gold, & T. Manning (Eds.), *Health promotion and interactive technology: Theoretical applications and future directions* (pp. 1–18). Mahwah, NJ: Lawrence Erlbaum Associates.

Sundar, S. S., Kalyanaraman, S., & Brown, J. (2003). Explicating website interactivity: Impression formation effects in political campaign sites. *Communication Research, 30,* 30–59.

World Health Organization. (2008). *The global burden of disease.* Geneva: WHO.

2

THE EMERGENCE OF eHEALTH APPLICATIONS

Sheana Bull

The advent of personal computers, the Internet, and mobile phones has been accompanied by inventive approaches to using technology for health promotion and disease prevention, which, according to Wantland, Portillo, Holzemer, Slaughter, and McGhee (2004), increased more than sevenfold in the years between 1996 and 2003. Over 75% of U.S. adults access the Internet and over 82% of those aged 18–64 use cell phones. We have unprecedented opportunities to reach people to facilitate their adoption of healthy behaviors and help improve health outcomes using technology (Fox, 2010).

In this chapter we introduce key historical events related to the emergence of eHealth applications. We will present the reader with information on key historical events and selected examples of innovations that have been introduced over time, followed by examples of the prime advantages of using eHealth applications. Many innovations in eHealth are addressed in greater detail in subsequent chapters, where readers can consider the benefits and drawbacks of each. We will then consider specific challenges we face in implementing eHealth applications, as well as future opportunities we anticipate. Table 2.1 in this chapter offers selected examples of studies discussed in the text, with detail on sample, design, and main study findings.

Origins of the Computer and Internet

Technological computing dates as far back as 1938 when Konrad Zuse, a construction engineer, was credited with creating electronic calculators, although the first consumer computers were not available until the early 1970s. A predecessor to the Internet called ARPAnet (Advanced Research Projects Agency network) was designed in 1969, originally for military use to create a network of geographically dispersed computers. ARPAnet was a catalyst for new inventions such as email, local area networks (LAN), and ultimately NSFnet (National Science Foundation network), which linked together supercomputers and was the immediate precursor to the modern Internet (Bellis, n.d.).

Origins of Bulletin Boards and User Groups

One feature of the Internet is the use of bulletin boards or discussion groups—known more commonly today as threaded discussions. Discussion groups originated from an idea of Internet-based discussion groups generated by students at Duke University in 1980 (Lueg & Fisher, 2003). They wanted to generate a way to share information about various topics on what they labeled USENET, where posts were sequentially stored on servers. USENET evolved over time into Internet forums and threaded discussions. Today, Internet users find threaded discussions for hundreds if not thousands of topics. People can rely on this approach to learn more about a subject (e.g., how to train your new puppy) from others who share interest in the topic and who don't necessarily have a commercial motive to engage with them.

Early Examples of Health-Related Research and Health Promotion on Bulletin Boards and Chat Rooms

In 1982, postings appeared on a USENET group encouraging persons in the group to review a recent publication of *Morbidity Mortality Weekly Report (MMWR)*; these postings offer early evidence that USENET forums could be used to direct conversation and discussion to health topics, in this case, HIV/AIDS (Bennett & Glasgow, 2009). Some of the earliest work in the technology and health area documented the use of chat rooms for solicitation of sex partners; Bull and McFarlane (2000) observed that clients in the Denver Public Health Sexually Transmitted Disease (STD) Clinic who were infected with syphilis had named sex partner contacts whom they originally met online. This work led to publication of evidence suggesting online sex partner seeking was a potential risk behavior associated with STDs (McFarlane, Bull, & Rietmeijer, 2000) and to another publication that was among the first to document the use of email as an approach to identify sex partner contacts who had been exposed to syphilis in an effort to get them in for treatment (Klausner, Wolf, Fischer-Ponce, Zolt, & Katz, 2000).

In 2002, Eysenbach, Powell, Kuss, and Sa reported on the widespread attraction to and use of chat rooms to discuss numerous health-related topics among lay persons. McFarlane, Kachur, Klausner, Roland, and Cohen (2005) have documented the popularity of using chat rooms for health education and outreach related to HIV prevention, although none of these efforts has been subjected to a formal evaluation for efficacy.

As mentioned, evidence emerged during the 1990s and early 2000s documenting use of chat rooms as a common means to solicit sex partners (Rhodes,

Diclemente, Cecil, Hergenrather, & Yee, 2002; Ross, Rosser, & Stanton, 2004; Rosser et al., 2009). In response, many AIDS service organizations (ASOs) and other community-based organizations serving men who have sex with men (MSM) generated guidelines and strategies for how to use chat rooms as an educational tool in HIV prevention. The Centers for Disease Control and Prevention (CDC) produced guidelines for using chat rooms for health education about prevention and treatment of STDs, including human immunodeficiency virus (HIV) (Mc-Farlane et al., 2005). These guidelines include important considerations for health promoters, such as (1) making a detailed profile to demonstrate your affiliation with a health promotion group or organization providing prevention services; (2) making decisions about how to engage with chatters (e.g., should you wait for them to contact you, or can you actively engage them?); and (3) following strict professional guidelines, including responding with information and clarification and not engaging in any inflammatory or reactionary chat.

Advantages of eHealth Applications

The Use of Technology to Standardize and Tailor Computerized Health Promotion Materials

A prime motivation for using technology for health promotion has been to standardize program materials and to make materials more relevant to individual users through tailoring (see chapter 8 of this volume). An abundant literature exists on use of expert systems; one can write algorithms that will allow different material and content delivery based on inputs from the user. Early and ongoing work on tailoring shows that it increases the "self-relevance" of print material for subjects, such that material is more likely to be read, comprehended, and remembered, and subsequently produce significant behavior change (Hawkins, Kreuter, Resnicow, Fishbein, & Dijkstra, 2008; Kreuter & Wray, 2003; Kroeze, Werkman, & Brug, 2006; Noar, Benac, & Harris, 2007; Noar, Harrington, & Aldrich, 2009) across a wide variety of behavioral outcomes (e.g., smoking cessation, diet and nutrition, cancer screening). Tailoring in the computer environment was one of the early applications employed in eHealth, and a recent meta-analysis of 88 interventions using computer tailoring to address smoking, diet, mammography, and physical activity demonstrates it to be a robust and consistently successful approach (Krebs, Prochaska, & Rossi, 2010).

In addition to the benefits achieved through tailoring, standardization of program material delivered through computers means that health promotion programs can be delivered consistently. Standardization also facilitates the use of the same format each time. Unlike face-to-face program delivery, whose success may hinge on the personality of a health educator or the relationship between individuals in a program, this type of standardization means that success in program delivery is not dependent on these variables (Kreuter & Wray, 2003; Kroeze, Werkman, & Brug, 2006).

Examples of tailoring using the Internet are shown in Table 2.1. A pilot program tested with 200 Latinos in the Denver metropolitan area explored using computer kiosks to tailor feedback related to physical activity, nutrition, and smoking behaviors based on user-specific information about these behaviors. The program showed promise in increasing consumption of fruits and vegetables and physical activity, but did not document any changes in smoking behaviors (Leeman-Castillo, Beaty, Raghunath, Steiner, & Bull, 2010). A study conducted in Belgium across multiple worksites used tailored messages related to reduction in fat consumption. Researchers offered users access to a computer kiosk in the workplace where they could input personal information on dietary practices and receive feedback that was personally tailored to help them reduce fat consumption. Those receiving tailored information were better able to reduce total fat consumption compared to those receiving generic nontailored information (De Bourdeaudhuij, Stevens, Vandelanotte, & Brug, 2007).

The CHESS program (Comprehensive Health Enhancement Support System) developed by researchers in Wisconsin is a comprehensive computer-based system that offers patients with varied diagnoses (e.g., breast cancer, HIV) a variety of important functions. These include opportunities to (1) communicate with providers via email and online chat, (2) participate in threaded discussions with other users, (3) access information about their condition through links to online resources, and (4) complete needs assessments (Gustafson et al., 2002). Needs assessments offer opportunities for patients to input data on behavior and receive tailored feedback to facilitate decision making, adherence, and planning for care. Breast cancer patients have been shown to have higher levels of awareness of breast cancer when obtaining tailored information (Gustafson et al., 2002).

The Activ-O-Meter program offers users tailored feedback on their individual level of physical activity. Persons regularly log their physical activity either manually or through tools such as pedometers and cyclometers; when tested with adolescent school children across six countries in Europe, this program was shown to increase moderate physical activity and cycling for transportation (De Bourdeaudhuij et al., 2010).

Social Support in Health Promotion

Table 2.1 highlights several studies focused on use of technology to facilitate social support. The aforementioned CHESS program not only incorporates tailoring to personalize materials, it is among the best researched programs demonstrating the efficacy of using online social support to facilitate healthy outcomes. Gustafson et al. (2001, 2005) were able to show that women with a breast cancer diagnosis were eager to log on to social support groups in a short-term period following diagnosis to exchange comments online with other women who also had breast cancer and exchange stories, discuss experiences with treatment, and obtain advice for how to manage their disease.

Table 2.1 Selected examples of research using technology for health promotion

Authors	Sample	Design	Results	Conclusions
Standardizing and tailoring materials				
Leeman–Castillo, Beaty, Raghunath, Steiner, & Bull (2010)	200 Latinos in Denver, Colorado with diverse educational backgrounds; 70% female; 50% native Spanish speakers	Pilot test of the feasibility, acceptability, and potential for positive behavior change of the LUCHAR Kiosk, an interactive program with tailored feedback on nutrition, physical activity, and smoking behavior	Findings showed significant increases in fruit and vegetable consumption and physical activity among all participants (no controls in study)	LUCHAR is feasible and acceptable; needs to be tested for efficacy in an RCT
De Bourdeaudhuji, Stevens, Vandelanotte, & Brug (2007)	337 participants from six different Belgian companies	RCT involving six companies randomly assigned to one of two intervention groups, or a control group to test benefits of a tailored Internet education	The computer-tailored intervention group proved to be more effective in regulating/reducing total fat intake than the generic or control group	Computer-tailored interventions can be effective for behavior change
De Bourdeaudhuji et et al. (2010)	675 12–17-year-olds in six European countries	A group-level RCT that exposed intervention participants to tailored feedback on their individual level of physical activity	Intervention group reported higher levels of moderate and vigorous physical activity and higher levels of cycling for transport compared to the control group	Effects sustained at three months; one of the largest trials of an online physical activity program showing positive and sustained effects

(*Continued*)

Table 2.1 (*Continued*)

Authors	Sample	Design	Results	Conclusions
Online social support and social networking				
Webber, Tate, & Quintiliani (2008)	20 female university employees of diverse age and academic background	Pilot testing feasibility of motivational Internet-based online group and controls for weight loss	Weight loss was experienced by both intervention and control groups	The use of motivational interviewing in online groups for weight loss is acceptable and feasible. Effects of program for weight loss not demonstrated
Glasgow, Boles, McKay, Feil, & Barrera Jr. (2003)	320 type II diabetes patients, equally divided between men and women	RCT comparing a user-friendly diabetes self-anagement website to website access plus a tailored self-management tool, and a peer support group online	All conditions improved from baseline on behavioral, psychosocial, and some biological outcomes	Showed positive effects from an interactive website but no additional benefits with tailored information or peer support
Engagement through games and interactive elements				
Brown et al. (1997)	59 8–16-year-olds with diabetes	RCT testing efficacy of playing an educational video game on diabetes	Participants playing the video had better diabetes-related self-efficacy, communication with parents about diabetes, and self-management than those in the control group. No changes between groups on HbA1C levels	Gaming can be an effective tool for self-management behaviors related to diabetes for youth

Beale, Kato, Marin-Bowling, Guthrie, & Cole (2007)	375 adolescent and young adult cancer patients	RCT testing effects of *Re-Mission*, a video game on cancer-related knowledge	Cancer-related knowledge increased over time in both groups but was significantly higher among those playing *Re-Mission*	Gaming can be an effective tool for education about and retention of cancer-related knowledge

Technology used to enhance or extend face-to-face health promotion

Downer, Meara, & Da Costa (2005)	2,151 patients who had a scheduled appointment at the hospital (C = 769, R = 1,382)	RCT targeting patients who had appointments who gave their cell phone numbers in order to increase attendance rates for appointments	The failure to attend rate was significantly lower in the intervention versus control group.	The ease, low cost, and feasibility for large-scale customizable messages suggest cell phone reminders may be a suitable means of improving patient attendance
Vidrine, Arduino, Lazev, & Gritz (2006)	95 racially diverse HIV positive smokers with history of drug use from an inner-city AIDS clinic in Texas	RCT exploring efficacy of eight cell phone counseling sessions to controls	Intervention group experienced significantly greater reductions in anxiety, depression, and significantly greater increases in self-efficacy and were five times more likely to abstain from smoking at three months	Cell phones can be effective in addressing some factors for smoking cessation in people living with AIDS, which could also impact medical adherence

(Continued)

Table 2.1 (*Continued*)

Authors	Sample	Design	Results	Conclusions
Mobile phones				
Rodgers et al. (2005)	1,705 smokers from New Zealand	RCT exploring efficacy of personalized text messages to provide smoking cessation advice, support, and distraction versus control group	More participants had quit at six weeks in the intervention in comparison to the control group	Being affordable, personalized, age-appropriate, and not location dependent, use of text messages to assist in smoking cessation potentially offers a new way to help young smokers to quit
Patrick et al. (2009)	65 participants; both genders included, primarily white population	RCT exploring efficacy of personalized text and picture messages sent two to five times daily, printed materials, and brief monthly phone calls from a health counselor versus receiving monthly printed materials on weight control	The intervention group lost more weight than the comparison after adjusting for time, sex, and mean age	Text messages are promising for weight loss. Further studies are needed with a larger sample size and a longer intervention period
Cole-Lewis & Kershwa (2010)	2,425 patients across 12 studies	Review article exploring overall effects of using cell phones for disease prevention	All studies showed high rates of retention; significant effects in five of 12 with trends to significance in four studies	Cell phones have promise for promotion of healthy eating, physical activity and smoking cessation

Broad reach

Winett, Anderson, Wojcik, Winett, & Bowden (2007)	RCT comparing wait list controls to either an Internet-based program on physical activity and nutrition (GTH-only) or the GTH enhanced with participation in a church-based support group (GTH Plus)	GTH-plus and GTH-only increased fiber and fruit and vegetable intake and number of daily steps. GTH-plus also decreased fat intake	Participants in the GTH-plus and GTH-only made more behavioral changes than controls. The results suggest supports in socially mediated Internet interventions for behavior change
1,071 participants; 1/4 African American; male and female			
Christensen, Griffiths, & Korten (2002)	Descriptive study of the effects of Mood Gym, an online cognitive behavioral therapy for young adults	Both anxiety and depression scores decreased significantly as individuals progressed through Mood Gym	Suggests we can have widespread access to a useful tool for CBT; still need RCT to establish efficacy
1,503 Web users in Australia			
Bull, Pratte, Whitesell, Rietmeijer, & McFarlane (2009)	RCT testing exposure to didactic, text-based information on HIV prevention to tailored information delivered by role models of same gender and race/ethnicity (Youthnet)	Youthnet participants showed an increase in norms related to condom use, which in turn was associated with a very small increase in use of condoms or contraception	Study reach was high, participation limited to lower risk groups; effects were very small, suggesting greater program intensity is needed
1,398 Internet users aged 18–24; primarily white			
Graham, Cobb, Raymond, Sill, & Young (2007)	Intent to treat study of Quit Net, an Internet based smoking cessation program	Quit rates ranged from 13% to 43%	Program was effective at reaching geographically dispersed employees and in promoting cessation and preventing relapse
1,776 IBM employees accessing worksite computer-based program			

In addition to support for breast cancer self-management, researchers have explored the use of technology to facilitate social support for other healthy behavior. Webber, Tate, and Quintiliani (2008) showed that participation in an online support group and motivational interviewing intervention contributed to weight loss among users, although there was not a significant difference between online users and those in a control group in this pilot study. Similarly, Glasgow, Boles, McKay, Feil, and Barrera (2003) showed that the use of chat rooms is feasible, but they weren't able to demonstrate that added social support contributed to changes in health-related behaviors to manage diabetes (see Table 2.1). Social support is reemerging in the examination of the effects of using social media such as Facebook, MySpace, and Twitter for health promotion. This is discussed in more detail below.

Challenges with eHealth Applications

The Digital Divide

The concept of a digital divide emerged early on in the history of the Internet. The National Institute of Technology Assessment (NITA) published a report in 1999 documenting a racial, ethnic, and income gap between persons who had access to the Internet and those who did not, with poor persons and persons of color less likely to have access to both computers and the Internet (Gustafson, Robinson, Ansley, Adler, & Brennan, 1999). While data show that a disparity in access to and use of the Internet among racial and ethnic minorities (called the "digital divide") is shrinking in the United States, some argue that it persists among elderly, non-English speakers, and those with the lowest incomes (Lenhart & Horrigan, 2003; Lorence, Park, & Fox, 2006). Much of the detail on Internet access, use, and the digital divide has been reported by PEW Internet and American Life, an organization dedicated to regular reporting on the evolution of technology use in the United States (Boase, Horrigan, Wellman, & Rainie, 2006; Horrigan, 2007; Horrigan, 2008a; Lenhart, Ling, Campbell, & Purcell, 2010).

Making Health Promotion Engaging with Technology

Evidence from early health promotion efforts shows the importance of engagement for participant retention. As a result, we need to keep content interesting, updated, and interactive to ensure people will stay engaged in sessions and use technology over time (Glasgow et al., 2003).

Researchers have long recognized the value of using entertainment as an education tool. The use of engaging content has been shown to be effective for enhancing memory and retention of knowledge (Erk et al., 2003; Gray, Braver, & Raichle, 2002; Svirko & Mellanby, 2008). Media and entertainment have been utilized with success to raise consciousness about health and social issues and to impact health behaviors (Maibach, Flora, & Nass, 1991; Rogers, 1995; Rogers et al., 1999).

Miguel Sabido is well known in Mexico and internationally as a pioneer in entertainment-education for developing a series of six *telenovelas,* or Spanish-language soap operas, in Mexico to promote family planning. The first program, called *Acompaname* (Accompany Me), was linked to a 23% increase in the purchase of contraceptive supplies and a 33% increase in the use of national family planning services in Mexico (Population Media Center, 2009). The success of entertainment-education may be due in part to the reliance on culturally popular mechanisms such as storytelling. Storytelling has also been shown to have efficacy for teaching African American women about breast health and for increasing awareness of cervical cancer and screening among Native American women (Hodge, Fredericks, & Rodriguez, 1996; Williams-Brown, Baldwin, & Bakos, 2002).

With the emergence of YouTube and other video sharing sites online, the possibility of using video online for health promotion has arrived. In Colorado, researchers are working with youth at a local middle school to develop short (30-second) public service announcements (PSAs) and videos (one to three minutes long) about sun protection that they will then post on the Web and track "hits" (viewings) in an effort to understand how to generate popular interest in a health behavior video-based intervention (L. Crane, personal communication, October 1, 2010).

Emerging Opportunities for eHealth Applications

Social Media and Social Networking

The term *Web 2.0* became common in 2004, when sites began incorporating "social media" that allowed users to chat, blog, and interact with each other online. These activities encompassed under the Web 2.0 term were largely available before the term was coined; however, with the emergence of the Web 2.0 concept came more explicit recognition that the Internet was now a place where people could interact not only with the computer, but with other people as well—in real or delayed time. Social media sites have grown in popularity since they emerged in the early part of this century. Recent reports from PEW Internet and American Life indicate that almost three-quarters of teens and young adults aged 18–29 use social networking sites and just under half of adults over 29 use them (Lenhart et al., 2010).

Social networking sites offer promise for health promotion. If we can reach individuals online, we also now have the potential to reach people within their social network via sites such as MySpace and Facebook. There is empirical evidence dating from 2007 suggesting the likely importance of studying the relationships between social networks and health, when Christakis and Fowler demonstrated that persons enrolled in the Framingham Heart Study experienced more obesity over a 32-year period if they had a close friend or relative who was also obese (Christakis & Fowler, 2007). The emergence of online social networks suggests we can study this phenomenon in the virtual world also.

Currently, efforts are underway to utilize Facebook to deliver HIV prevention messages and to evaluate the results. This study, sponsored by the National Institute of Nursing Research, is exploring not only whether delivering content in this medium is effective but also, perhaps more important, whether users of the program can influence others in their social networks to change behaviors and/or adopt healthy sexual practices. Users are invited to join the study and are randomly assigned to become a member of the HIV Prevention activities through the "Just/Us" Facebook page or a control page on Facebook dedicated to sharing non–health-related news targeting young adults. All participants see content relevant to their group each time they open up their Facebook page—content such as quizzes, links to videos and games, and threaded discussions on specific topics (e.g., conversations on how to disclose your sexual history to a new partner). At the time of this writing, we had completed enrolling a sample of 1,588 persons, and data collection continued with study participants through the spring of 2011. Results are expected soon.

Gaming

Technology offers new opportunities for the use of interactive and entertaining content to engage users and enhance their learning. An example of how this can be achieved is computer gaming (see Lieberman, this volume). About 53% of all American adults play video games on different consoles including computers, portable gaming devices, cell phones, handheld devices, and online (Lenhart, Jones, & Macgill, 2008). The most popular gaming device for young adults is gaming consoles, which often simulate real-world environments. An estimated 75% of 18- to 29-year-olds play games on consoles and about 68% use computers, the second most popular gaming device for this population. Younger adults are more likely to play games on the Internet than older adults: 43% of adults between the ages of 18 and 29 play games online, whereas 26% of people ages 30–49 do so. More than half of adults—59%—play at least a few times a week. Those who play multiplayer games (such as *World of Warcraft*) play much more frequently—89% play at least a few times a week and 49% play every day or almost every day (Lenhart et al., 2008). Internet simulations that are similar to games have great potential for reaching a young at-risk population.

Table 2.1 offers two examples of games related to health that have been tested for efficacy. One study tested a video game to enhance self-management of diabetes, and although the game wasn't effective in reducing HbA1C levels for participants, it did help with self-efficacy for diabetes management (Brown et al., 1997). Another tested the efficacy of *Re-Mission,* a game for cancer patients, and showed it to be effective in increasing cancer-related knowledge (Beale et al., 2007).

In order to increase access to and utilization of gaming for health promotion, researchers have looked to the Internet as a platform for game delivery. "Second Life" (SL) is a virtual world that offers users opportunities to create an avatar (see Fox, this volume) and interact in real time with others online. Computer scientists and health researchers are exploring opportunities to deliver health promotion content using this medium (Second Life, 2010). Kamel Boulos, Hetherington, and Wheeler (2007) describe a "nutrition game" allowing users in SL to learn about the impact that fast food has on health and offers experiments with different eating styles. SL also has programs in action for listening to heart sounds (called cardiac auscultation) where visitors can test their skills identifying different types of heart murmurs through sound. More research needs to be done regarding increased engagement and participation in online games through SL, but it has been shown that better participation can be encouraged through purposeful and authentic online activity (Kamel Boulos et al., 2007).

AIDS.gov collaborated with funders to develop a virtual community library and resource center in a video game. This is a program developed to improve awareness of AIDS and HIV and to provide resources to those diagnosed with the disease, as well as friends and family members of those diagnosed. The CDC has also developed programs in SL, with the intention of engaging SL users through interactive tools to influence healthy behaviors. Areas in SL are called "islands," and the CDC island offers "walking kiosks" that inform users on many different health topics (Kamel Boulos, Ramloll, Jones, & Toth-Cohen, 2008).

Technology to Enhance Privacy and Extend Clinical Services

An advantage afforded by technology is that of privacy. Using technology for collection of sensitive health behavior data (e.g., sexual risk behavior, drug and alcohol use) may offer improved disclosure (Turner et al., 1998). In addition, people can now access elements of their health records online, and investigations are ongoing to facilitate use of the personal health record (PHR) for increased self-care and shared patient-provider decision making (Detmer, Bloomrosen, Raymond, & Tang, 2008).

The field of telemedicine offers numerous examples of ways to extend care to rural populations, to enhance and supplement care delivery, and to support clinical service delivery in resource-poor areas. (Because our focus in this chapter is on health promotion specifically, we will not discuss delivery of health care via technology, per se; however, there are numerous resources related to telemedicine that summarize the evidence of efficacy and discuss potential for technology-delivered health services [Ekeland, Bowes, & Flottorp, 2010; Turner, 2003].) These advantages aside, there is also substantial concern over *loss* of privacy through technology. Hackers, viruses, and lax security could all lead to loss of privacy and exposure of sensitive personal information. Later in the chapter, we will address cautions related to security systems and expectations we can realistically hold about privacy online. Here we consider opportunities that exist to enhance and extend clinical services.

Hybrid health promotion programs that expand face-to-face efforts can include "booster" sessions—for example, using something as simple as an email from a provider to a participant in a group-level diabetes self-management program. People could meet with a provider and then be linked to social support online in an effort to reinforce positive behavior change. Consider the "buddy" system, linking people to others online trying to adopt a specific behavior. Buddies can offer testimonials or personal stories, for example, to encourage and support others in behavior change efforts.

Table 2.1 lists examples of how technology has been linked to clinical care for improved health promotion. Perhaps the simplest example is that of Downer, Meara, and De Costa (2005) who used text messaging on cell phones to effectively increase appointment adherence. More intensive interventions using technology to facilitate and extend clinical care include effective efforts to use phone-based counseling to facilitate smoking cessation among persons with HIV (Vidrine et al., 2006).

The Use of Cell Phone Technology for Health Promotion

As technology continues to evolve, we have seen a tremendous increase in the use of handheld devices and cell phones in daily life across diverse populations. While cell phones were technically used as early as 1946, they didn't become available to consumers until 1967. Early cell phones were heavy and large—about the size of a shoebox; users could only make calls within a single cell area, and their phone numbers were tied to the base station in that area. The first truly portable phones were available in 1983, and the relatively lower cost of building cell towers has contributed to their widespread adoption worldwide. Increasing advancements in technology make phones cheaper and more portable, with higher speeds for accessing and downloading data, voice, and text. Some estimates are that ownership is over 75% in the United States and even higher than 100% in other industrialized countries, where people have more than one phone (Tech-FAQ, 2011).

Cell phones offer voice capabilities for making and receiving telephone calls, short message service (SMS, also known as text messaging), access to the Internet, and storage of files, photos, and music. Cell phones with these capabilities have been dubbed *smartphones,* and their adoption has been steadily increasing in recent years. In the United States, estimates are that 75% of youth ages 12–17 and 90% of those aged 18–29 have cell phones. More than 70% youth with phones use text messaging, and 54% text daily (Lenhart et al., 2010). A full 65% of cell phone–using youth use smartphones to access the Internet. African Americans' use of mobile phones equals or surpasses that of white Americans and is almost universal among teens and young adults (Horrigan, 2008b). A recent survey found cell ownership is higher among blacks and Latinos than whites and that minority cell owners take advantage of a greater range of phone features than white cell users—including smartphone features (Smith, 2010).

Numerous studies have been published that show the promise of this medium (see Abroms, Padmanabhan, & Evans; Fjeldsoe, Miller, & Marshall, this volume; also see Table 2.1). For example, Rodgers et al. (2005) have demonstrated that using text messages with smokers can be effective in increasing quit rates, and Patrick et al. (2009) have demonstrated the efficacy of using text messaging, picture messages, and brief phone calls for increased weight loss. A systematic review of 12 studies—seven of which were RCTs—using mobile phones for disease prevention efforts demonstrated that phones can be used effectively to reach participants and have positive effects on nutrition, physical activity, and smoking behaviors (Cole-Lewis & Kershsaw, 2010).

Conclusion

The broad field of eHealth has emerged and evolved rapidly, and it has significant implications for health promotion and health behavior change. In recent decades we have developed a strong understanding of the potential for technology to reach large numbers of people (see Table 2.1), and we are increasingly aware of the best practices in balancing reach with targeting our desired audiences. We have effectively used computers to develop algorithms and deliver tailored information, we can standardize health promotion content to ensure delivery of consistent and high quality messages, and we have begun to consider how to best engage audiences with material that they can enjoy. We have utilized computers and computer kiosks, the Internet, and cell phones to deliver our health promotion programs, and we are increasing our efforts to link face-to-face programs with technology-based programs to extend and enhance health promotion.

With the advancements in technology and eHealth applications, however, we recognize important cautions. First, technology has limited ability to establish rapport and trust; although we have an opportunity to explore how we might use technology to enhance and extend existing relationships, we should not rely on technology to establish the levels of trust that may be needed for excellent delivery of education and care. Second, while stand-alone health technology programs have demonstrated efficacy, we must take care not to replace effective face-to-face programs with technological facsimiles. Any adaptation of efficacious face-to-face interventions needs to be evaluated to determine if efficacy can be replicated online; furthermore, if something "works" in real life, decisions about migrating programs to the virtual world should be made carefully, balancing participant preference with program cost and utility, for example. Third, maintenance of privacy and security are critical through eHealth applications. Recently, media have drawn attention to the amount of personal information that is potentially available about people who use social networking sites, along with terms of service that may or may not make explicit social networking site ownership of any online post. While people may be aware of limitations to privacy online, we cannot assume they are, and we must maintain high standards of disclosure and transparency about how we handle data, who has access to such information, and how we will ensure security using the most up-to-date standards from the field of Internet technology (IT). Not only must developers of such applications apply the most high quality security available, but they must also carefully communicate to users what privacy risks still exist when one engages with a program that asks for personal health information.

We look forward to the coming decades in the field of eHealth where we anticipate a growth in understanding of how to best use social media and networking sites for our work; how to tap into the potential of (increasingly sophisticated) cell phones for health promotion and disease prevention; and how to better and more consistently link technology into face-to-face clinical, institutional, and community-based efforts to promote health. We anticipate that current efforts to develop an evidence base for stand-alone eHealth applications will be realized, and we will generate wide reaching best practices for the field. We anticipate being able to improve our own evaluation methods to more quickly assess efficacy and disseminate effective programs more widely. We also anticipate as-of-yet undiscovered technological applications will offer additional opportunities to use technology in relevant and engaging ways to continually contribute to improvements in health and well-being.

References

Bellis, M. (n.d.). Inventors of the modern computer: The first freely programmable computer invented by Konrad Zuse. *About.com*. Retrieved July 11, 2011, from: http://inventors.about.com/library/weekly/aa050298.htm.

Bennett, G. G., & Glasgow, R. E. (2009). The delivery of public health interventions via the Internet: Actualizing their potential. *Annual Review of Public Health, 30,* 273–292.

Boase, J., Horrigan, J. B., Wellman, B., & Rainie, L. (2006). The strength of Internet ties: The Internet and email aid users in maintaining their social networks and provide pathways to help when people face big decisions. *Pew Internet & American Life Project.* Retrieved January 25, 2006, from: http://www.pewinternet.org/~/media//Files/Reports/2006/PIP_Internet_ties.pdf.pdf.

Brown, S. J., Lieberman, D. A., Gemeny, B. A., Fan, Y. C., Wilson, D. M., & Pasta, D. J. (1997). Educational video game for juvenile diabetes: Results of a controlled trial. *Informatics for Health and Social Care, 22,* 77–89.

Bull, S. S., & McFarlane, M. (2000). Soliciting sex on the Internet: What are the risks for sexually transmitted diseases and HIV? *Sexually Transmitted Diseases, 27,* 545–550.

Bull, S., Pratte, K., Whitesell, N., Rietmeijer, C., & McFarlane, M. (2009). Effects of an Internet-based intervention for HIV prevention: The Youthnet trials. *AIDS and Behavior, 13,* 474–487.

Christakis, N. A., & Fowler, J. H. (2007). The spread of obesity in a large social network over 32 years. *New England Journal of Medicine, 357,* 370–379.

Christensen, H., Griffiths, K. M., & Korten, A. (2002). Web-based cognitive therapy: Analysis of site usage and changes in depression and anxiety scores. *Journal of Medical Internet Research, 4,* e3.

Cole-Lewis, H., & Kershsaw, T. (2010). Text messaging as a tool for behavior change in disease prevention and management. *Epidemiologic Reviews, 32,* 56–69.

De Bourdeaudhuij, I., Maes, L., De Henauw, S., De Vriendt, T., Moreno, L. A., Kersting, M., et al. (2010). Evaluation of a computer-tailored physical activity intervention in adolescents in six European countries: The Activ-O-Meter in the HELENA intervention study. *Journal of Adolescent Health, 46,* 458–466.

De Bourdeaudhuij, I., Stevens, V., Vandelanotte, C., & Brug, J. (2007). Evaluation of an interactive computer-tailored nutrition intervention in a real-life setting. *Annals of Behavioral Medicine, 33,* 39–48.

Detmer, D., Bloomrosen, M., Raymond, B., & Tang, P. (2008). Integrated personal health records: Transformative tools for consumer-centric care. *BMC Medical Informatics and Decision Making, 8,* 45–58.

Downer, S. R., Meara, J. G., & Da Costa, A. C. (2005). Use of SMS text messaging to improve outpatient attendance. *Medical Journal of Australia, 183,* 366–368.

Ekeland, A. G., Bowes, A., & Flottorp, S. (2010). Effectiveness of telemedicine: A systematic review of reviews. *International Journal of Medical Informatics, 79,* 736–771.

Erk, S., Kiefer, M., Grothe, J., Wunderlich, A. P., Spitzer, M., & Walter, H. (2003). Emotional context modulates subsequent memory effect. *NeuroImage, 18,* 439–447.

Eysenbach, G., Powell, J., Kuss, O., & Sa, E-R. (2002). Empirical studies assessing the quality of health information for consumers on the World Wide Web: A systematic review. *Journal of the American Medical Association, 287,* 2691–2700.

Fox, S. (2010, July 8). Generations online and the social life of health information. *Pew Internet & American Life Project.* Retrieved July 11, 2011, from: http://www.slideshare.net/PewInternet/fox-nlm-july2010.

Glasgow, R. E., Boles, S. M., McKay, H. G., Feil, E. G., & Barrera Jr., M. (2003). The D-Net diabetes self-management program: Long-term implementation, outcomes, and generalization results. *Preventive Medicine, 36,* 410–419.

Graham, A. L., Cobb, N. K., Raymond, L., Sill, S., & Young, J. (2007). Effectiveness of an Internet-based worksite smoking cessation intervention at 12 months. *Journal of Occupational and Environmental Medicine, 49,* 821–828.

Gray, J. R., Braver, T. S., & Raichle, M. E. (2002). Integration of emotion and cognition in the lateral prefrontal cortex. *Proceedings of the National Academy of Sciences of the United States of America, 99,* 4115–4120.

Gustafson, D. H., Hawkins, R. P., Boberg, E. W., McTavish, F., Owens, B., Wise, M., et al. (2002). CHESS: 10 years of research and development in consumer health informatics for broad populations, including the underserved. *International Journal of Medical Informatics, 65,* 169–177.

Gustafson, D. H., Hawkins, R., Pingree, S., McTavish, F., Arora, N. K., Mendenhall, J., et al. (2001). Effect of computer support on younger women with breast cancer. *Journal of General Internal Medicine, 16,* 435–445.

Gustafson, D. H., McTavish, F. M., Stengle, W., Ballard, D., Hawkins, R., Shaw, B. R., et al. (2005). Use and impact of eHealth system by low-income women with breast cancer. *Journal of Health Communication, 10,* 195–218.

Gustafson, D. H., Robinson, T. N., Ansley, D., Adler, L., & Brennan, P. F. (1999). Consumers and evaluation of interactive health communication applications. *American Journal of Preventative Medicine, 16,* 23–29.

Hawkins, R. P., Kreuter, M., Resnicow, K., Fishbein, M., & Dijkstra, A. (2008). Understanding tailoring in communicating about health. *Health Education Research, 23,* 454–466.

Hodge, F. S., Fredericks, L., & Rodriguez, B. (1996). American Indian women's talking circle: A cervical cancer screening and prevention project. *Cancer, 78,* 1592–1597.

Horrigan, J. B. (2007, May 7). A typology of information and communication technology users. *Pew Internet & American Life Project*. Retrieved January 2, 2010, from: http://www.pewinternet.org/~/media//Files/Reports/2007/PIP_ICT_Typology.pdf.pdf.

Horrigan, J. (2008a, March 5). Seeding the cloud: What mobile access means for usage patterns and online content. *Pew Internet & American Life Project*. Retrieved April 10, 2008, from: http://www.pewinternet.org/Reports/2008/Seeding-The-Cloud-What-Mobile-Access-Means-for-Usage-Patterns-and-Online-Content.aspx.

Horrigan, J. (2008b, May 5). Mobile access to data and information. *Pew Internet & American Life Project*. Retrieved April 10, 2008, from: http://www.pewinternet.org/Press-Releases/2008/Mobile-Access-to-Data-and-Information.aspx.

Kamel Boulos, M. N., Hetherington, L., & Wheeler, S. (2007). Second Life: An overview of the potential of 3-D virtual worlds in medical and health education. *Health Information and Libraries Journal, 24,* 233–245.

Kamel Boulos, M. N., Ramloll, R., Jones, R., & Toth-Cohen, S. (2008). Web 3D for public, environmental and occupational health: Early examples from Second Life. *International Journal of Environmental Research and Public Health, 5,* 290–317.

Kato, P. M., & Beale, I. L. (2006). Factors affecting acceptability to young cancer patients of a psychoeducational video game about cancer. *Journal of Pediatric Oncology Nursing, 23,* 269–275.

Klausner, J. D., Wolf, W., Fischer-Ponce, L., Zolt, I., & Katz, M. H. (2000). Tracing a syphilis outbreak through cyberspace. *Journal of the American Medical Association, 284,* 447–449.

Krebs, P., Prochaska, J., & Rossi, J. (2010). A meta-analysis of computer-tailored interventions for health behavior change. *Preventive Medicine, 51,* 214–221.

Kreuter, M. W., & Wray, R. J. (2003). Tailored and targeted health communication: Strategies for enhancing information relevance. *American Journal of Health Behavior, 27,* S227–S232.

Kroeze, W., Werkman, A., & Brug, J. (2006). A systematic review of randomized trials on the effectiveness of computer-tailored education on physical activity and dietary behaviors. *Annals of Behavioral Medicine, 31,* 205–223.

Leeman-Castillo, B., Beaty, B., Raghunath, S., Steiner, J., & Bull, S. (2010). LUCHAR: Using computer technology to battle heart disease among Latinos. *American Journal of Public Health, 100,* 272–275.

Lenhart, A., & Horrigan, J. B. (2003). Re-visualizing the digital divide as a digital spectrum. *IT & Society, 1,* 23–39.

Lenhart, A., Jones, S., & Macgill, A. R. (2008, December 7). Adults and video games. *Pew Internet & American Life Project*. Retrieved July 25, 2009, from: http://www.pewinternet.org/Reports/2008/Adults-and-Video-Games.aspx.

Lenhart, A., Ling, R., Campbell, S., & Purcell, K. (2010, April 20). Text messaging explodes as teens embrace it as a vital form of daily communication with friends. *Pew Internet & American Life Project*. Retrieved August 10, 2010, from: http://www.pewinternet.org/Reports/2010/Teens-and-Mobile-Phones/Chapter-2/Part-1.aspx.

Lorence, D. P., Park, H., & Fox, S. (2006). Racial disparities in health information access: Resilience of the digital divide. *Journal of Medical Internet Systems, 30,* 241–249.

Lueg, C., & Fisher, D. (Eds.) (2003). *From Usenet to CoWebs: Interacting with social information spaces*. London: Springer.

Maibach, E., Flora, J. A., & Nass, C. (1991). Changes in self-efficacy and health behavior in response to a minimal contact community health campaign. *Health Communication, 3,* 1–15.

McFarlane, M., Bull, S., & Rietmeijer, C. A. (2000). The Internet as a newly emerging risk environment for sexually transmitted diseases. *Journal of the American Medical Association, 284,* 443–446.

McFarlane, M., Kachur, R., Klausner, J. D., Roland, E., & Cohen, M. (2005). Internet-based health promotion and disease control in the 8 cities: Successes, barriers, and future plans. *Sexually Transmitted Diseases, 32,* S60–S64.

Noar, S. M., Benac, C. N., & Harris, M. S. (2007). Does tailoring matter? Meta-analytic review of tailored print health behavior change interventions. *Psychological Bulletin, 133,* 673–693.

Noar, S. M., Harrington, N., & Aldrich, R. (2009). The role of message tailoring in the development of persuasive health communication messages. *Communication Yearbook, 33,* 72–133.

Patrick, K., Raab, F., Adams, M. A., Dillon, L., Zabinski, M., Rock, C. L., et al. (2009). A text message–based intervention for weight loss: Randomized controlled trial. *Journal of Medical Internet Research, 11,* e1.

Population Media Center. (2009, June 5). *Sex Sells: A Tiny Nonprofit Uses Mass Media to Encourage Family Planning.* Retrieved July 15, 2011, from: http://www.populationmedia. org/2009/06/05/sex-sells-a-tiny-nonprofit-uses-mass-media-to-encourage-family-planning/.

Rhodes, S. D., Diclemente, R. J., Cecil, H., Hergenrather, K. C., & Yee, L. J. (2002). Risk among men who have sex with men in the United States: A comparison of an Internet sample and a conventional outreach sample. *AIDS Education and Prevention, 14,* 41–50.

Rodgers, A., Corbett, T., Bramley, D., Riddell, T., Wills, M., Lin R. B., et al. (2005). Do u smoke after txt? Results of a randomised trial of smoking cessation using mobile phone text messaging. *Tobacco Control, 14,* 255–261.

Rogers, E. M. (1995). *Diffusion of innovations* (4th ed.). New York: Free Press.

Rogers, E. M., Vaughan, P. W., Swalehe, R. M. A., Rao, N., Svenkerud, P., & Sood, S. (1999). Effects of an entertainment-education radio soap opera on family planning behavior in Tanzania. *Studies in Family Planning, 30,* 193–211.

Ross, M. W., Rosser, B. R., & Stanton, J. (2004). Beliefs about cybersex and Internet-mediated sex of Latino men who have Internet sex with men: Relationships with sexual practices in cybersex and in real life. *AIDS Care, 16,* 1002–1011.

Rosser, B. R. S., Miner, M. H., Bockting, W. O., Ross, M. W., Konstan, J., Gurak, L., et al. (2009). HIV risk and the Internet: Results of the Men's INTernet Sex (MINTS) Study. *AIDS and Behavior, 13,* 746–756.

Second Life [Computer software]. (2010). San Francisco: Linden Lab. Retrieved July 11, 2011, from: http://secondlife.com/?lang=en-US.

Smith, A. (2010, July 7). Mobile access 2010. *Pew Internet & American Life Project.* Retrieved August 10, 2010, from: http://pewinternet.org/Reports/2010/Mobile-Access-2010/Summary-of-Findings.aspx.

Svirko, E., & Mellanby, J. (2008). Attitudes to e-learning, learning style and achievement in learning neuroanatomy by medical students. *Medical Teacher, 30,* e219–e227.

Tech-FAQ. (2011). *History of cell phones.* Retrieved January 11, 2011, from: http://www. tech-faq.com/history-of-cell-phones.html.

Turner, C. F., Ku, L., Rogers, S. M., Lindberg, L. D., Pleck, J. H., & Sonerstein, F. L. (1998). Adolescent sexual behavior, drug use, and violence: Increased reporting with computer survey technology. *Science, 280,* 867–873.

Turner, J. (2003). Expanding healthcare into virtual environments. In T. Thompson, A. Dorsey, K. Miller, & R. Parrott (Eds.), *Handbook of health communication* (pp. 515–536). Mahwah, NJ: Lawrence Erlbaum Associates.

Vidrine, D. J., Arduino, R. C., Lazev, A. B., & Gritz, E. R. (2006). A randomized trial of a proactive cellular telephone intervention for smokers living with HIV/AIDS. *AIDS, 20,* 253–260.

Wantland, D. J., Portillo, C. J., Holzemer, W. L., Slaughter, R., & McGhee, E. M. (2004). The effectiveness of Web-based vs. non-Web-based interventions: A meta-analysis of behavioral change outcomes. *Journal of Medical Internet Research, 6,* e40.

Webber, K. H., Tate, D. F., & Quintiliani, L. M. (2008). Motivational interviewing in Internet groups: A pilot study for weight loss. *Journal of the American Dietetic Association, 108,* 1029–1032.

Williams-Brown, S., Baldwin, D. M., & Bakos, A. (2002). Storytelling as a method to teach African American women breast health information. *Journal of Cancer Education, 17,* 227–230.

Winett, R. A., Anderson, E. S., Wojcik, J. R., Winett, S. G., & Bowden, T. (2007). Guide to health: Nutrition and physical activity outcomes of a group-randomized trial of an Internet-based intervention in churches. *Annals of Behavioral Medicine, 33,* 251–261.

3

INTERACTIVITY

Conceptualizations, Effects, and Implications

Deborah S. Chung

Interactivity has been called the "hallmark of the digital medium" (Online News Association, 2003), and some have referred to it as the single most important quality that distinguishes newer digital media from traditional forms of communication (Sundar, 2007). Interactivity fundamentally challenges existing models of communication and blurs the lines between mass and interpersonal, sender and receiver, and traditional and new media. Because of its unique appeal with qualities that extend and enhance user experiences and lead to more audience empowerment, interactivity has attracted the attention of many scholars from a broad range of disciplines, including communication (Chan-Olmsted & Park, 2000; Greer & Mensing, 2006; Massey & Levy, 1999; Schultz, 1999), political science (Stromer-Galley, 2000; Stromer-Galley & Foot, 2002), business/marketing (Aikat, 2000; Ha & James, 1998), and health contexts (Lustria, 2007; McMillan, 2002; Noar, Clark, Cole, & Lustria, 2006). Although scholars have defined interactivity in multiple ways, and the debate continues regarding its locus, key characteristics, and consequences, many scholars concur that interactivity influences individuals' cognition, attitudes, and behaviors.

The Internet and various interactive informational tools have increasingly become a major resource for individuals seeking information, including those seeking health information, and thus, the effective implementation of interactive applications for health promotion has become a topic of considerable discussion. Audiences are now able to take more active roles in their health information consumption experiences as content is presented through websites, online support networks, various eHealth applications/mobile health communication devices, and electronic health records (Neuhauser & Kreps, 2010).

Today 61% of American adults seek health information online—a growth from 25% almost a decade ago (Fox & Jones, 2009). The development of extensive Web 2.0 tools has also expanded users' options for actively seeking information. For example, mobile devices draw audiences into health-related discussions through easy-to-use interactive technologies. A majority of individuals involved in seeking health-related information also consume user-generated content that is motivated by a search for timely, relevant information catered to individuals' specific needs. Forty-one percent of Americans have read someone else's commentary or experiences regarding medical issues on blogs, news groups, or other websites (Fox & Jones, 2009). Thus, health consumers are utilizing various interactive tools in order to meet their specific health care and information needs.

Interactivity has also been identified as the communication attribute with the greatest potential to enhance health promotion (Rice, 2001; Street & Rimal, 1997). Thus, the concept of interactivity in such contexts is highly relevant; furthermore, interactivity has broad implications for consumers because varying interactive features also extend different kinds of user activities through specific interactive functions (Chung, 2008). The present chapter seeks to examine the current state of interactivity literature and summarize key definitional models of interactivity. In the examination, three types of interactivity are presented (interactivity as a medium characteristic, interactivity as a user-centered concept, and interactivity as personalization and customization) with implications for appropriate implementation strategies within health communication contexts.

Defining the Concept: What Is Interactivity?

The dominant mass communication paradigm is based on Shannon and Weaver's (1949) model, which describes communication as a sequential process for information sharing. Starting with a communication source that produces or selects a message, the model describes how the message is subsequently transmitted by a signal through a channel that carries the signal to a receiver who then transforms the signal back to the destination. Rogers (1986) refers to this model as "the single most important turning point in the history of communication science" (pp. 86–87).

Bordewijk and van Kaam's (1986) four-part typology of information asserts that the key to interactivity is control—who controls and produces the information and who controls the distribution of information in terms of timing and subject matter. McQuail (1994) refines this model and states the key is where the control resides—with a central provider or with an individual user. He further makes distinctions between different patterns of communication: allocution (transmission), conversation, consultation, and registration. Allocution represents one-way traditional mass media, such as real-time radio or television, whereas conversation is akin to interpersonal communication. A consultation communication pattern takes place when the consumer makes a request to the information provider for specific information, and a registration communication pattern may represent central registration systems typically available in many organizations for record keeping and information gathering through surveillance. Each represents distinct information traffic patterns.

However, new information and communication technologies (ICTs) with interactive capabilities enable various types of communication directionality, including one-to-one communication, such as email; one-to-few/many and few-to-few communication, such as chats; and many-to-many communication, such as user forums (Morris & Ogan, 1996). This change in possible directional flow of messages between sender and receiver is a key distinction between new and traditional forms of media. Particularly in mediated communication interfaces, such as the computer, interactivity is a foundational characteristic. As Sundar, Xu, and Bellur (2010) state, interactivity transforms a system into a communication medium through the elicitation of user interaction with the interface. Thus, interactivity in essence is a set of system affordances that allows users to manipulate the source, message, channel, and receiver combinations.

Such changes in communication flow imply that the audience may take on more active roles as agents of communication. These observations have significant implications for traditional mass communication theories (Delwiche, 2005; Roberts, Wanta, & Dzwo, 2002; Thelwall, Byrne, & Goody, 2007) because the traditional information providers, or gatekeepers of information, have been distinct from the receivers of information—those who have been left out of the process of being able to manipulate the content or form of communication. Through interactivity, however, audiences are afforded an increased sense of agency because they have a greater influence on the communication process and their information consumption experiences. Sundar (2008) defines agency as "the degree to which the self feels that he/she is a relevant actor in the CMC [computer-mediated communication] situation . . . it is the extent of manipulability afforded by the interface to assert one's influence over the nature and course of the interaction" (p. 61). Agency allows users to feel involved as active participants engaged in the communication process.

Additionally, interactivity can extend and emulate mediated face-to-face communication experiences. Thus, through interactive interfaces, users can be said to share many of the assumptions of Schudson's (1978) "conversational ideal," such as receiving continuous feedback, engaging in multichannel communication, participating in spontaneous utterances when desired, assuming both sender and receiver roles, and engaging in a more or less egalitarian communication setting. In sum, interactivity can be discussed within the realm of directionality of communication, agency of the communicators involved, and mutual discourse between participants.

Types of Interactivity and Their Traits

Over the last three decades, interactivity has been discussed in various ways. Among them, as Rafaeli and Ariel (2007) summarize, representative conceptualizations describing interactivity include synchronicity (Liu & Shrum, 2002; Steuer, 1995; Van Dijk, 1999), control (Jensen, 1998; Lieb, 1998; Neuman, 1991; Rogers,

1995), speed (Lombard & Ditton, 1997), participation (Dyson, 1993), choice (Ha & James, 1998), hypertextuality (Sundar, Kalyanaraman, & Brown, 2003), responsiveness (Heeter, 1989; Rafaeli, 1988; Rafaeli & Sudweeks, 1997), and experience (Bucy, 2004a; Laurel, 1991). Some definitions take on a functional approach (Steuer, 1995; Sundar, 2004), whereas others take on a user approach (Rogers, 1995; Williams, Rice, & Rogers, 1988). Other models combine both perspectives (Ha & James, 1998; Heeter, 1989).

Among the various definitional models of interactivity, however, there is general agreement in conceptualizing interactivity through the distinction between medium interactivity and human interactivity (Bucy, 2004a; Chung & Yoo, 2008; Lee, 2000; Outing, 1998; Schultz, 1999; Stromer-Galley, 2000, 2004), although foci of key characteristics vary within each discussion. Additionally, some scholars have discussed human interactivity as being more interactive (and more critical) than medium interactivity (Chung & Yoo, 2008; Outing, 1998; Schultz, 1999; Stromer-Galley, 2000), while others have denounced such conceptualizations (e.g., Rafaeli, 1988). Medium interactivity, also known as content or product interactivity, generally refers to communication between users and technology with a focus on the technical aspects of a medium enabling users to carry out certain activities. Human interactivity, also known as process, interpersonal, or user-to-user interactivity, focuses on mediated human interactions often dealing with issues of role, power, and ritual (Stromer-Galley, 2004). This distinction is by no means a neat classification because numerous models exist that employ both user and medium approaches (e.g., Chung & Yoo, 2008; Deuze, 2003; Heeter, 1989; McMillan, 2002). In fact, definitions that incorporate both perspectives dominate the literature. This illustrates the challenge of conceptualizing and operationalizing this construct, which has been a continual problem. Interactivity is often considered to be a multidimensional construct leading to various user experiences and outcomes.

Despite the definitional frustration and confusion, the following section presents the different types (and levels) of interactivity within prominent conceptualizations that may lead to a helpful general understanding of interactivity. Indeed, certain models offer a better fit depending on medium, context, and user.

Interactivity as Medium Characteristic: Choice, Selectivity, Navigability, and Modality

Definitions focusing on interactivity as a medium characteristic discuss the technological attributes of interactivity and the functionality of features. Some researchers have used the term control (Bordewijk & van Kaam, 1986; Rogers, 1995), although this concept may be considered overly broad and may be too inclusive of a wide range of user activities.

Implicit in this discussion are issues of increased audience choice or selectivity and navigability. Heeter (1989) claims a medium is more interactive if it allows extensive choice options to the user. This results in increased selectivity for control over the communication process (Massey & Levy, 1999). Navigation of a website, for example, also becomes nonlinear, with control given to the user. The importance of choice is also reflected in Ha and James's (1998) and Massey and Levy's (1999) models of interactivity. For example, Ha and James studied early business websites and proposed choice as a critical dimension of interactivity that leads to potentially unrestrained navigation. Deuze (2003) also points to navigational interactivity as facilitating users with structured ways to peruse online content through hyperlinks that move the users forward and backward, back to top, and so on.

In illustrating central choice options offered through technological features, Steuer's model (1995) may be considered the most representative within this classification. In his exploration of concepts aiding virtual reality (VR), Steuer identified vividness and interactivity as concepts that define telepresence—the state of feeling present, or immersed, in a mediated environment. Steuer defines interactivity as the extent to which the medium allows the participant to modify the content or form of a mediated environment in real time and specifies three characteristics: speed, range, and mapping. *Speed* refers to real-time responses. Real-time input and output is most similar to interpersonal communication and is therefore considered ideal in this model. The goal is to create input that allows change to the mediated environment fast enough to avoid lag time. Here, feedback is not sufficient; the feedback must be immediate to deliver a realistic experience. *Range* refers to the number of choices available to alter the mediated environment. The wider the range, the more choices available and the more a user will feel able to control the mediated environment. Thus, the user may feel a sense of empowerment. *Mapping* refers to how similar or dissimilar, as well as how natural or unnatural, a mediated representation is in relation to physical reality. The more similar it is, the more immersed a user will feel. Steuer's definition of interactivity focuses on the user's ability to work with the technology. His model may be most helpful in understanding interactivity in VR settings. While incorporating users into his definition, Steuer's true focus for his model is the technology.

Within this tradition of focusing on technological attributes, a discussion of modality has also been given prime attention. Through the computer and digital media tools, information can be presented in various formats, including video, audio, and multimedia. Sundar et al. (2010) report that while a single modality used to be associated with a particular medium, modern day technologies make convergence of multiple modalities possible within a single medium, furthering the depth of information presentation and its reception. In addition, interactive tools give rise to new modalities (Sundar et al., 2010) that not only cater to our senses, such as sight and sound, but further extend those capabilities. Modality can be extended in clicking activity (e.g., hyperlinks), mouse-over behaviors, scrolling, and even zooming. Thus, users can now experience information within a single modality, multiple modalities, or back and forth between modalities (Sundar et al., 2010). Such varying modal presentations offer a diversity of user experiences.

Thus, within this classification, there may exist lower and higher levels of medium interactivity. For example, information presented with fewer choice options by offering users a limited number of hyperlinks or limited ways to experience a story (e.g., single modality or text-only interfaces) may be considered to be low in medium interactivity. On the other hand, information presented with multiple-choice options (e.g., multiple links to various topics) with various ways to navigate an interface (e.g., click, scroll, hover, zoom) or information provided through multiple converged modalities (e.g., text, audio, video) with the ability to switch among varied modes of content may be considered as offering users a higher level of medium interactivity.

Previous eHealth studies have used various types of medium interactive features in their interventions. For example, in order to create a rich multimedia environment that would facilitate user engagement, Buller et al. (2008) integrated audio narration, sound effects, graphics, animation, and music. This contextual setting was provided to deliver relevant nonverbal information that would aid in learning and improve message credibility. Matano et al. (2007) also used colorful graphics, computer animation, artwork, and various links to online resources in their study of an interactive Web-based intervention for reducing alcohol consumption.

Interactivity as User Centered: Reciprocal User Exchange, Mutual Discourse/Dialogue, Democratic Deliberation

Interpersonal communication contexts, or face-to-face communication settings, have often been deemed the standard of interactivity. Various user interfaces and digital media tools and their content presentations have been evaluated based on how closely they resemble such communication formats (Walther & Burgoon, 1992). Some scholars have challenged this observation (Rafaeli, 1988; Schudson, 1978), yet numerous definitional models have integrated some form of user-to-user or person-to-person interactivity into their conceptualizations, such as reciprocal communication exchanges, conversation, responsiveness, and continuous feedback. For example, Rice and Williams (1984) state that the key to interactivity is the exchange between sender and receiver. Heeter (1989) recognizes "responsiveness to user" and "facilitation of interpersonal communication" as key dimensions within her multidimensional model. Ha and James (1998), too, include "reciprocal communication" as one of their dimensions of interactivity.

Several practitioners and scholars, including Outing (1998), Schultz (1999), Stromer-Galley (2000), and Chung (2008), have focused on human interactivity in particular. The focus on human interactivity could be attributed to high hopes in the participatory potential and democratic promises of online communication settings since scholars have long criticized the one-way paradigm of traditional media. Media critics have argued that the mass media have largely produced messages independent from their audiences (Habermas, 1962; Schultz, 1999). Critics also have lamented the lack of opportunities for citizen dialogue and intense political discussion (that may lead to democratic deliberation) available through traditional media channels (Barber, 1984; Habermas, 1996).

Interactivity, however, affords audiences with an increased sense of agency to have a greater influence on the communication process and information consumption experiences by allowing both horizontal (between users) and vertical (between users and journalists/public figures) communication. Such mediated user interactions also happen in more egalitarian communication contexts. Stromer-Galley (2000) describes computer-mediated human interaction as allowing senders and receivers of information to exchange communication roles and offer feedback to each other. She claims that human interactivity is more interactive because it provides two-way communication exchange between the communicator (source) and the audience, which provides the foundation for public deliberation. Human interactivity, thus, may facilitate an environment for communication that is the key to Habermas's (1984) theory of the public sphere, where citizens can converse with the guarantee of freedom of assembly and express their opinions according to the standards of critical reasoning. In these environments, conversation, communication, and lively debate are open to all—in principle. Accordingly, the goals of human interactivity are not only to increase discussion but also to increase quality discussion. Ideal human interactivity should not only allow the potential for increased interpersonal communication opportunities but also allow the potential for richer, quality dialogue.

The immediacy of information or real-time message delivery through interactive technologies, much like that experienced in face-to-face interpersonal communication, has been underscored (e.g., Steuer, 1995) in discussions of medium interactivity. The focus here, however, is on extended communication exchanges. In this context both synchronous and asynchronous exchanges further reciprocal communication. Rather than emphasizing the timeliness of information, some scholars (e.g., Downes & McMillan, 2000) have identified the convenience of communication afforded through interactive technologies. Users are able to initiate a communication on the basis of when they wish to carry out that exchange. The ability for users to determine when they desire to communicate further extends users' agency and control because they can choose to communicate in a more timely fashion or postpone further communication exchanges for the time being. In other words, users can determine when they wish to perform as sender or receiver of information and have the ability to role play as they please. Such time flexibility is illustrated in email communications, message boards, and user forum discussions.

One of the most widely used definitions of interactivity by communication scholars is Rafaeli's (1988) model of interactivity as responsiveness, which focuses on discourse and the relatedness of sequential messages (Rafaeli, 1988; Rafaeli & Ariel, 2007). Rafaeli studied the communication exchanges among asynchronous, multi-participant public discussion groups. While his original study (1988) predates the Web, his exploration of interactivity has contributed to the communication field as well as computer science, sociology, and informatics. Rafaeli and Sudweeks (1997) define interactivity as "the extent to which messages in a sequence relate to each other and especially the extent to which later messages recount the relatedness of earlier messages."

Rafaeli (1988) makes three distinctions: two-way communication, reactive communication, and fully interactive communication. Two-way communication occurs once messages are delivered both ways, but this form of communication is not considered interactive. Two individuals talking at each other do not necessarily lead to a build up of conversation or a progress of information. Reactive communication occurs when there is semi-interactivity present. This communication requires that later messages respond to previous messages. Fully interactive communication occurs when later messages respond to a sequence of previous messages.

This model delineates strict criteria and is rather exclusive in its qualifications for achieving full levels of interactivity. Additionally, while not discussed in his model, time appears to play a role in reaching fully interactive settings because the act of referencing and building related messages cannot be achieved instantaneously. Thus, full interactivity, from this perspective, is an almost unattainable ideal (Bucy, 2004a).

Overall, within Rafaeli's (1988) classification, there also may exist lower and higher levels of human interactivity on the basis of the explanations above. For example, lower human interactivity communication contexts may offer opportunities for mutual discourse, but the discussion may not build up or the context may be peripheral to the central topic of the forum, and only a few users may be involved. However, when there is a back and forth of content exchanges that moves a discussion forward in a meaningful way among numerous individuals, then higher levels of human interactivity have been achieved.

There are many reports regarding the positive effects of human interactivity applied to online health contexts. For example, P. N. Schultz, Stava, Beck, and Vassilopoulou-Sellin (2003) created and examined an online message board that provided timely information about different types of cancer, treatments, and research results. After analyzing data available on the message board over a 16-month period, the team reported that message boards served as useful tools for sharing information with others who had similar conditions, sharing their experiences about their treatment, and providing social support. In a study addressing cancer patients and their companions, Chung and Kim (2008) examined the relationship between various blogging activities and gratifications of using blogs. They found that posting comments on others' blogs positively predicted information-sharing gratifications. The feedback mechanism of blogs appears to function as a source for information distribution and transaction among cancer patients and their companions. Active blogging practices in which users can post comments and exchange views were found to offer more useful blogging experiences for cancer patients and their companions than passive blogging activity such as merely reading blog posts. Overall, the authors conclude that blogs have the potential to function as useful tools for cancer patients and their companions, particularly as a resource for emotion management and information sharing.

Perceived Interactivity

Within the user perspective of interactivity, the approach toward perceived interactivity has also gained considerable attention. Here, user perceptions are the unit of measure rather than structural features or message exchange processes. Proponents of this tradition believe that interactivity is a subjective experience (Bucy, 2004a; Kiousis, 2002; Laurel, 1991; McMillan & Hwang, 2002; Newhagen, Cordes, & Levy, 1995; Wu, 2005). As Rafaeli and Ariel (2007) note, "Even when research defines interactivity in a particular setting as high or low, users can subjectively have different feelings, experiences, or perceptions of interactivity of different levels of intensity" (p. 82).

For example, Laurel (1991) asserts that the key to the interactive experience is the feeling. "You either feel yourself to be participating in the ongoing action of the representation (*computer interface*) or you don't" (pp. 20–21). As a software designer and programmer, Laurel (1991) worked primarily on interactive fiction and fantasy for children and explored the human-computer relationship possible through new technologies. While studying interface design, she discovered that computer interfaces are much like theatres—direct manipulation and engagement arouses enthusiasm and the feeling of interactivity within a user/audience. When users are directly engaged, they become active and involved in the experience. They are no longer simply the passive audience. Laurel (1991) uses theatre as a metaphor for computers. In a theatre, the stage setting, the props, and the lighting all add to the "feeling" of the simulation. The theatre and computer interfaces are highly context dependent. In theater and graphical interfaces, the aim is to create environments that are realistic but different. While Laurel (1991) also identifies three features of interactivity—frequency, the number of times a user can interact within an interface; range, the number of choice options available; and significance, the choices that are meaningful and actually make a difference—she argues that the key is not these mechanical features but the true experience and feeling that the user undergoes in a simulation interface.

Thus, it is argued that users must psychologically perceive and sense that they can exert an influence on the communication context at hand before interactivity can be said to exist (Sundar et al., 2010). Some researchers have even suggested that the perception of interactivity is more critical than the actual existence of interactivity (Kalyanaraman & Sundar, 2006). For example, studies report that individuals assessed different levels of interactivity on websites when, in fact, they were the same (Lee, Lee, Kim, & Stout, 2004). Additionally, users may perceive a communication context to be highly interactive despite the absence of obvious signs of user agency (Newhagen et al., 1995). Furthermore, depending on skill level and savviness with the technology, users may perceive varying sets and levels of affordances offered by the interface presented (Norman, 1999). This underscores the importance of perceived versus actual interactivity.

As the focus of this volume is on eHealth applications, a perceptually driven definition of interactivity may not be practical. However, it would be critical to acknowledge the varied approaches toward different interactivity perspectives and the psychological nature of interactivity in order to fully apply its meaningfulness to the eHealth context.

A Little Bit of Both: Adaptability, Tailoring, and Personalization versus Customization

Interfaces that use characteristics of both medium and human interactivity have also been discussed in the literature (e.g., medium/human and human/medium interactivity from Chung, 2008; Chung & Yoo, 2008). These interfaces have also been called *adaptive interactivity,* allowing users' experiences to have consequences on site content (Deuze, 2003). Some scholars have also referred to the adaptability of new media tools as *personalization* or *customization* (Chung, 2008; Sundar & Marathe, 2010) and have even argued that this represents the most sophisticated form of interactivity (Guay, 1995). Shoemaker (1991) claims that customization alters gatekeeping capabilities of the traditional press by allowing users to function as informational sources (Sundar & Nass, 2001).

Chung (2008) identified two types of adaptive interactive features in her study of online news sites. The first type focuses on technological attributes that allow users to customize their news consumption experiences to their liking. Users input personal information (e.g., zip codes) regarding their interests to adjust content (e.g., weather information, movie choices) to their liking. The online site then programs itself to retain information about users' preferences. These interactive features can be deemed personalization options and are more a function of the technology. The second type of adaptive interactive feature allows users to submit their customized opinions or stories to the news sites, providing the audience with a sense of ownership. These features allow users to share and express their own perspectives and become actively involved in the creation of content because they must exert more effort to make use of these functions. These customization options share interpersonal communication qualities but do not necessarily facilitate human-to-human communication.

Sundar and Marathe (2010) distinguish the above two types of adaptive interactivity as personalization and customization. The former is system initiated while the latter is user initiated. Some personalization systems are automatic and may gather user information both overtly and covertly. For example, overt personalization features may directly ask users about their zip codes or gender. Covert personalization involves the use of cookies in browsers. These systems may track users' browsing behavior and recommend products or other services. Both types of personalization require little or no direct user involvement and underscore the end result of the interactive experience (Sundar & Marathe, 2010).

In health communication, such processes are called tailoring (see chapter 8 of this volume), a strategy that involves the modification of information to meet the needs of a specific individual through the identification of distinct attributes of the user (Kreuter, 2000). Many studies in this domain indeed emphasize the relevance of resulting content (Hawkins, Kreuter, Resnicow, Fishbein, & Dijkstra, 2008) rather than the process of how that tailored content is delivered to the users. Scholars studying electronic commerce have also acknowledged the adaptive capabilities newer media systems bring since they can offer information according to user specifications (Rayport & Jaworski, 2001).

While the message recipients receive relevant information on the basis of their health needs and user attributes, some have suggested that personalized tailoring systems may not be as effective in empowering the recipients for three reasons: (1) The locus of control is situated in the information delivery system, (2) the user passively receives rather than actively solicits information, and (3) there is no guarantee that the user will find utility in the tailored messages (Sundar, Marathe, & Kang, 2009).

However, customization focuses on the process of adaptability. As Sundar and Marathe (2010) emphasize, the real innovation of adaptable experiences comes from the fact that audiences are now able to tailor content on their own rather than have that tailored content automatically delivered to them. Customization activities offer audiences a more active role in dictating information, whereas personalization/tailoring engages audiences only passively. Agency plays a central role here as audience members are able to act as sources of information and exert greater influence in the gatekeeping process (Sundar & Marathe, 2010).

Thus, within this classification, there exist lower and higher levels of adaptive interactivity. For example, a health website that only allows users to input information such as birthday and gender (on the basis of which the site automatically personalizes content) would be considered offering lower levels of adaptive interactivity. However, a site that allows visitors to input not only their own user attributes but also submit/publish customized stories or photos that were created by the users themselves would be considered offering higher levels of adaptive interactivity. Wikis, for example, allow users to actively perform source functions and also participate in creating content and, thus, would qualify as offering higher levels of adaptive interactivity.

The literature to date shows that many Web-based health interventions have generally not taken advantage of the various adaptive interactivity tools available. Sundar et al. (2009) found that only about half of the popular health sites included some form of customization option. They conclude that health websites still follow a transmission-oriented communication model despite the considerable potential offered by interactive technologies. In their review of safer sex websites, Noar et al. (2006) reported finding little evidence of tailoring risk reduction messages with interactive customization tools despite the opportunity to tailor messages to individuals' unique characteristics and needs. However, in a more recent study, Lustria, Cortese, Noar, and Glueckauf (2009) found promise in their review of computer-tailored, online behavioral intervention studies. They reported on the diversity of features and formats of the interventions, some offering complex, full-blown customized health programs. The authors found that message tailoring was generally achieved through a combination of feedback, personalization, and adaptation mechanisms.

More contemporary examples, such as the Wii *Fit* game (see Lieberman, this volume), make good use of adaptive tools, allowing various user personalization and customization options (Sundar et al., 2010). For example, by implementing the use of avatars (see Fox, this volume), participants may extend their personal identities through a computer interface. Users can modify their avatars' appearance by changing characteristics such as gender, facial appearance, hair, and body type. Individuals may also create personal user profiles by submitting specific information regarding their fitness needs.

Outcomes of Interactivity

In the discussions above, interactivity has generally been described as a positive quality with increasing levels of interactive functionality described as leading to more satisfying user experiences. However, studies have reported the complex and often problematic nature of interactive presentations and the consequences related to use of such features (Bucy, 2004b; Chung, 2008; Sundar, 2000; Sundar et al., 2003).

For example, literature has documented that too much interactivity may hinder learning (Bucy, 2004b; Sundar et al., 2003). With increased control, users may become overwhelmed with too many choice and selection options and experience information overload. Additionally, as interactivity facilitates various information presentation formats, the complexity of presentation also increases, potentially leading to disorientation. Interactive features may also require more patience, expertise, and cognitive resources of the user, which consequently would increase the likelihood of frustration and confusion and even reduce memory for news (Sundar, 2000). Thus, higher levels of interactivity may lead to negative cognitive and affective effects.

Unnava, Burnkrant, and Erevelles (1994) posit that each individual modality—text, picture, and audio—contains unique characteristics, and people encode this content when processing information. In the journalism context, adding pictures and graphics enhances memory for print and broadcast news (Findahl & Hoijer, 1981). In contrast, limited-capacity information processing theory argues that media messages delivered through multiple modalities are cognitively complex and may overload the processing system (Lang, 2000). Future research should further examine the complex nature of multimodal presentations of information to better understand enhanced and reduced user learning and the subsequent affective effects of medium interactivity.

Additionally, while human interactivity may extend continuous feedback and discussion opportunities, information created by individuals and then shared by others may lead to the circulation of unverifiable, and sometimes inaccurate, information. Previous literature documents such concerns (e.g., Bernhardt, Lariscy, Parrott, Silk, & Felter, 2002; Pew Internet & American Life Project, 2000). Future research should seek to develop information flow monitoring and regulating mechanisms to ensure the veracity of information available through more fluid media tools (e.g., social media) because much is at stake through such information transactions among those who seek health information and interventions. Additionally, health care providers and experts may educate users with more sophisticated information search and filtering habits (Eysenbach, 2006).

Despite the above limitations, numerous studies support positive outcomes offered by interactivity. Tedesco (2007) found that there were significant increases in political information efficacy for individuals exposed to highly interactive Web features. These individuals were also more likely than those in the low interactive condition to say voting was important. Similarly, in the advertising and business disciplines, Ha and James (1998) demonstrated support for the positive effects of interactivity on engagement and relationship building between a company and its customers. Cho and Leckenby (1999) found that higher levels of interactivity resulted in favorable attitudes toward a target ad and brand and greater purchase intentions. Additionally, Teo, Oh, Liu, and Wei (2003) found that increased levels of website interactivity facilitated satisfaction, effectiveness, efficiency, value, and positive perceptions toward a site. More specifically, Kalyanaraman and Sundar (2006) found increased levels of personalized content translated into more positive attitudes of a Web portal and further prompted behavioral effects (e.g., browsing activity).

In the eHealth arena, Lustria (2007) also found that higher levels of interactivity (focusing on increased control, sensory stimulation, and synchronicity) led to greater comprehension of and more positive attitudes toward online health content. Iverson, Howard, and Penney (2008) examined patients' online health-seeking behaviors and found that more than half of the patients reported changing behaviors after being exposed to information online. Patients also were more actively involved in their health-seeking habits, such as asking more questions during physician visits and making self-directed behavioral changes.

Moreover, Shahab and McEwen (2009) conducted a meta-analysis of interactive interventions for smoking cessation and found online interventions, compared with those that were not online (such as untailored written material), were acceptable to users and of superior efficacy to other wide-reach interventions. Their report also suggests that online interventions may have similar efficacy to face-to-face interventions. Noar, Black, and Pierce (2009) reviewed computer technology–based HIV prevention interventions targeting condom use among at-risk populations. They found that computer technology-based interventions focused on condom use behavior yielded statistically significant protective effects. They also found interventions to result in reduced frequency of sexual behavior and incident STD and reduced number of sexual partners. They conclude that computer-delivered interventions have similar efficacy compared to more traditional human-based interventions. In addition, Baranowski, Buday, Thompson, and Baranowski (2008) examined studies on video games that promoted health-related behavioral change. Overall, they found positive health changes from participating in video games, including dietary change, motivation for increased physical activity, fewer hospitalizations, increased knowledge, and more internal control. The authors note that role-playing may increase the personal stake of the player in the outcome of the game as it provides an immersive environment. The report recommends game designers to structure various interactive options to provide relevant feedback for participant-made choices.

Implications for eHealth Applications

Altogether, interactivity is an important characteristic of contemporary digital tools and must be considered carefully for effective and appropriate implementation in health promotion strategies. I conclude this chapter with four key observations. First, as more and more individuals seek health information through ubiquitous interactive tools, a proper understanding of interactivity and its implementation through various interactive features is critical for developing meaningful eHealth applications. That is, interface designers and those interested in eHealth interventions should familiarize themselves with the interactivity literature because it provides baseline knowledge regarding various conceptualizations leading to specific operationalization and implementations. Second, as communication directionality may be manipulated, with users taking on more active roles as participants and sources in the communication process and extending reciprocal communication capabilities, the effective application of interactive tools will be key to engaging users in making healthier behavioral changes. For example, it may be worth focusing on the intended audience rather than the information delivery system and allowing users to take on more active roles in eHealth interventions. Third, depending on the context in which information is communicated and shared, different types of interactivity with unique traits may be more successful in developing messages and user interfaces. For instance, while there exists a wide range of interactive tools, specific technologies may lead to unique types and levels of user engagement. Finally, the possible social and psychological consequences of interactivity should also be considered when creating eHealth applications since research has demonstrated that there are tradeoffs users make with varying outcomes on cognition, attitudes, and behavior. A reasonable level and amount of medium interactive options may be recommended over overtly highly interactive environments.

Conclusion

The concept of interactivity offers exciting opportunities in the design of eHealth applications. Further investigation into the effects of interactivity is needed as more and more individuals depend on online services and interactive tools. It would be beneficial to gain a proper understanding of interactivity—its potential, consequences, and drawbacks—to more appropriately and effectively address user needs. The implementation of these tools may offer more meaningful and potentially empowering user experiences for those seeking health information and healthy behavioral changes.

References

Aikat, D. (2000). A new medium for organizational communication: Analyzing Web content characteristics of Fortune 500 companies. *Electronic Journal of Communication, 10*(1&2). Retrieved December 2007 from: http://shadow.cios.org:7979/journals/EJC/010/1/010111.html.

Baranowski, T., Buday, R., Thompson, D. I., & Baranowski, J. (2008). Playing for real: Video games and stories for health-related behavioral change. *American Journal of Preventive Medicine, 34*, 74–82.

Barber, B. (1984). *Strong democracy: Participatory politics for a new age.* Berkeley: University of California Press.

Bernhardt, J. M., Lariscy, R. A., Parrott, R. L., Silk, K. J., & Felter, E. M. (2002). Perceived barriers to Internet-based health communication on human genetics. *Journal of Health Communication, 7*, 325–340.

Bordewijk, J., & van Kaam, B. (1986). Towards a new classification of teleinformation services. *Inter Media, 14*, 16–21.

Bucy, E. (2004a). Interactivity in society: Locating an elusive concept. *The Information Society, 20*, 373–383.

Bucy, E. (2004b). The interactivity paradox: Closer to the news but confused. In E. Bucy & J. Newhagen (Eds.), *Media access: Social and psychological dimensions of new technology use* (pp. 47–72). Mahwah, NJ: Lawrence Erlbaum Associates.

Buller, D. B., Borland, R., Woodall, W. G., Hall, J. R., Hines, J. M., Burris-Woodall, P., et al. (2008). Randomized trials on Consider This, a tailored, Internet-delivered smoking prevention program for adolescents. *Health Education & Behavior, 35*, 260–281.

Chan-Olmsted, S., & Park, J. (2000). From on-air to online world: examining the content and structures of broadcast TV stations' websites. *Journalism & Mass Communication Quarterly, 77*, 321–339.

Cho, C.-H., & Leckenby, J. D. (1999). Interactivity as a measure of advertising effectiveness: Antecedents and consequences of interactivity in Web advertising. In M. S. Roberts (Ed.), *Proceedings of the 1999 Conference of the American Academy of Advertising* (pp. 162–179). Gainesville: University of Florida.

Chung, D. S. (2008). Interactive features of online newspapers: Identifying patterns and predicting use of engaged readers. *Journal of Computer-Mediated Communication, 13*, 658–679. Retrieved October 2008 from http://www3.interscience.wiley.com/cgibin/fulltext/119414160/HTMLSTART.

Chung, D. S., & Kim, S. (2008). Blogging activity among cancer patients and their companions: Uses, gratifications and predictors of outcomes. *Journal of the American Society for Information Science and Technology, 59,* 297–306.

Chung, D. S., & Yoo, C. Y. (2008). Audience motivations for using interactive features: Distinguishing use of different types of interactivity on an online newspaper. *Mass Communication and Society, 11,* 375–397.

Delwiche, A. (2005). Agenda-setting, opinion leadership, and the world of Web logs. *First Monday, 10.* Retrieved March 2009 from: http://firstmonday.org/htbin/cgiwrap/bin/ojs/index.php/fm/article/view/1300/1220.

Deuze, M. (2003). The Web and its journalisms: Considering the consequences of different types of news media online. *New Media & Society, 5,* 203–230.

Downes, E. J., & McMillan, S. (2000). Defining interactivity: A qualitative identification of key dimensions. *New Media and Society, 2,* 157–179.

Dyson, E. (1993). Interactivity means "active" participation. *Computerworld, 27,* 33–34.

Eysenbach, G. (2006). The impact of the Internet on cancer outcomes. *CA: A Cancer Journal for Clinicians.* Retrieved October 30, 2006, from: http://caonline.amcancersoc.org/cgi/reprint/53/6/356.

Findahl, O., & Hoijer, B. (1981). Media content and human comprehension. In K. E. Rosengren (Ed.), *Advances in content analysis* (pp. 111–132). Beverly Hills, CA: Sage.

Fox, S., & Jones, S. (2009, June 11). *The social life of health information.* Retrieved March 2011, from: http://www.pewinternet.org/Reports/2009/8-The-Social-Life-of-Health-Information.aspx.

Greer, J., & Mensing, D. (2006). The evolution of online newspapers: A longitudinal content analysis, 1997–2003. In X. Li (Ed.), *Internet newspapers: The making of a mainstream medium* (pp. 13–32). Mahwah, NJ: Lawrence Erlbaum Associates.

Guay, T. (1995). *Web publishing paradigms.* Retrieved April 2004 from: http://www.faced.ufba.br/~edc708/biblioteca/interatividade/web%20paradigma/Paradigm.html.

Ha, L., & James, L. (1998). Interactivity reexamined: A baseline analysis of early business websites. *Journal of Broadcasting & Electronic Media, 42,* 457–474.

Habermas, J. (1962). *The structural transformation of the public sphere: An inquiry into a category of bourgeois society.* Cambridge, MA: MIT Press.

Habermas, J. (1984). *The theory of communicative action* (2 vols.) (T. McCarthy, Trans.). Boston: Beacon Press.

Habermas, J. (1996). *Between facts and norms: Contributions to a discourse theory of law and democracy.* Cambridge, MA: MIT Press.

Hawkins, R. P., Kreuter, M., Resnicow, K., Fishbein, M., & Dijkstra, A. (2008). Understanding tailoring in communicating about health. *Health Education Research, 23,* 454–466.

Heeter, C. (1989). Implications of new interactive technologies for conceptualizing communication. In J. L. Salvaggio & J. Bryant (Eds.), *Media use in the information age* (pp. 217–235). Hillsdale, NJ: Lawrence Erlbaum Associates.

Iverson, S. A., Howard, K. B., & Penney, B. K. (2008). Impact of Internet use on health-related behaviors and the patient-physician relationship: A survey-based study and review. *Journal of the American Osteopathic Association, 108,* 699–711.

Jensen, J. F. (1998). Interactivity: Tracing a new concept in media and communication studies. *Nordicom Review, 19,* 185–204.

Kalyanaraman, S., & Sundar, S. S. (2006). The psychological appeal of personalized online content in Web portals: Does customization affect attitudes and behavior? *Journal of Communication, 56*(1), 110–132.

Kiousis, S. (2002). Interactivity: A concept explication. *New Media & Society, 4,* 355–383.

Kreuter, M. W. (2000). Tailoring: What's in a name? *Health Education Research, 15,* 1–4.

Lang, A. (2000). The limited capacity model of mediated message processing. *Journal of Communication, 50*(1), 46–70.

Laurel, B. (1991). *Computers as theatre.* Reading, MA: Addison-Wesley.

Lee, J. S. (2000). *Interactivity: A new approach.* Paper presented at the Association for Education in Journalism and Mass Communication Conference, Phoenix, AZ, August 9–12.

Lee, S.-J., Lee, W.-N., Kim, H., & Stout, P. A. (2004). A comparison of objective characteristics and user perception of Web sites. *Journal of Interactive Advertising, 4.* Retrieved March 2011 from: http://jiad.org/article50.

Lieb, T. (1998). Interactivity on interactivity. *Journal of Electronic Publishing, 3.* Retrieved June 2005 from: http://www.press.umich.edu/jep/03–03/lieb0303html.

Liu, Y. P., & Shrum, L. J. (2002). What is interactivity and is it always such a good thing? Implications of definition, person and situation for the influence of interactivity on advertising effectiveness. *Journal of Advertising, 31,* 53–64.

Lombard, M., & Ditton, T. B. (1997). At the heart of it all: The concept of presence. *Journal of Computer-Mediated Communication, 3.* Retrieved October 2008 from: http://jcmc.indiana.edu/vol3/issue2/lombard.html.

Lustria, M. L. A. (2007). Can interactivity make a difference? Effects of interactivity on the comprehension of and attitudes toward online health content. *Journal of the American Society for Information Science and Technology, 58,* 766–776.

Lustria, M. L. A., Cortese, J., Noar, S. M., & Glueckauf, R. L. (2009). Computer-tailored health interventions delivered over the Web: Review and analysis of key components. *Patient Education and Counseling, 74,* 156–173.

Massey, B., & Levy, M. (1999). Interactivity, online journalism, and English-language Web newspapers in Asia. *Journalism & Mass Communication Quarterly, 76,* 138–151.

Matano, R. A., Koopman, C., Wanat, S. F., Winzelberg, A. J., Whitsell, S. D., Westrup, D., et al. (2007). A pilot study of an interactive website in the workplace for reducing alcohol consumption. *Journal of Substance Abuse Treatment, 32,* 71–80.

McMillan, S. J. (2002). A four-part model of cyber-interactivity: Some cyber-places are more interactive than others. *New Media and Society, 4,* 271–291.

McMillan, S. J., & Hwang, J.-S. (2002). Measures of perceived interactivity: An exploration of the role of direction of communication, user control, and time in shaping perceptions of interactivity. *Journal of Advertising, 31,* 29–42.

McQuail, D. (1994). *Mass communication theory: An introduction* (3rd ed.). Thousand Oaks, CA: Sage.

Morris, M., & Ogan, C. (1996). The Internet as mass medium. *Journal of Communication, 46*(1), 39–50.

Neuhauser, L., & Kreps, G. L. (2010). eHealth communication and behavior change: Promise and performance. *Social Semiotics, 20,* 7–24.

Neuman, W. R. (1991). *The future of the mass audience.* Cambridge. MA: Cambridge University Press.

Newhagen, J., Cordes, J. W., & Levy, M. (1995). Nightly @nbc.com: Audience scope and the perception of interactivity in viewer mail on the Internet. *Journal of Communication, 45*(3), 164–175.

Noar, S. M., Black, H. G., & Pierce, L. B. (2009). Efficacy of computer technology-based HIV prevention interventions: A meta-analysis. *AIDS, 23,* 107–115.

Noar, S. M., Clark, A., Cole, C., & Lustria, M. L. (2006). Review of interactive safer sex websites: Practice and potential. *Health Communication, 20,* 233–241.

Norman, D. A. (1999). Affordance, conventions, and design. *Interactions, 6,* 38–42.

Online News Association. (2003). *Digital journalism credibility study.* Miami, FL: Knight Foundation.

Outing, S. (1998). What exactly is "interactivity?" *E & P Interactive.* Retrieved January 1999 from: http://www.mediainfo.com/ephome/news/newshtm/stop/st120498.htm.

Pew Internet & American Life Project (2000, November 26). The online health care revolution: How the Web helps Americans take better care of themselves. Retrieved March 2011 from: http://www.pewinternet.org/Reports/2005/Health-Information-Online.aspx.

Rafaeli, S. (1988). Interactivity: From new media to communication. In R. Hawkins, J. Wiemann, & S. Pingree (Eds.), *Advancing communication science: Merging mass and interpersonal processes* (pp. 110–134). Newbury Park, CA: Sage.

Rafaeli, S., & Ariel, Y. (2007). Assessing interactivity in computer-mediated research. In A. N. Joinson, K. Y. A. McKenna, T. Postmes, & U.-D. Reips (Eds.), *The Oxford Handbook of Internet Psychology* (pp. 71–88). Oxford University Press.

Rafaeli, S., & Sudweeks, F. (1997). Networked interactivity. *Journal of Computer-Mediated Communication, 2.* Retrieved October 2008 from: http://jcmc.indiana.edu/vol2/issue4/rafaeli.sudweeks.html.

Rayport, J. F., & Jaworski, B. J. (2001). *E-commerce.* New York: McGraw-Hill/Irwin.

Rice, R. E. (2001). The Internet and health communication: A framework of experiences. In R. E. Rice & J. E. Katz (Eds.), *The Internet and health communication* (pp. 5–46). Thousand Oaks, CA: Sage.

Rice, R. E., & Williams, F. (1984). Theories old and new: The study of new media. In R. E. Rice & Associates (Eds.), *The new media: Communication, research and technology* (pp. 55–80). Beverly Hills, CA: Sage.

Roberts, M., Wanta, W., & Dzwo, T.-H. (2002). Agenda setting and issue salience online. *Communication Research, 29,* 452–465.

Rogers, E. M. (1986). *Communication technology: The new media in society.* New York: Free Press.

Rogers, E. M. (1995). *Diffusion of innovations* (4th ed.). New York: Free Press.

Schudson, M. (1978). The ideal of conversation in the study of mass media. *Communication Research, 5,* 320–329.

Schultz, P. N., Stava, C., Beck, M. L., & Vassilopoulou-Sellin, R. (2003). Internet message board use by patients with cancer and their families. *Clinical Journal of Oncology Nursing, 7,* 663–667.

Schultz, T. (1999). Interactive options in online journalism: A content analysis of 100 U.S. newspapers. *Journal of Computer-Mediated Communication, 5*(1). Retrieved October 2008 from: http://jcmc.indiana.edu/vol5/issue1/schultz.html.

Shahab, L., & McEwen, A. (2009). Online support for smoking cessation: A systematic review of the literature. *Addiction, 104,* 1792–1804.

Shannon, C., & Weaver, W. (1949). *The mathematical theory of communication.* Urbana: University of Illinois Press.

Shoemaker, P. J. (1991). *Communication concepts 3: Gatekeeping.* Newbury Park, CA: Sage.

Steuer, J. (1995). Defining virtual reality: Dimensions determining telepresence. In F. Biocca & M. R. Levy (Eds.), *Communication in the age of virtual reality* (pp. 33–56). Hillsdale, NJ: Lawrence Erlbaum Associates.

Street, R. L., & Rimal, R. (1997). Health promotion and interactive technology: A conceptual foundation. In R. L. Street, W. Gold, & T. Manning (Eds.), *Health promotion and interactive technology: Theoretical applications and future directions* (pp. 1–18). Mahwah, NJ: Lawrence Erlbaum Associates.

Stromer-Galley, J. (2000). On-line interaction and why candidates avoid it. *Journal of Communication, 50*(4), 111–132.

Stromer-Galley, J. (2004). Interactivity-as-product and interactivity-as-process. *The Information Society, 20,* 391–394.

Stromer-Galley, J., & Foot, K. A. (2002). Citizen perceptions of online interactivity and implications for political campaign communication. *Journal of Computer-Mediated Communication, 8.* Retrieved February 2007 from: http://jcmc.indiana.edu/vol8/issue1/stromerandfoot.html.

Sundar, S. (2000). Multimedia effects on processing and perception of online news: A study of picture, audio, and video downloads. *Journalism & Mass Communication Quarterly, 77,* 480–499.

Sundar, S. S. (2004). Theorizing interactivity's effects. *Information Society, 20,* 385–389.

Sundar, S. S. (2007). Social psychology of interactivity in human-website interaction. In A. N. Joinson, K. Y., A. McKenna, T. Postmes, & U.-D. Reips (Eds.), *The Oxford Handbook of Internet Psychology* (pp. 89–102). Oxford University Press.

Sundar, S. S. (2008). Self as source: Agency and customization in interactive media. In E. Konijn, S. Utz, M. Tanis, & S. Barnes (Eds.), *Mediated interpersonal communication* (pp. 58–74). New York: Routledge.

Sundar, S. S., Kalyanaraman, S., & Brown, J. (2003). Explicating website interactivity: Impression formation effects in political campaign sites. *Communication Research, 30,* 30–59.

Sundar, S. S., & Marathe, S. S. (2010). Personalization vs. customization: The importance of agency, privacy and power usage. *Human Communication Research, 36,* 298–322.

Sundar, S. S., Marathe, S., & Kang, H. (2009, November). *Beyond tailoring: Customization in health websites.* Paper presented at the 95th annual convention of the National Communication Association, Chicago, IL.

Sundar, S. S., & Nass, C. (2001). Conceptualizing sources in online news. *Journal of Communication, 51*(1), 52–72.

Sundar, S. S., Xu, Q., & Bellur, S. (2010). Designing interactivity in media interfaces: A communications perspective. *Proceedings of the 28th International Conference on Human Factors in Computing Systems* (CHI'10), 2247–2256.

Tedesco, J. C. (2007). Examining Internet interactivity effects on young adult political information efficacy. *American Behavioral Scientist, 50,* 1183–1194.

Teo, H. H., Oh, L. B., Liu, C., & Wei, K. K. (2003). An empirical study of the effects of interactivity on Web user attitude. *International Journal of Human-Computer Studies, 58,* 281–305.

Thelwall, M., Byrne, A., & Goody, M. (2007). Which types of news story attract bloggers? *Information Research, 12.* Retrieved June 2008 from: http://informationr.net/ir/12–4/paper327.html.

Unnava, H. R., Burnkrant, R. E., & Erevelles, S. (1994). Effects of presentation order and communication modality on recall and attitude. *Journal of Consumer Research, 21,* 481–490.

Van Dijk, J. (1999). *The network society: Social aspects of new media* (L. Spoorenberg Trans.). Thousand Oaks, CA: Sage.

Walther, J. B., & Burgoon, J. K. (1992). Relational communication in computer-mediated interaction. *Human Communication Research, 19,* 50–88.

Williams, F., Rice, R., & Rogers, E. M. (1988). *Research methods and the new media.* New York: Free Press.

Wu, G. (2005). The mediating role of perceived interactivity in the effect of actual interactivity on attitude toward the website. *Journal of Interactive Advertising, 5,* 29–39.

eHealth Applications

4

INTERNET-BASED INTERVENTIONS FOR HEALTH BEHAVIOR CHANGE

David B. Buller and Anna H. L. Floyd

Sonia has been a smoker since she was 15. Now, at 45, she wants to quit. This isn't the first time she has tried, but she has never succeeded. Last month, she asked her doctor for advice. Congratulating her, the doctor gave Sonia a self-help manual on quitting. After reading the manual at home, Sonia had questions, but reaching the doctor without an appointment was difficult. Sonia decided to try nicotine patches and called her state's telephone quit line. Unfortunately, Sonia's work and child care responsibilities kept getting in the way of her telephone counseling appointments. Sonia needed a quit service that was available when she could use it, did not feel judgmental, would tailor counseling to her circumstances, would keep her motivated, and enable her to ask people around her for support. Sonia's sister told her about an Internet website that helped smokers quit and was available free from her health plan. It sounded like just what she needed.

The rapid growth of the Internet was one of the most remarkable innovations that shaped the first decade of the twenty-first century. By 2009, 74% of American adults had access to the Internet (Rainie, 2010). As the Internet grew more accessible in U.S. schools, workplaces, and homes, many people like Sonia turned to it for advice when faced with a health problem. In 2009, 61% of American adults looked for health information online, up from 25% just nine years prior (Fox & Jones, 2009). The Internet's ubiquity, interactivity, and multimedia features presented rich, engaging, and sophisticated health communication opportunities.

In this chapter, we discuss research on Internet-based interventions (IBIs) designed to improve health. These interventions are primarily self-guided, interactive Web-based programs, created with the goals of assisting users to make behavior changes that will prevent disease, monitor health status, and/or improve response to clinical treatment. Many IBIs tailor information and support

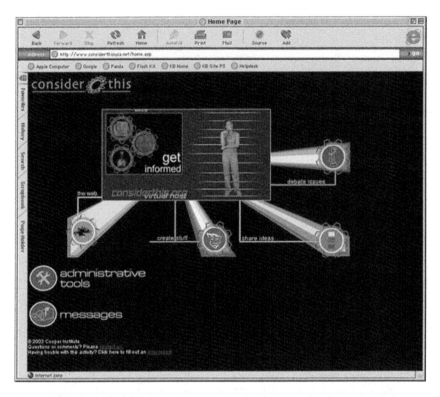

Figure 4.1 Internet-based intervention to prevent smoking uptake

either by self-navigation or through interactive feedback. Most make use of multimedia components (i.e., images, video, audio [Glasgow, 2009; Ritterband, Thorndike, Cox, Kovatchev, & Gonder-Frederick, 2009]). This is the kind of intervention that someone like Sonia may find appealing. Fortunately, IBIs have shown success, and the increasing ubiquity of the Internet along with improvements in usability promise to benefit children and adults across a variety of health behaviors.

The sophistication of IBIs has expanded as the reach of the Internet has exploded and the software for authoring and administering websites has increased in complexity and power. The first IBIs relied primarily on flat text-based presentation with shallow navigation that could be delivered over slow dial-up modems (Buller, Woodall, et al., 2008). Now, IBIs deliver bandwidth-intensive graphics, animation, and video and fast real-time, personalized content to create a rich, engaging multimedia experience. With the advent of new platforms (e.g., smartphones and tablet computers), wireless networks, and communication features (e.g., text messaging and social media), the latest IBIs can deliver interactive health communication when users want it, where they want it, and on whatever device they want it.

Our research group has developed and evaluated IBIs over the past decade. For instance, we developed a website to prevent smoking uptake by adolescents

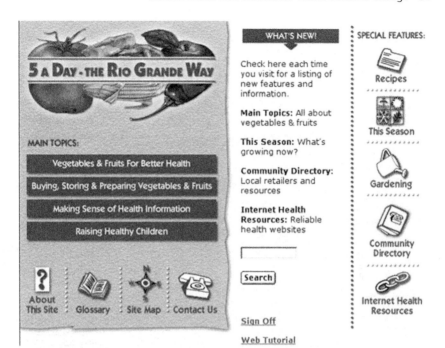

Figure 4.2 Internet-based intervention to improve nutrition

(Figure 4.1) that contained 72 interactive activities in six learning modules integrated by a video host whose presentation was tailored to adolescents' experiences with smoking (Buller, Borland, et al., 2008). We created a website to help adults increase their consumption of fruits and vegetables (Figure 4.2). Due to bandwidth limitations, the website's architecture was a series of Web pages on benefits of these foods, how to purchase and prepare them, and how to increase acceptability by the family; graphics and content relevant to the local communities complemented the primary text (Buller, Woodall, et al., 2008). We have also created IBIs that provided technical assistance and training and supported communication among local tobacco activists (Figure 4.3) (Buller, Young, et al., 2011) and assisted smokers in quitting by providing them with an expert personalized online counseling system (Figure 4.4). Most recently, we pilot tested a smartphone program that works in concert with the smoking cessation IBI.

Advantages and Limitations of Internet-Based Interventions for Health Communication

The Internet can be an ideal medium for delivery of interventions to improve health. To the benefit of the user, it can be a dynamic, engaging, multimedia channel that provides real-time on-demand access to an unprecedented wealth of information. IBIs can overcome barriers created by distance, disability, and

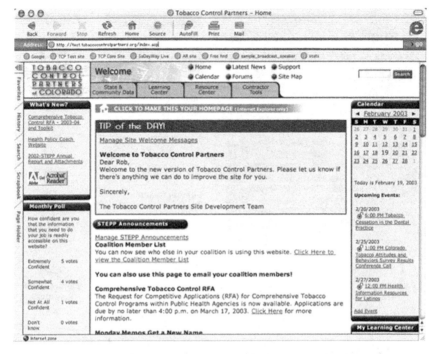

Figure 4.3 Internet-based intervention to assist local tobacco control coalitions

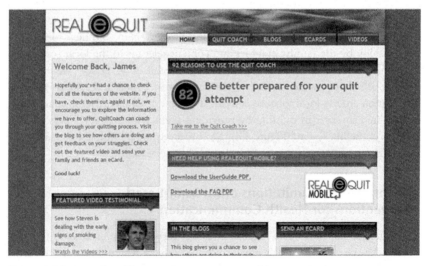

Figure 4.4 Internet-based intervention to support smoking cessation

stigma (Griffiths, Lindenmeyer, Powell, Lowe, & Thorogood, 2006). Handheld smartphones and tablet computers (e.g., iPad) have substantially expanded Internet accessibility for Americans (see Abroms, Padmanabhan, & Evans, this volume). These are the kind of benefits that someone like Sonia might find appealing—which could ultimately improve her ability to use such a program and receive its benefits. To the benefit of interventionists, IBIs can be easily and cheaply updated and modified. Health care providers may enjoy their apparent effect in reducing demands on other hospital services (e.g., general inquiries, routine examinations, or outpatient visits [Miyasaka, Suzuki, Sakai, & Kondo, 1997]). Finally, researchers may find useful the ease with which IBIs can be evaluated, with online surveys and unobtrusive tools to monitor participants' usage (Danaher & Seeley, 2009).

With these advantages, the Internet can deliver low-cost interventions (Tate, Finkelstein, Khavjou, & Gustafson, 2009), at least after the relatively large costs of constructing them are paid. Fixed costs (e.g., server maintenance, updating of programs) change very little in response to the number of participants, and variable costs (e.g., staff time to monitor program) are small, unless one includes opportunity cost to individuals in using IBIs or the number of users expands considerably (Meenan et al., 2009). Our website that supported local tobacco control coalitions in Colorado exemplified this low cost. An economic downturn reduced tax revenues, causing the state government to cut funding for coalitions. However, the website remained active at no cost to coalitions, the defunded coalitions continued to use it, and members reported that their coalitions continued to function well. The very low cost of administering the website appeared to compensate for the loss of funding (Buller, Young, et al., 2011).

One of the defining features of IBIs is their interactivity; that is, their ability to "talk with" users by collecting information and adjusting content, resources, and advice to be personally relevant and appropriate (Burgoon et al., 2000; Heeter, 1989; Rice & Katz, 2003; Rogers & Albritton, 1995). Interactivity distinguishes IBIs from other mass-mediated interventions such as televised public service announcements. Interactivity in IBIs can be as simple as navigation bars used to forage for information or as complicated as an expert system that tailors advice to meet users' expressed motivations and readiness to change. Interactivity should appeal to users but whether it facilitates or impedes IBIs depends on its qualities, the communication objectives, and users (Burgoon et al., 2000; Walther, 1996). One study (Hurling, Fairley, & Dias, 2010) using three types of interactivity in a physical activity IBI confirmed that interactivity can increase user engagement; improve exercise expectations, user satisfaction, and self-perception of fitness; and achieve greater actual exercise compared with an online intervention without interactivity or with no-treatment controls.

However, interactivity comes with a price. Complex, interactive sites can be difficult and time consuming to navigate and require users to learn how to use them. This we heard from leaders of community tobacco control coalitions who received the rich website we built with learning modules, several communication tools, and a large variety of online resources (Buller, Young, Bettinghaus, Maloy, et al., in press). Websites that use expert tailoring systems to personalize content often require users to complete initial assessments (and update them). It is conceivable that this extra work might frustrate some users, especially those not very motivated from the outset to change their behavior.

The advantages of using the Internet have undoubtedly contributed to the rapid growth of IBIs, but three shortcomings could undermine their effectiveness. First, there is an overwhelming number of websites and IBIs, which can make finding a useful IBI difficult. Second, it is not always easy for users to determine the source and credibility of online information, and credibility can be compromised in interventions that allow users to contribute content. Users seem to prioritize opinions of friends and family over scientific research findings, evaluate whether comments come from users that seem "like them," and appraise apparent utility when selecting IBIs (Metzger, Flanagin, & Medders, 2010; Wang, Walther, Pingree, & Hawkins, 2008). Third, the actual extent of privacy on the Internet is a potential problem. The much-touted ability to tailor content to users will be undermined if privacy policies do not meet users' expectations, as illustrated by the public outcry of Facebook users to its changes in privacy policies (Boyd & Hargittai, 2010). In addition, database security risks must be minimized, especially when collecting highly personal clinical and genetic information.

Topics and Target Populations for Internet-Based Interventions

IBI applications have been designed on an assortment of health issues, from management and treatment of chronic disease, to coping with mental illness and stress, to primary and secondary prevention of risk behavior, to general well-being (Table 4.1). They have been evaluated with a variety of populations, including healthy individuals and patients. Several studies have also been conducted with children and college students, and some studies have enrolled adult employees through worksites (Table 4.2).

Theoretical Basis for Internet-Based Interventions

Researchers generally take one of three approaches to theoretical guidance for IBIs. On a most basic level, many researchers simply do not appear to consider theoretical models in their published reports. Other researchers do not utilize a certain theory but take a well-accepted method of therapeutic intervention (which may be theoretically based) and apply it in an Internet context. For example, several IBIs have made use of cognitive behavior therapy to aid patients with tinnitus (Andersson, Stromgren, Strom, & Lyttkens, 2002) or eating disorders

Table 4.1 Health topics of Internet-based interventions

Topic	Sample studies
Alcohol abuse treatment	Cunningham, Wild, Cordingley, Van Mierlo, & Humphreys, 2009; Linke, Murray, Butler, & Wallace, 2007
Alcohol or drug abuse prevention	Neighbors, Lee, Lewis, Fossos, & Walter, 2009; Schwinn, Schinke, & Di Noia, 2010
Asthma management	Finkelstein, Cabrera, & Hripcsak, 2000; Homer et al., 2000
Back pain management	Lorig et al., 2002
Bereavement or grief treatment	Van der Houwen, Schut, Van den Bout, Stroebe, & Stroebe, 2010; Wagner & Maercker, 2007
Brain injury treatment	Bergquist et al., 2009; Egan, Worrall, & Oxenham, 2005
Depression management	Atherton-Naji, Hamilton, Riddle, & Naji, 2001
Diabetes management	Feil, Glasgow, Boles, & McKay, 2000; Glasgow, Barrera Jr., McKay, & Boles, 1999; McKay, Glasgow, Feil, Boles, & Barrera, 2002; Tate, Jackvony, & Wing, 2003; Tsang et al., 2001
Eating disorders and healthy body images	Celio, et al., 2000; Heinicke, Paxton, McLean, & Wertheim, 2007; Paxton et al., 2007; Robinson & Serfaty, 2001; Winzelberg, et al., 2000; Zabinski, et al., 2001
General well-being	Mitchell, Stanimirovic, Klein, & Vella-Brodrick, 2009
Good parenting	Salonen, Kaunonen, Astedt-Kurki, Jarvenpaa, & Tarkka, 2008
HIV management	Gustafson et al., 1999
Nutrition education	Baranowski et al., 2003; Buller, Woodall, et al., 2008; Glasgow et al., 1999; Oenema, Brug, & Lechner, 2001; Prochaska, Zabinski, Calfas, Sallis, & Patrick, 2000; Thompson et al., 2009
Panic disorder management	Carlbring, Ekselius, & Andersson, 2003
Quality of life of breast cancer and HIV patients	Gustafson et al., 1999; Gustafson et al., 2001; Rolnick et al., 1999; Winzelberg et al., 2003
Physical activity	Bosak, Yates, & Pozehl, 2009; Prochaska et al., 2000
Smoking prevention	Balmford, Borland, & Benda, 2008; Buller, Borland, et al., 2008; Myung, McDonnell, Kazinets, Seo, & Moskowitz, 2009
Support for parents of low-birth weight babies in neonatal intensive care units	Gray et al., 2000
Technical assistance for community tobacco control activists	Buller, Young, et al., 2011
Tinnitus management	Andersson et al., 2002; Krishna et al., 2003

(Continued)

Table 4.1 (*Continued*)

Topic	Sample studies
Tobacco cessation counseling	Fisher, Severson, & Hripcsak, 2001; Stoops, et al., 2009; Woodruff, Edwards, Conway, & Elliott, 2001
Weight management	Tate, Wing, & Winett, 2001; Tate et al., 2003

Table 4.2 Study populations for Internet-based interventions

Population	Sample studies
Healthy individuals	Balmford et al., 2008; Baranowski et al., 2003; Billipp, 2001; Buller, Woodall, et al., 2008; Buller, Borland, et al., 2008; Buller et al., 2011; Celio et al., 2000; Dunton et al., 2008; Fisher et al., 2001; Graham, Cobb, Raymond, Sill, & Young, 2007; Gray et al., 2000; Harvey-Berino et al., 2002; Heinicke et al., 2007; Jago et al., 2006; Neighbors et al., 2009; Oenema et al., 2001; Prochaska et al., 2000; Salonen et al., 2008; Sciamanna, et al., 2002; Steele, Mummery, & Dwyer, 2007, Tate et al., 2001, 2003; Winzelberg et al., 2000; Woodruff et al., 2001; Zabinski et al., 2001
Patients	Andersson et al., 2002; Atherton-Naji et al., 2001; Bosak et al., 2009; Carlbring et al., 2003; Egan et al., 2005; Feil, Noell, Lichtenstein, Boles, & McKay, 2003; Finkelstein et al., 2000; Glasgow et al., 1999; Gustafson et al., 1999, 2001; Homer et al., 2000; Krishna et al., 2003; Lorig et al., 2002; McKay, King, Eakin, Seeley, & Glasgow, 2001; McKay et al., 2002; Robinson & Sefarty 2001; Rolnick et al., 1999; Tsang et al., 2001; Winzelberg et al., 2003.
Children	Jago et al., 2006; Thompson et al., 2009
Teens	Buller, Young, et al., 2008; Neighbors et al., 2009; Schwinn et al., 2010
College students	Celio et al., 2000; Zabinski et al., 2001
Employees	Graham et al., 2007; Oenema et al., 2001

(Paxton, McLean, Gollings, Faulkner, & Wertheim, 2007), motivational interviewing to help teenagers quit smoking (Woodruff, Edwards, Conway, & Elliott, 2001), supportive-expressive group therapy for women with breast cancer (Winzelberg et al., 2003), or self-expressive writing and writing therapy for bereavement (Pennebaker & Beall, 1986; Van der Houwen et al., 2010). Still other researchers explicitly describe their interventions' theoretical underpinnings. Here, a variety of theories have been used. To illustrate, some researchers have used the transtheoretical model (Prochaska, Redding, & Evers, 2005) to assess users' readiness to change and then tailor personalized feedback to users, for instance, to help increase physical activity (Dunton & Robertson, 2008), while others have employed social cognitive theory (Bandura, 1986) to guide online content that enhances self-efficacy, for example, for dietary change (Baranowski et al., 2003; Thompson et al., 2009).

Ritterband et al. (2009) proposed an Internet intervention model describing nine components in effectively deploying IBIs. These components encompass characteristics of the user, environmental factors, website use, support, website characteristics, behavior change, mechanisms of change, symptom improvement, and treatment maintenance. This model is an organizing framework but not really an explanatory one, so an understanding of IBIs requires using several theories to explain its components.

In our own research, we have created IBIs guided by theoretical models as well as best practices in health behavior change. We used diffusion of innovations theory to design a nutrition education website (Buller, Woodall, et al., 2008) and social cognitive theory to construct websites to prevent smoking uptake (Buller, Borland, et al., 2008) and to help smokers quit. This latter website also incorporated principles of motivational readiness to quit. We relied on the Centers for Disease Control and Prevention's (CDC) best practices in community tobacco control to guide the technical assistance website for local tobacco control coalitions (Buller, Young, et al., 2011; Buller et al., in press).

Much more theoretical development is needed to explain other IBI model components. A current theoretical challenge for IBIs is to understand how users engage with them to ensure that IBIs reach their intended audience. Theories pertaining to information seeking (Afifi & Weiner, 2004) and media use (Beaudoin & Thorson, 2004) may prove useful. Likewise, social ecological models could be considered for explanation of how users' information seeking processes and reactions to IBIs are influenced by individuals' circumstances (McKay et al., 2001). However, there is nothing unique about these models. Many of their predictions would be applicable to interventions delivered offline, too. It appears that effective IBIs will arise from a multitheoretical approach (see Hurling et al., 2010, for an example).

Health Effects of Internet-Based Interventions

Meta-analyses and systematic reviews of IBIs show that they can produce positive treatment outcomes, reduce symptoms, and improve participants' quality of life (Griffiths & Christensen, 2007; Kuhl, Sears, & Conti, 2006; Ritterband & Tate, 2009; Saperstein, Atkinson, & Gold, 2007). Generally speaking, these summaries show that when compared to a no-treatment group, participants receiving IBIs almost invariably show better improvements (Myung, et al., 2009; Stinson, Wilson, Gill, Yamada, & Holt, 2009; Van den Berg, Schoones, & Vliet Vlieland, 2007). For example, IBIs have improved adherence to asthma interventions among children (Jan et al., 2007), decreased restricted activity days among asthma patients (Joseph et al., 2007), and improved social and physical functioning among cardiovascular patients (Delgado, Costigan, Wu, & Ross, 2003; Dew et al., 2004). IBIs have also shown success at increasing weight loss (Saperstein et al), reducing depression and anxiety symptoms (Griffiths & Christensen), controlling recurrent pain among children (Hicks, von Baeyer, & McGrath, 2006), and improving asthma symptoms among asthma patients (Jan et al.; Krishna et al., 2003). One of the areas where results appear more equivocal is in physical activity (Napolitano et al., 2003; Plotnikoff, McCargar, Wilson, & Loucaides, 2005; Vandelanotte, Spathonis, Eakin, & Owen, 2007; Van den Berg et al., 2006, 2007).

The success of IBIs may be attributable to their positive impact on theoretical mediators of health behavior change. To illustrate, IBIs improved health-related knowledge (Griffiths & Christensen, 2007), self management skills (Jan et al., 2007), quality of life (Kuhl et al., 2006; White et al., 2004), social support (Gustafson et al., 2001), social norms and self-efficacy (Schwinn et al., 2010), and progress along stages of motivational readiness to change (Vandelanotte et al., 2007). However, few studies directly tested mediation. One study that did test for mediators failed to find hypothesized mediation of a weight loss IBI by program adherence, self-efficacy, and parental adherence (White et al.), but another found that the effectiveness of an IBI to reduce twenty-first birthday binge drinking was mediated by perceived norms for drinking (Neighbors et al., 2009). In our study of an IBI to prevent smoking uptake, the program's success was mediated by improvements in smoking norms (Buller, Borland, et al., 2008).

Current and Future Dissemination Potential for Internet-Based Interventions

The real promise of IBIs for individuals like Sonia will only be realized when they are translated from the research bench and taken to scale to reach the populations in need (Glasgow et al., 1999). At the introduction of the Internet, access and computer aptitude presented barriers to disseminating IBIs (Kalichman, Weinhardt, Benotsch, & Cherry, 2002; McKay et al., 2002). The more educated, younger and middle-aged populations, whites, males, and suburban dwellers were the first to embrace the Internet (U.S. Department of Commerce & National Telecommunications and Information Administration, 1999), and early websites, such as our nutrition education website for rural adults, could only deliver simple content features on low-bandwidth dial-up modems. Fortunately, many of these early disparities have all but disappeared as the majority of Americans are now online (Smith, 2010). In fact, Internet access is nearly universal in schools (Wells & Lewis, 2006), and two-thirds of homes have broadband access (Smith). Almost no gap in Internet access exists by gender (Smith), and older

(Madden, 2010) and minority populations are experiencing some of the highest rates of new adoption (Smith). What may be more problematic currently than demographic differences is regional variation in Internet access (Spooner, 2003), due especially to poor or no broadband service in certain areas (Saint, 2010). IBIs made available over a smartphone platform may be one way to reach potential users in regionally Internet-poor locations, if high quality cellular phone service is available (see Abroms, Padmanabhan, & Evans, and Fjeldsoe, Miller, & Marshall, this volume).

A second challenge is to ensure that populations who could benefit from IBIs will locate and use them. Many IBIs are used by just a small proportion of users. Even in research projects, where study participants have agreed to visit IBIs, a substantial number rarely if ever use them, and the amount of use per participant varies widely. For example, in a review of seven IBIs for alcohol interventions, an estimated 12% to 60% of websites' visitors made use of the available intervention assessments (Vernon, 2010). Likewise, a review of physical activity IBIs showed that exposure to the online programs was low and decreased as the interventions progressed (Vandelanotte et al., 2007). A similar decline in use over the intervention period was reported for a weight loss IBI (Tate et al., 2001). We, too, have seen low and declining use in our evaluations of IBIs.

Gaining the attention of users is becoming a great challenge with the fragmentation of the Internet where social media, such as social networking sites, shared videos, blogs, and tweets rival older email functions, and many individuals are using programs that aggregate and customize online information (i.e., smartphone applications), often for a fee (Anderson & Wolff, 2010). Thus, careful consideration of how and over what online channel IBIs are implemented is essential because low use can undermine intervention effectiveness, as has been clearly demonstrated by dose-response trends (i.e., greater use of IBIs is associated with improved health behavior outcomes) (Baranowski et al., 2003; Buller, Borland, et al., 2008; Buller, Woodall, et al., 2008; Doshi, Patrick, Sallis, & Calfas, 2003; Funk et al., 2010; Graham et al., 2007; Leslie, Marshall, Owen, & Bauman, 2005; Manwaring et al., 2008; Vandelanotte et al., 2007). Achieving use of particular online features in IBIs, not just overall use, is also an important consideration. For instance, viewing recipes on our website promoting fruits and vegetables was related to larger improvements in diets (Buller, Woodall, et al., 2008). Use of a quit date expert system was related to increased smoking cessation in another study (Graham et al., 2007). Low use is of particular concern when it occurs within groups that might benefit most. Participant use of our nutrition education website was lower among younger adults, Hispanic adults, and adults with less Internet experience, groups who might be expected to have fewer health resources. This raised concerns that the intervention did not address existing health inequities (Buller & Woodall, in press).

Second-Generation Research on Internet-Based Interventions

One could say that the research on IBIs is entering a new generation. First-generation research explored whether IBIs could be developed, were usable, and could improve health-related behavior. Now, researchers have begun addressing "second-generation" questions about IBIs. Among the most notable new directions in research are the following:

- **Effectiveness of Components and Features of IBIs:** Early evaluations tested the effectiveness of entire IBIs, which were usually multifaceted. Exactly which content, feature, and/or message is responsible for intervention success is only now being examined (Lustria, Cortese, Noar, & Glueckauf, 2009; Noar, Harrington, & Aldrich, 2009; Ritterband et al., 2009; Strecher, 2007).
- **Strategies to Improve Use of IBIs:** More theoretical and empirical focus is needed on how users decide which IBIs to visit and how they use them (Eysenbach, 2005; Ritterband et al., 2009). Some studies have used material incentives (Marcus et al., 2007) and email reminders (Schwinn et al., 2010; Woodall et al., 2007). Another consideration is how content interests and needs affect use. For instance, across three nutrition education websites, we observed that recipes were used by middle-aged and older, but not college-aged adults (Buller, Buller, Liu, & Kane, 2010). Magee, Ritterband, Thorndike, Cox, and Borowitz (2009) found in a study of an IBI for pediatric encopresis that parental worry over their child's health was associated with higher use. Intermediary organizations such as schools, employers, and health insurers may help distribute IBIs (Buller, Young, Fisher, & Maloy, 2006) through established communication channels and with resources to support ongoing maintenance of them (Dearing, Maibach, & Buller, 2006).
- **Cost and Cost-effectiveness of IBIs:** Information is needed on the costs of developing and deploying IBIs (Meenan et al., 2009) and confirming their cost advantage (Tate et al., 2009). One study found that IBIs have similar outcomes as face-to-face interventions (Ritterband et al., 2009). If IBIs prove less costly than face-to-face interventions (Tate et al., 2009), their comparable effectiveness will yield a better cost per user ratio, which may make them attractive for controlling spiraling health care costs.
- **Role of IBIs in Health Equity:** Health equity remains an essential area of research on IBIs. Their potential to reduce geographic and social barriers are chief advantages (e.g., they seem ideal for helping the elderly feel less isolated [Fokkema & Knipscheer, 2007] and improve their well-being [Shapira, Barak, & Gal, 2007]), but research is needed on factors that promote use among the groups who can most benefit from IBIs and reduce barriers to this use.
- **Integration of Internet Delivery Platforms:** The emergence of multiple platforms for accessing the Internet raises interesting questions regarding

how to best use desktop and laptop computers, smartphones, tablet computers, Internet television, and other emerging Internet technologies to deliver IBIs. We are currently testing a smartphone application to extend a smoking cessation website, focusing on how smokers use the application, whether they will use both the application and the website (and on what platform), as well as whether it moves them toward quitting.

- **Online Recruitment to Studies of IBIs:** The ubiquity of the Internet makes a large majority of Americans available to be recruited to studies evaluating IBIs, regardless of their geographic location. Online recruiting methods have the potential to influence the timeline, selection biases, study costs, and validity of experiments. Research is just now emerging on this important methodological issue (Buller, Meenan, et al., in press; Graham, Milner, Saul, & Pfaff, 2008; Koo & Skinner, 2005; Lieberman, 2008; Ramo, Hall, & Prochaska, 2010).

The Internet continues to revolutionize the media environment for health communication. Research in the past decade confirming that IBIs can be delivered over the Internet and successfully change behaviors that improve health provides an incomplete understanding of this important new intervention channel. Additional research is needed to develop and apply theoretical models explaining how these interventions are effective and can be disseminated to improve the health of Sonia and all Americans.

References

Afifi, W. A., & Weiner, J. L. (2004). Toward a theory of motivated information management. *Communication Theory, 14,* 167–190.

Anderson, C., & Wolff, M. (2010, August 17). The Web is dead: Long live the Internet. *WIRED.* Retrieved May 23, 2011, from: http://www.wired.com/magazine/2010/08/ff_webrip/all/1.

Andersson, G., Stromgren, T., Strom, L., & Lyttkens, L. (2002). Randomized controlled trial of Internet-based cognitive behavior therapy for distress associated with tinnitus. *Psychosomatic Medicine, 64,* 810–816.

Atherton-Naji, A., Hamilton, R., Riddle, W., & Naji, S. (2001). Improving adherence to antidepressant drug treatment in primary care: A feasibility study for a randomized controlled trial of educational intervention. *Primary Care Psychiatry, 7,* 61–67.

Balmford, J., Borland, R., & Benda, P. (2008). Patterns of use of an automated interactive personalized coaching program for smoking cessation. *Journal of Medical Internet Research, 10,* e54.

Bandura, A. (1986). *Social foundations of thought and action: A social cognitive theory.* Englewood Cliffs, NJ: Prentice Hall.

Baranowski, T., Baranowski, J. C., Cullen, K. W., Thompson, D. I., Nicklas, T., Zakeri, I. E., et al. (2003). The Fun, Food, and Fitness Project (FFFP): The Baylor GEMS pilot study. *Ethnicity & Disease, 13,* S30-S39.

Beaudoin, C. E., & Thorson, E. (2004). Testing the cognitive mediation model: The roles of news reliance and three gratifications sought. *Communication Research, 31,* 446–471.

Bergquist, T., Gehl, C., Mandrekar, J., Lepore, S., Hanna, S., Osten, A., et al. (2009). The effect of Internet-based cognitive rehabilitation in persons with memory impairments after severe traumatic brain injury. *Brain Injury, 23,* 790–799.

Billipp, S. H. (2001). The psychosocial impact of interactive computer use within a vulnerable elderly population: A report on a randomized prospective trial in a home health care setting. *Public Health Nursing, 18,* 138–145.

Bosak, K. A., Yates, B., & Pozehl, B. (2009). Feasibility of an Internet physical activity intervention. *Western Journal Nursing Research, 31,* 648–661.

Boyd, D., & Hargittai, E. (2010, August 2). Facebook privacy settings: Who cares? *First Monday.* Retrieved May 23, 2011, from: http://www.uic.edu/htbin/cgiwrap/bin/ojs/index.php/fm/article/view/3086/2589.

Buller, D. B., Borland, R., Woodall, W. G., Hall, J. R., Hines, J. M., Burris-Woodall, P., et al. (2008). Randomized trials on Consider This, a tailored, Internet-delivered smoking prevention program for adolescents. *Health Education & Behavior, 35,* 260–281.

Buller, D. B., Buller, M. K., Liu, X., & Kane, I. (2010, June). *Trends in selective exposure by adults to online nutrition content across four Web-based programs.* 12th International Conference on Language and Social Psychology. Brisbane, Queensland, Australia.

Buller, D. B., Meenan, R., Severson, H., Halperin, A., Edwards, E., & Magnusson, B. (in press). Comparison of four recruiting strategies in a smoking cessation trial. *American Journal of Health Behavior.*

Buller, D. B., & Woodall, W. G. (in press). 5 a day, the Rio Grande Way: Internet intervention and health inequities in the Upper Rio Grande Valley. In G. Kreps & M. Dutta (Eds.), *Reducing health disparities: Communication intervention.* New York: Peter Lang Publishing.

Buller, D. B., Woodall, W. G., Zimmerman, D. E., Slater, M. D., Heimendinger, J., Waters, E., et al. (2008). Randomized trial on the 5 a day, the Rio Grande Way Website, a Web-based program to improve fruit and vegetable consumption in rural communities. *Journal of Health Communication, 13,* 230–249.

Buller, D. B., Young, W. F., Bettinghaus, E. P., Borland, R., Walther, J. B., Helme, D., et al. (2011). Continued benefits of a technical assistance website to local tobacco control coalitions during a state budget shortfall. *Journal of Public Health Management and Practice, 17,* E10-E19.

Buller, D. B., Young, W. F., Bettinghaus, E. P., Maloy, J. A., Andersen, P. A., Borland, R., et al. (in press). Tobacco control partners: A website providing online technical assistance to local tobacco control coalitions. In S. Esrock, J. Hart, & K. Walker (Eds.), *Talking tobacco: Interpersonal, organizational, and mediated messages.* New York: Peter Lang Publishing.

Buller, D. B., Young, W. F., Fisher, K. H., & Maloy, J. A. (2006). The effect of endorsement by local opinion leaders and testimonials from teachers on the dissemination of a Web-based smoking prevention program. *Health Education Research, 22,* 609–618.

Burgoon, J. K., Bonito, J., Bengtsson, B., Ramirez, A., Dunbar, N. E., & Miczo, N. (2000). Testing the interactivity model: Communication processes, partner assessments, and the quality of collaborative work. *Journal of Management Information Systems, 16,* 35–38.

Carlbring, P., Ekselius, L., & Andersson, G. (2003). Treatment of panic disorder via the Internet: A randomized trial of CBT vs. applied relaxation. *Journal of Behavior Therapy and Experimental Psychiatry, 34,* 129–140.

Celio, A. A., Winzelberg, A. J., Wilfley, D. E., Eppstein-Herald, D., Springer, E. A., Dev, P., et al. (2000). Reducing risk factors for eating disorders: Comparison of an Internet- and a classroom-delivered psychoeducational program. *Journal of Consulting and Clinical Psychology, 68,* 650–657.

Cunningham, J. A., Wild, T. C., Cordingley, J., van Mierlo, T., & Humphreys, K. (2009). A randomized controlled trial of an Internet-based intervention for alcohol abusers. *Addiction, 104,* 2023–2032.

Danaher, B. G., & Seeley, J. R. (2009). Methodological issues in research on Web-based behavioral interventions. *Annals of Behavioral Medicine, 38,* 28–39.

Dearing, J. W., Maibach, E., & Buller, D. (2006). A convergent diffusion and social marketing approach for disseminating proven approaches to physical activity promotion. *American Journal of Preventive Medicine, 31,* S11–S23.

Delgado, D. H., Costigan, J., Wu, R., & Ross, H. J. (2003). An interactive Internet site for the management of patients with congestive heart failure. *Canadian Journal of Cardiology, 19,* 1381–1385.

Dew, M. A., Goycoolea, J. M., Harris, R. C., Lee, A., Zomak, R., Dunbar-Jacob, J., et al. (2004). An Internet-based intervention to improve psychosocial outcomes in heart transplant recipients and family caregivers: Development and evaluation. *Journal of Heart and Lung Transplantation, 23,* 745–758.

Doshi, A., Patrick, K., Sallis, J. F., & Calfas, K. (2003). Evaluation of physical activity web sites for use of behavior change theories. *Annals of Behavioral Medicine, 25,* 105–111.

Dunton, G. F., & Robertson, T. P. (2008). A tailored Internet-plus-email intervention for increasing physical activity among ethnically-diverse women. *Preventive Medicine, 47,* 605–611.

Egan, J., Worrall, L., & Oxenham, D. (2005). An Internet training intervention for people with traumatic brain injury: Barriers and outcomes. *Brain Injury, 19,* 555–568.

Eysenbach, G. (2005). The law of attrition. *Journal of Medical Internet Research, 7,* e11.

Feil, E. G., Glasgow, R. E., Boles, S., & McKay, H. G. (2000). Who participates in Internet-based self-management programs? A study among novice computer users in a primary care setting. *Diabetes Education, 26,* 806–811.

Feil, E. G., Noell, J., Lichtenstein, E., Boles, S. M., & McKay, H. G. (2003). Evaluation of an Internet-based smoking cessation program: Lessons learned from a pilot study. *Nicotine & Tobacco Research, 5,* 189–194.

Finkelstein, J., Cabrera, M. R., & Hripcsak, G. (2000). Internet-based home asthma tele-monitoring: Can patients handle the technology? *Chest, 117,* 148–155.

Fisher, K. J., Severson, H. H., & Hripcsak, G. (2001). Using interactive technology to aid smokeless tobacco cessation. *American Journal of Health Education, 32,* 332–342.

Fokkema, T., & Knipscheer, K. (2007). Escape loneliness by going digital: A quantitative and qualitative evaluation of a Dutch experiment in using ECT to overcome loneliness among older adults. *Aging & Mental Health, 11,* 496–504.

Fox, S., & Jones, S. (2009). *The social life of health information.* Washington, DC: Pew Research Center. Retrieved May 23, 2011, from: http://www.pewinternet.org/~/media//Files/Reports/2009/PIP_Health_2009.pdf.

Funk, K. L., Stevens, V. J., Appel, L. J., Bauck, A., Brantley, P. J., Champagne, C. M., et al. (2010). Associations of Internet website use with weight change in a long-term weight loss maintenance program. *Journal of Medical Internet Research, 12,* e29.

Glasgow, R. E. (2009). Enhancing the scientific foundation of Internet intervention research. *Annals of Behavioral Medicine, 38,* 46–47.

Glasgow, R. E., Barrera, M., Jr., McKay, H. G., & Boles, S. M. (1999). Social support, self-management, and quality of life among participants in an Internet-based diabetes support program: A multi-dimensional investigation. *Cyberpsychology & Behavior, 2,* 271–281.

Graham, A. L., Cobb, N. K., Raymond, L., Sill, S., & Young, J. (2007). Effectiveness of an Internet-based worksite smoking cessation intervention at 12 months. *Journal of Occupational & Environmental Medicine, 49,* 821–828.

Graham, A. L., Milner, P., Saul, J. E., & Pfaff, L. (2008). Online advertising as a public health and recruitment tool: Comparison of different media campaigns to increase demand for smoking cessation interventions. *Journal of Medical Internet Research, 10,* e50.

Gray, J. E., Safran, C., Davis, R. B., Pompilio-Weitzner, G., Stewart, J. E., Zaccagnini, L. et al. (2000). Baby CareLink: Using the Internet and telemedicine to improve care for high-risk infants. *Pediatrics, 106,* 1318–1324.

Griffiths, F., Lindenmeyer, A., Powell, J., Lowe, P., & Thorogood, M. (2006). Why are health care interventions delivered over the Internet? A systematic review of the published literature. *Journal of Medical Internet Research, 8,* e10.

Griffiths, K. M., & Christensen, H. (2007). Internet-based mental health programs: A powerful tool in the rural medical kit. *Australian Journal of Rural Health, 15,* 81–87.

Gustafson, D. H., Hawkins, R., Boberg, E., Pingree, S., Serlin, R. E., Graziano, F., et al. (1999). Impact of a patient-centered, computer-based health information/support system. *American Journal of Preventive Medicine, 16,* 1–9.

Gustafson, D. H., Hawkins, R., Pingree, S., McTavish, F., Arora, N. K., & Mendenhall, J. (2001). Effect of computer support on younger women with breast cancer. *Journal of General Internal Medicine, 16,* 435–445.

Harvey-Berino, J., Pintauro, S., Buzzell, P., DiGiulio, M., Casey, G. B., Moldovan, C., et al. (2002). Does using the Internet facilitate the maintenance of weight loss? *International Journal of Obesity, 26,* 1254–1260.

Heeter, C. (1989). *Implication of new interactive technologies for conceptualizing communication.* Hillsdale, NJ: Lawrence Erlbaum Associates.

Heinicke, B. E., Paxton, S. J., McLean, S. A., & Wertheim, E. H. (2007). Internet-delivered targeted group intervention for body dissatisfaction and disordered eating in adolescent girls: A randomized controlled trial. *Journal of Abnormal and Social Psychology, 35,* 379–391.

Hicks, C. L., von Baeyer, C. L., & McGrath, P. J. (2006). Online psychological treatment for pediatric recurrent pain: A randomized evaluation. *Journal of Pediatric Psychology, 31,* 724–736.

Homer, C., Susskind, O., Alpert, H. R., Owusu, C., Schneider, L., Rappaport, L. A., et al. (2000). An evaluation of an innovative multimedia educational software program for asthma management: Report of a randomized, controlled trial. *Pediatrics, 106,* 210–215.

Hurling, R., Fairley, B. W., & Dias, M. B. (2010). Internet-based exercise intervention systems: Are more interactive designs better? *Psychology and Health, 21,* 757–772.

Jago, R., Baranowski, T., Baranowski, J. C., Thompson, D., Cullen, K. W., Watson, K., et al. (2006). Fit for Life Boy Scout badge: Outcome evaluation of a troop and Internet intervention. *Preventive Medicine, 42,* 181–187.

Jan, R. L., Wang, J. Y., Huang, M. C., Tseng, S. M., Su, H. J., & Liu, L. F. (2007). An Internet-based interactive telemonitoring system for improving childhood asthma outcomes in Taiwan. *Telemedicine Journal and E-Health, 13,* 257–268.

Joseph, C. L., Peterson, E., Havstad, S., Johnson, C. C., Hoerauf, S., Stringer, S., et al. (2007). A Web-based, tailored asthma management program for urban African-American high school students. *American Journal of Respiratory and Critical Care Medicine, 175,* 888–895.

Kalichman, S. C., Weinhardt, L., Benotsch, E., & Cherry, C. (2002). Closing the digital divide in HIV/AIDS care: Development of a theory-based intervention to increase Internet access. *AIDS Care, 14,* 523–537.

Koo, M., & Skinner, H. (2005). Challenges of Internet recruitment: A case study with disappointing results. *Journal of Medical Internet Research, 7,* e6.

Krishna, S., Francisco, B. D., Balas, E. A., Konig, P., Graff, G. R., & Madsen, R. W. (2003). Internet-enabled interactive multimedia asthma education program: A randomized trial. *Pediatrics, 111,* 503–510.

Kuhl, E. A., Sears, S. F., & Conti, J. B. (2006). Internet-based behavioral change and psychosocial care for patients with cardiovascular disease: A review of cardiac disease-specific applications. *Heart Lung, 35,* 374–382.

Leslie, E., Marshall, A. L., Owen, N., & Bauman, A. (2005). Engagement and retention of participants in a physical activity website. *Preventive Medicine, 40,* 54–59.

Lieberman, D. Z. (2008). Evaluation of the stability and validity of participant samples recruited over the Internet. *Cyberpsychology and Behavior, 11,* 743–745.

Linke, S., Murray, E., Butler, C., & Wallace, P. (2007). Internet-based interactive health intervention for the promotion of sensible drinking: Patterns of use and potential impact on members of the general public. *Journal of Medical Internet Research, 9,* e10.

Lorig, K. R., Laurent, D. D., Deyo, R. A., Marnell, M. E., Minor, M. A., & Ritter, P. L. (2002). Can a back pain e-mail discussion group improve health status and lower health care costs? A randomized study. *Archives Internal Medicine, 162,* 792–796.

Lustria, M. L., Cortese, J., Noar, S. M., & Glueckauf, R. L. (2009). Computer-tailored health interventions delivered over the Web: Review and analysis of key components. *Patient Education and Counseling, 74,* 156–173.

Madden, M. (2010). *Older adults and social media.* Washington, DC: Pew Research Center. Retrieved May 23, 2011, from: http://pewinternet.org/Reports/2010/Older-Adults-and-Social-Media.aspx

Magee, J. C., Ritterband, L. M., Thorndike, F. P., Cox, D. J., & Borowitz, S. M. (2009). Exploring the relationship between parental worry about their children's health and usage of an Internet intervention for pediatric encopresis. *Journal of Pediatric Psychology, 34,* 530–538.

Manwaring, J. L., Bryson, S. W., Goldschmidt, A. B., Winzelberg, A. J., Luce, K. H., Cunning, D., et al. (2008). Do adherence variables predict outcome in an online program for the prevention of eating disorders? *Journal of Consulting and Clinical Psychology, 76,* 341–346.

Marcus, B. H., Lewis, B. A., Williams, D. M., Dunsiger, S., Jakicic, J. M., Whiteley, J. A., et al. (2007). A comparison of Internet and print-based physical activity interventions. *Archives of Internal Medicine, 167,* 944–949.

McKay, H. G., Glasgow, R. E., Feil, E. G., Boles, S. M., & Barrera, M. (2002). Internet-based diabetes self-management and support: Initial outcomes from the diabetes network project. *Rehabilitation Psychology, 47,* 31–48.

McKay, H. G., King, D., Eakin, E. G., Seeley, J. R., & Glasgow, R. E. (2001). The diabetes network Internet-based physical activity intervention: A randomized pilot study. *Diabetes Care, 24,* 1328–1334.

Meenan, R., Stevens, V. J., Funk, K., Bauck, A., Jerome, G., Lien, L., et al. (2009). Development and implementation cost analysis of telephone- and Internet-based interventions for the maintenance of weight loss. *International Journal of Technology Assessment in Health Care, 25,* 400–410.

Metzger, M. J., Flanagin, A. J., & Medders, R. B. (2010). Social and heuristic approaches to credibility evaluation online. *Journal of Communication, 60*(3), 413–439.

Mitchell, J., Stanimirovic, R., Klein, B., & Vella-Brodrick, D. (2009). A randomized controlled trial of a self-guided Internet intervention promoting well-being. *Computers in Human Behavior, 25,* 749–760.

Miyasaka, K., Suzuki, Y., Sakai, H., & Kondo, Y. (1997). Interactive communication in high-technology home care: Videophones for pediatric ventilatory care. *Pediatrics, 99*, e1.

Myung, S. K., McDonnell, D. D., Kazinets, G., Seo, H. G., & Moskowitz, J. M. (2009). Effects of Web- and computer-based smoking cessation programs: Meta-analysis of randomized controlled trials. *Archives of Internal Medicine, 169*, 929–937.

Napolitano, M. A., Fotheringham, M., Tate, D., Sciamanna, C., Leslie, E., Owen, N., et al. (2003). Evaluation of an Internet-based physical activity intervention: A preliminary investigation. *Annals of Behavioral Medicine, 25*, 92–99.

Neighbors, C., Lee, C. M., Lewis, M. A., Fossos, N., & Walter, T. (2009). Internet-based personalized feedback to reduce 21st-birthday drinking: A randomized controlled trial of an event-specific prevention intervention. *Journal of Consulting and Clinical Psychology, 77*, 51–63.

Noar, S. M., Harrington, N. G., & Aldrich, R. S. (2009). The role of message tailoring in the development of persuasive health communication messages. In C. S. Beck (Ed.), *33 Communication Yearbook* (pp. 72–133). New York: Routledge.

Oenema, A., Brug, J., & Lechner, L. (2001). Web-based tailored nutrition education: Results of a randomized controlled trial. *Health Education Research, 16*, 647–660.

Paxton, S. J., McLean, S. A., Gollings, E. K., Faulkner, C., & Wertheim, E. H. (2007). Comparison of face-to-face and Internet interventions for body image and eating problems in adult women: An RCT. *International Journal of Eating Disorders, 40*, 692–704.

Pennebaker, J. W., & Beall, S. K. (1986). Confronting a traumatic event: Toward an understanding of inhibition and disease. *Journal of Abnormal Psychology, 95*, 274–281.

Plotnikoff, R. C., McCargar, L. J., Wilson, P. M., & Loucaides, C. A. (2005). Efficacy of an e-mail intervention for the promotion of physical activity and nutrition behavior in the workplace context. *American Journal of Health Promotion, 19*, 422–429.

Prochaska, J. J., Zabinski, M. F., Calfas, K. J., Sallis, J. F., & Patrick, K. (2000). PACE+: Interactive communication technology for behavior change in clinical settings. *American Journal of Preventive Medicine, 19*, 127–131.

Prochaska, J. O., Redding, C. A., & Evers, K. E. (2005). The transtheoretical model and stages of change. In K. Glanz, B. K. Rimer, & F. M. Lewis (Eds.), *Health Behavior and Health Education* (pp. 60–66). San Francisco, CA: Jossey-Bass.

Rainie, L. (2010). *Internet broadband and cell phone statistics.* Washington, DC: Pew Internet & American Life Project. Retrieved May 23, 2011, from: http://www.pewinternet.org/Reports/2010/Internet-broadband-and-cell-phone-statistics.aspx.

Ramo, D. E., Hall, S. M., & Prochaska, J. J. (2010). Reaching young adult smokers through the Internet: Comparison of three recruitment mechanisms. *Nicotine & Tobacco Research, 12*, 768–775.

Rice, R. E., & Katz, J. E. (2003). *The Internet and health communication: Experiences and expectations.* Thousand Oaks, CA: Sage.

Ritterband, L. M., & Tate, D. F. (2009). The science of Internet interventions. *Annals of Behavioral Medicine, 38*, 1–3.

Ritterband, L. M., Thorndike, F. P., Cox, D. J., Kovatchev, B. P., & Gonder-Frederick, L. A. (2009). A behavior change model for Internet interventions. *Annals of Behavioral Medicine, 38*, 18–27.

Robinson, P. H., & Serfaty, M. A. (2001). The use of e-mail in the identification of bulimia nervosa and its treatment. *European Eating Disorders Review, 9*, 182–193.

Rogers, E. M., & Albritton, M. M. (1995). Interactive communication technologies in business organizations. *Journal of Business Communication, 32*, 177–195.

Rolnick, S. J., Owens, B., Botta, R., Sathe, L., Hawkins, R., Cooper, L., et al. (1999). Computerized information and support for patients with breast cancer or HIV infection. *Nursing Outlook, 47,* 78–83.

Saint, N. (2010, July 27). The 10 U.S. counties stuck in the dial-up dark ages. *Business Insider.* Retrieved May 23, 2011, from: http://www.businessinsider.com/us-counties-broadband-access-2010–7.

Salonen, A. H., Kaunonen, M., Astedt-Kurki, P., Jarvenpaa, A. L., & Tarkka, M. T. (2008). Development of an Internet-based intervention for parents of infants. *Journal of Advanced Nursing, 64,* 60–72.

Saperstein, S. L., Atkinson, N. L., & Gold, R. S. (2007). The impact of Internet use for weight loss. *Obesity Reviews, 8,* 459–465.

Schwinn, T. M., Schinke, S. P., & Di Noia, J. (2010). Preventing drug abuse among adolescent girls: Outcome data from an Internet-based intervention. *Prevention Science, 11,* 24–32.

Sciamanna, C. N., Lewis, B., Tate, D., Napolitano, M. A., Fotheringham, M., & Marcus, B. H. (2002). User attitudes toward a physical activity promotion website. *Preventive Medicine, 35,* 612–615.

Shapira, N., Barak, A., & Gal, I. (2007). Promoting older adults' well-being through Internet training and use. *Aging & Mental Health, 11,* 477–484.

Smith, A. (2010). *Home broadband 2010.* Washington, DC: Pew Research Center. Retrieved May 23, 2011, from: http://pewinternet.org/~/media//Files/Reports/2010/Home%20broadband%202010.pdf.

Spooner, T. (2003). *Internet use by region in the United States.* Retrieved May 23, 2011, from: http://www.pewinternet.org/Reports/2003/Internet-Use-by-Region-in-the-US/Summary-of-Findings.aspx.

Steele, R., Mummery, W. K., & Dwyer, T. (2007). Using the Internet to promote physical activity: A randomized trial of intervention delivery modes. *Journal of Physical Activity & Health, 4,* 245–260.

Stinson, J., Wilson, R., Gill, N., Yamada, J., & Holt, J. (2009). A systematic review of Internet-based self-management interventions for youth with health conditions. *Journal of Pediatric Psychology, 34,* 495–510.

Stoops, W. W., Dallery, J., Fields, N. M., Nuzzo, P. A., Schoenberg, N. E., Martin, C. A., et al. (2009). An Internet-based abstinence reinforcement smoking cessation intervention in rural smokers. *Drug and Alcohol Dependence, 105,* 56–62.

Strecher, V. (2007). Internet methods for delivering behavioral and health-related interventions (eHealth). *Annual Review of Clinical Psychology, 3,* 53–76.

Tate, D. F., Finkelstein, E. A., Khavjou, O., & Gustafson, A. (2009). Cost effectiveness of Internet interventions: Review and recommendations. *Annals of Behavioral Medicine, 38,* 40–45.

Tate, D. F., Jackvony, E. H., & Wing, R. R. (2003). Effects of Internet behavioral counseling on weight loss in adults at risk for type 2 diabetes: A randomized trial. *Journal of the American Medical Association, 289,* 1833–1836.

Tate, D. F., Wing, R. R., & Winett, R. A. (2001). Using Internet technology to deliver a behavioral weight loss program. *Journal of American Medical Association, 285,* 1172–1177.

Thompson, D., Baranowski, T., Baranowski, J., Cullen, K., Jago, R., Watson, K., et al. (2009). Boy Scout 5-a-day Badge: Outcome results of a troop and Internet intervention. *Preventive Medicine, 49,* 518–526.

Tsang, M. W., Mok, M., Kam, G., Jung, M., Tang, A., Chan, U., et al. (2001). Improvement in diabetes control with a monitoring system based on a hand-held, touch-screen electronic diary. *Journal of Telemedicine and Telecare, 7,* 47–50.

U.S. Department of Commerce & National Telecommunications and Information Administration. (1999). *Falling through the Net: Defining the digital divide; Fact sheet: Native Americans lacking information resources.* Washington, DC: U.S. Department of Commerce. Retrieved May 23, 2011, from: http://www.ntia.doc.gov/ntiahome/fttn99/contents.html.

Vandelanotte, C., Spathonis, K. M., Eakin, E. G., & Owen, N. (2007). Website-delivered physical activity interventions: A review of the literature. *American Journal of Preventive Medicine, 33,* 54–64.

Van den Berg, M. H., Ronday, H. K., Peeters, A. J., le Cessie, S., Van der Giesen, F. J., Breedveld, F. C., et al. (2006). Using Internet technology to deliver a home-based physical activity intervention for patients with rheumatoid arthritis: A randomized controlled trial. *Arthritis and Rheumatism, 55,* 935–945.

Van den Berg, M. H., Schoones, J. W., & Vliet Vlieland, T. P. (2007). Internet-based physical activity interventions: A systematic review of the literature. *Journal of Medical Internet Research, 9,* e26.

Van der Houwen, K., Schut, H., Van den Bout, J., Stroebe, M., & Stroebe, W. (2010). The efficacy of a brief Internet-based self-help intervention for the bereaved. *Behavior Research and Therapy, 48,* 359–367.

Vernon, M. L. (2010). A review of computer-based alcohol problem services designed for the general public. *Journal of Substance Abuse Treatment, 38,* 203–211.

Wagner, B., & Maercker, A. (2007). A 1.5-year follow-up of an Internet-based intervention for complicated grief. *Journal of Traumatic Stress, 20,* 625–629.

Walther, J. (1996). Computer-mediated communication: Impersonal, interpersonal, and hyperpersonal interaction. *Communication Research, 23,* 3–43.

Wang, Z., Walther, J. B., Pingree, S., & Hawkins, R. P. (2008). Health information, credibility, homophily, and influence via the Internet: Websites versus discussion groups. *Health Communication, 23,* 358–368.

Wells, J., & Lewis, L. (2006). *Internet access in U.S. public schools and classrooms: 1994–2005.* Washington DC: National Center for Education Statistics. Retrieved May 23, 2011, from: http://nces.ed.gov/pubs2007/2007020.pdf.

White, M. A., Martin, P. D., Newton, R. L., Walden, H. M., York-Crowe, E. E., Gordon, S. T., et al. (2004). Mediators of weight loss in a family-based intervention presented over the Internet. *Obesity Research, 12,* 1050–1059.

Winzelberg, A. J., Classen, C., Alpers, G. W., Roberts, H., Koopman, C., Adams, R. E., et al. (2003). Evaluation of an Internet support group for women with primary breast cancer. *Cancer, 97,* 1164–1173.

Winzelberg, A. J., Eppstein, D., Eldredge, K. L., Wilfley, D., Dasmahapatra, R., Dev, P., et al. (2000). Effectiveness of an Internet-based program for reducing risk factors for eating disorders. *Journal of Consulting and Clinical Psychology, 68,* 346–350.

Woodall, W. G., Buller, D. B., Saba, L., Zimmerman, D., Waters, E., Hines, J. M., et al. (2007). Effect of emailed messages on return use of a nutrition education website and subsequent changes in dietary behavior. *Journal of Medical Internet Research, 9,* e27.

Woodruff, S. I., Edwards, C. C., Conway, T. L., & Elliott, S. P. (2001). Pilot test of an Internet virtual world chat room for rural teen smokers. *Journal of Adolescent Health, 29,* 239–243.

Zabinski, M. F., Pung, M. A., Wilfley, D. E., Eppstein, D. L., Winzelberg, A. J., Celio, A., et al. (2001). Reducing risk factors for eating disorders: Targeting at-risk women with a computerized psychoeducational program. *International Journal of Eating Disorders, 29,* 401–408.

5

VIRTUAL INTERACTIVE INTERVENTIONS FOR REDUCING RISKY SEX

Adaptations, Integrations, and Innovations

Lynn Carol Miller, Paul Robert Appleby, John L. Christensen, Carlos Godoy, Mei Si, Charisse Corsbie-Massay, Stephen J. Read, Stacy Marsella, Alexandra N. Anderson, and Jennifer Klatt

> I met him at a house party given by friends of friends. He was so hot, I was attracted to him immediately. We danced and as we talked about ourselves I found myself more and more attracted to him. After a few drinks I decided to stay at his place for the night. We were naked and I was really caught up in the moment and just didn't want to think about using a condom—or anything else, but a little voice kept saying, "Are you kidding, anal sex without a condom...you know how dangerous that is, tell him you want to play safe, right now."

Most virtual interactive interventions designed to change risky sexual behaviors involve adapting an existing conventional interpersonal or group intervention into a computer-generated version. For example, there might be a classroom-based intervention with modules on learning how to use a condom correctly or how to negotiate safer sex; these modules could be adapted to be conducted virtually (e.g., with video or a game) instead of face to face. Increasingly, however, developments in virtual interactive technologies are enabling features that allow us to move beyond adaptation and inspire theoretically and empirically based intervention integrations and innovations. In such cases, the user can be part of virtual narratives, like the realistic one depicted above in which self-regulation enhancing interventions interrupt and alter more automatic risky decisions.

We begin our chapter on virtual interactive interventions with a definition of the term, and then we provide an example of one such intervention, SOLVE

(Socially Optimized Learning in Virtual Environments). After using this example to illustrate the potential advantages of this approach, we briefly review the work of other researchers in this domain. Because there have been a number of recent reviews of interactive approaches (e.g., Noar, Black, & Pierce, 2009; Noar, Clark, Cole, & Lustria, 2006; Noar, Pierce, & Black, 2010), we focus primarily on those that have been found in randomized trials to be efficacious for reducing risky sexual behavior. We exclude studies that do not evaluate interactive interventions (e.g., Scholes et al., 2003 [subjects' answers to computer-based questions yielded magazine-style printouts, a noninteractive format]), and we exclude digital games that do not simulate an interpersonal communication (e.g., *Pos or Not*, 2009 [users guess whether a photo is of a person with HIV or not]; *Shagland*, 2011 [digital characters chase condoms]). Finally, we conclude our chapter by discussing the effectiveness, dissemination, and cumulative science advancement potential of virtual interactive interventions.

Virtual Interactive Interventions Defined

Virtual interactive interventions are defined as interventions delivered over the Web or a computer (including interactive videos and computer games) that involve a social interaction with real or perceived others with the aim of optimizing users' healthier choices (Appleby, Godoy, Miller, & Read, 2008; Read et al., 2006). Individuals, particularly younger ones, at risk for contracting STIs/HIV may be most responsive to such computer mediated interactive interventions (Appleby et al., 1996; Miller, Christensen, Appleby, Read, & Corsbie-Massay, 2010; Read et al., 2006). Interactivity "can be defined as the degree to which a communication technology can create a mediated environment in which participants can communicate (one-to-one, one-to-many, and many-to-many), both synchronously and asynchronously, and participate in reciprocal message exchanges. With regard to human users, it additionally refers to their ability to perceive the experience as a simulation of interpersonal communication" (Kiousis, 2002, p. 372; see also Noar et al., 2006).

Socially Optimized Learning in Virtual Environments (SOLVE): An Example

Our SOLVE intervention begins by putting the target population—men who have sex with men (MSM)—in an interactive virtual environment in which, unlike with passive media such as videos alone, users' choices affect how the scenario unfolds. The scenarios are designed to simulate typical narratives and choice points (e.g., using alcohol or not, using methamphetamine or not, successfully negotiating safer sex with one's partner or failing to do so) leading up to sexual risk taking (i.e., unprotected anal sex). The sexual scenario begins with preparation for the date (e.g., ensuring condoms are fresh and available). Later, the user seeks a partner at a club in the "hooking up" phase, when he chats up and ultimately finds an attractive partner. After going home with his partner, the user negotiates safer sex in the partner's apartment and bedroom before having sex. Building on this narrative base, the intervention components are designed to optimize the learning of self-regulated safer sexual choices in challenging risk contexts.

Advantages and Illustrations of This Approach for Health Communication: Cognitive and Affective Aspects of Decision Making

Virtual interactive interventions can often readily be adapted from effective interventions designed for individual or one-on-one counseling interventions (for reviews, see Fisher & Fisher, 1998, and Peterson & DiClemente, 2000). Interventions whose designs have been guided by theory have been associated with stronger behavioral outcome effects (e.g., Webb, Joseph, Yardley, & Michie, 2010). The three most extensively used theories for Internet delivery (Webb et al., 2010) have been the transtheoretical model (TTM; Prochaska & DiClemente, 1984), the theory of reasoned action/planned behavior (TPB; Ajzen, 1991; Fishbein & Ajzen, 1975), and Bandura's social cognitive theory (SCT; Bandura, 1989). Related models (e.g., information motivation behavioral skills model [IMB]; Fisher, Fisher, Bryan, & Misovich, 2002) and the AIDS risk reduction model (Catania, Kegeles, & Coates, 1990) incorporate and integrate components from other theories. Although these theoretical approaches differ, collectively they have focused almost exclusively on more deliberative, conscious, and cognitive aspects of behavior change (e.g., changing cognitions and the balance of pros and cons for the behavior, enhancing skills and self-efficacy, enhancing motivation, enhancing intentions to engage in the behavior, etc.). They tend to neglect more affective-based aspects. SOLVE, however, considers both.

In terms of the more cognitively focused theories, SOLVE models how to negotiate safer sex with one's partner even when he resists condom use (Appleby, Miller, & Rothspan, 1999; Edgar, Freimuth, & Hammond, 1988) and features "guides" who narrate the story of a romantic couple and provide feedback regarding safer sex to the user. Scenes of the couple model how to negotiate safer sex as well as correct condom use in a sex-positive, playful, and erotic way (e.g., "I have condoms, all colors, flavors, and sizes!"). More unique modules (e.g., methamphetamine [MA] and HIV risk), during which MSM learn how to perform refusal skills and in which their beliefs about MA are challenged by the guides, were added because methamphetamine use is associated with increased sexual risk taking in the target population (Appleby, Briano, et al., 2010).

Evaluations of SOLVE show that MSM in the intervention, compared to those in the control group, develop enhanced skills and perceived self-efficacy in negotiating safer sex (Appleby, Miller, & Christensen, 2010). SOLVE also significantly changes key cognitions (e.g., Ajzen, 1991; Ajzen & Fishbein, 1980; Bandura, 1994;

Beck, 1970) that have also been found to predict risky sexual behaviors (e.g., Fisher & Fisher, 1992; Peterson & DiClemente, 2000). For example, guides discuss the consequences of HIV infection (e.g., "Even though there are treatments for HIV, they don't work for everyone and the side effects are no picnic") and the link between behavior and immediate and long-term negative outcomes (e.g., "You don't want to break out in a case of herpes right before your cousin Lupe's quinceañera"; "You can get HIV whether you're the top or the bottom").

Unlike other virtual interactive interventions, SOLVE also addresses the affect-based route to decision making (Bechara, Damasio, Tranel, & Damasio, 1997; Miller et al., 2009, 2010; Read et al., 2006; see Figure 5.1). Given research on state-dependent learning (Bowers & Forgas, 2000), activating sexual arousal with virtual scenarios and choices of sexual behavior (e.g., mutual masturbation, anal intercourse) might better simulate real-life risky sexual decision-making challenges. SOLVE has been designed to do this and, in fact, has been shown to significantly enhance sexual arousal compared to a control (Miller, Appleby, & Read, 2011). Virtual interventions designed to interrupt and change risky behavior under more emotionally similar conditions might then be more effective than interventions not designed for such situations. As we review below, SOLVE also has shown such effects.

A range of emotional obstacles to safer sex in the context of sexual decision making (e.g., sexual arousal, desire for an attractive man) may activate other emotions (e.g., shame) based on prior emotional experience (Damasio, 1994). For example, MSM often experience stigma and shame associated with their sexual

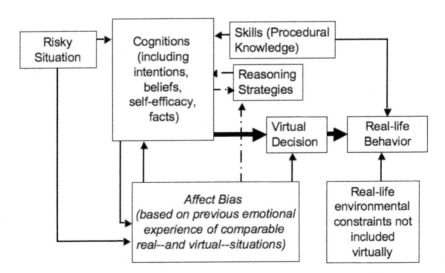

Figure 5.1 SOLVE conceptual model for reducing sexual risk taking

orientation (Balsam & Mohr, 2007; Herek, 2002). Such emotions, unaddressed, may more automatically increase the probability of engaging in sexual risks (Appleby, Briano, et al., 2010; Tangney & Dearing, 2002). To reduce stigma associated with MSM's sexual orientation, SOLVE interactive video interventions offer two innovative design features: (1) they are "sex positive" and (2) they incorporate strategies (see narrative self-regulatory circuitry in the next section) designed to change self-regulation capacity to reduce sexual risk taking (Read et al., 2006). In SOLVE, MSM's feelings of shame were significantly reduced by the intervention (the first intervention to do so). Furthermore, changes in shame significantly predicted reduction in unprotected receptive intercourse over three months (Christensen, Miller, & Appleby, 2010).

Narrative Self-Regulatory Circuitry

To enhance self-regulation, guides respond immediately if users make a risky choice in the narrative (e.g., unsafe sex). Guides provide what developmental psychologists, based on the work of Vygotsky (Berk & Winsler, 1995), refer to as scaffolding, or the temporary support that the teacher provides to the learner until that learner can self-regulate his or her own learning. The guides in SOLVE do this virtually through an Interrupt-Challenge-Acknowledgment-Provide (ICAP) sequence. That is, they *interrupt* more automatic risky choices, *challenge* those choices and beliefs, reward safer decisions, and use appropriate loss- and gain-framed messages to focus MSM on considering the future consequences of their actions (Appleby et al., 2005). Guides then *acknowledge* MSM's emotions, motives, and beliefs that may be conflicting (e.g., desire and shame). Here guides may read the affective cues of self and other; interpret and make inferences about cause, effect, or intent of one's own or the other's behavior; and clarify self and other goals, emotions, and beliefs. Then, guides *provide* a reframing of the situation and a set of strategies that grapple with conflicting beliefs, emotions, and motivations and help keep MSM safer (Read et al., 2006).

Users can then choose to make the same decision or an alternative less risky choice, and those decisions are recorded by the program. At the end of the intervention, guides provide a recap of individual MSM's choices with positive reinforcement for safer choices. For risky choices, they provide alternative scenes to model how safer choices could have been made. In short, SOLVE affords theory-based intervention integration across both cognitive and affective-based theories of decision making to better optimize risk reduction.

Virtual Interventions: Engaging and Responsive

Virtual environments can be particularly engaging (e.g., Woolf-King, Maisto, Carey, & Vanable, 2009) and can enhance intervention effectiveness (Zhang, Zhou, Briggs, & Nunamaker Jr., 2006). In some virtually interactive interventions (e.g.,

Read et al., 2006), users do not merely observe the actions of others and make choices regarding what intervention components to see in what order (as in Downs et al., 2004); instead, they make a series of choices that affect actors' behaviors and how the scenario unfolds. Users identify with the characters and come closer to owning the decisions. This significantly enhances participant engagement in the intervention compared to a condition in which MSM passively observe characters' modeling choices, without making active choices for the characters (Miller et al., 2009).

Virtual interventions also are responsive to users, primarily through tailoring of program responses to user input. Tailored interventions (see chapter 8 of this volume) have been shown to be more effective than nontailored interventions (Salovey, 2005). Virtual environments can make it easier to tailor responses not only to a given individual's preexisting characteristics (e.g., Kiene & Barta, 2006; Mackenzie et al., 2007) but also to their prior behavioral responses within the virtual intervention itself (Read et al., 2006). In addition, in interactive technologies, optional mentoring is possible when the user desires it. This allows the user to ask for advice or seek out help when making decisions about safer sex or alcohol and drug use, for example, further tailoring the experience to the user's needs. In SOLVE, this optional mentoring was available at a variety of choice points (e.g., whether to get alcohol, whether to buy methamphetamine, deciding what type of sex to have, deciding how to negotiate safer sex).

Achieving a Better Understanding of Active Change Components

With multicomponent interventions, researchers typically use a randomized controlled trial (RCT) to assess how the overall intervention compares to a control condition. These studies are called *summative assessments*. But, in developing an intervention, it is often difficult to test which components are likely to be effective or not, for whom, at which point, and under what circumstances. Virtual interactive interventions can address this need by using small portions of the interactive narrative and systematically manipulating intervention messages and components to assess users' behavioral intentions. For example, in SOLVE, we recently tested and found that the effectiveness of a message depended on whether the user's immediately preceding choice was risky or safer (Christensen, Miller, Appleby, Read, & Corsbie-Massay, 2009).

Improved Intervention Delivery and Dissemination

Virtual interactive interventions have greater potential for improved delivery and dissemination. In terms of delivery, for example, interventionists do not need to be trained and available to perform the intervention; this can greatly reduce costs of implementation. Additionally, virtual interactive interventions afford exactly the same responses given user choices for each user, enhancing the fidelity and reducing errors in intervention delivery or "slippage in message delivery" that can happen with HIV counselors (Appleby et al., 1996). Once the virtual interactive intervention has been developed, it can be rapidly disseminated to clinics (e.g., via DVD) or even more rapidly disseminated over the Web (Webb et al., 2010) to a given individual within or outside of a clinical context.

This means that at-risk individuals who typically cannot or do not frequent clinics or other sites of traditional intervention delivery (e.g., rural populations and MSM who choose not to socialize in the mainstream gay community) can still receive interventions and do so at their convenience. The Internet is a safe environment in which to learn about sexual negotiation skills, facts about HIV prevention, and risk factors associated with HIV such as the use of methamphetamine (Appleby, Miller, et al., 2010). A variety of interactive interventions involving changing risky sexual behavior are already being delivered and evaluated over the Web (Noar et al., 2006). Interactive interventions offer great promise for combining interpersonal efficacy with mass media's reach (Cassell, Jackson, & Cheuvront, 1998).

Are Virtual Interactive Interventions for Reducing Risky Sex Effective?

A recent meta-analysis of Internet use to promote changes in health behavior found 85 studies in which interventions were Web delivered, experimentally tested, and included a behavioral outcome (Webb et al., 2010). This study found small but significant effects. Only two of the studies included sexual outcome variables, however, and only one of those examined behaviors. Noar et al. (2006) identified 21 interactive safer sex websites; however, it is unclear if these sites have been evaluated for their efficacy.

Regarding sexual decision making, recent reviews of evaluated virtual interactive interventions indicate that these interventions can be efficacious (e.g., Noar et al., 2009). Interventions tested for efficacy have been applied to a variety of target populations, including younger adolescents (e.g., Downs et al., 2004; Lightfoot, Comulada, & Stover, 2007), older adolescents and adults (Bull, Pratte, Whitesell, Rietmeijer, & McFarlane, 2009; Redding et al., 2004; Roberto, Zimmerman, Carlyle, & Abner, 2007), college students (Kiene & Barta, 2006), at-risk females ages 13–35 (Peipert et al., 2008; Scholes et al., 2003), and prison populations (Martin, O'Connell, Inciardi, Surratt, & Maiden, 2008). Interventions also have been developed around HIV status and for MSM. For example, Gilbert et al. (2008) developed an interactive intervention for HIV-positive individuals, and Rosser et al. (2010) developed an intervention for HIV-positive and HIV-negative MSM. Finally, our SOLVE research teams developed and evaluated two interventions for HIV-negative MSM. The first team created an interactive CD-ROM appropriate for a general MSM sample (Appleby et al., 1996; Miller & Murphy, 1999; Read et al.,

2006). The second team created three DVDs: one targeting African American MSM, another for Latino MSM, and the third for Caucasian MSM (Appleby et al., 2008; Miller et al., 2010). We briefly describe the efficacy of a sample of these sexual decision-making interventions below.

Forestalling sexual debut in adolescents through interactive interventions has met with some success. Downs et al. (2004) evaluated the impact of a stand-alone interactive video (IAV) STD intervention on adolescent females. Comparing intervention to control participants, they found that those in the IAV condition were more likely to be abstinent in the first three months following the intervention, more likely to experience fewer condom failures in the next three months, and less likely to have been exposed to an STD six months after enrollment. Roberto et al. (2007) reported similar effects for an intervention tested in two public schools (one intervention and one control). Results indicated that students in the experimental school were less likely to initiate sexual activity and had greater condom negotiation self-efficacy. (Because individual participants were not randomly assigned to condition, however, questions about the independence of these data points within the two schools and the interpretation of these findings must be raised.) Studying somewhat older participants, Kiene and Barta (2006) found that sexually active undergraduates in the interactive intervention versus control condition reported significantly more condom use over four weeks.

For about-to-be-released prison populations, Martin et al. (2008) found that an experimental DVD-delivered HIV prevention intervention resulted in significantly more protected sex 90 days postintervention among experimental group participants than standard intervention control group participants. Gilbert et al. (2008) designed an interactive "video doctor" for HIV-positive patients that was found in an RCT over three and six months to reduce patients' numbers of sexual partners.

For SOLVE among MSM populations, Read et al. (2006) found that, compared to MSM who received standard-of-care one-on-one counseling only, MSM in an experimental group who also received the CD interactive video (SOLVE-IAV) reported more protected and less unprotected anal sex over three months. More recently, funded by the National Institute of Allergy and Infectious Diseases (NIAID), we developed three separate DVD interactive videos (one for each risk population of African American, Latino, and Caucasian MSM) and tested them for efficacy in an RCT over three months (Appleby et al., 2008; Miller et al., 2010). Results showed that the videos reduced unprotected receptive and insertive anal sex over time, but only for younger (18–24) and not older (25–30) MSM. Rosser et al. (2010) conducted an RCT of an interactive intervention targeting MSM (HIV-positive and HIV-negative) over the Web and found that at three months (but not subsequently) there were significant differences between the intervention and control group in the number of men with whom research participants had risky sex. These findings suggest that interactive interventions can reduce risky sexual behaviors in high-risk populations, including prisoners and MSM, and that, for the latter group at least, they can be efficaciously delivered via the Web.

Contexts for Virtual Interventions for Reducing Risky Sex

Virtual interventions have been tested for efficacy in a variety of contexts. Some interventions have been tested in a controlled laboratory setting (Kiene & Barta, 2006; Miller et al., 2010). Others have been tested in various field settings such as school environments for adolescents (Lightfoot et al., 2007; Roberto et al., 2007), health care settings (Appleby et al., 1996; Bull et al., 2009; Downs et al., 2004; Gilbert et al., 2008; Peipert et al., 2008; Read et al., 2006; Redding et al., 2004), and prison settings (Martin et al., 2008). Increasingly, researchers have not only recruited participants for laboratory and field studies over the Web but also have conducted interventions over the Web as well (e.g., Bull et al., 2009; Davidovich, 2006; Rosser et al., 2010).

Most virtual interventions were designed as stand-alone interventions (e.g., Bull et al., 2009; Davidovich, 2006; Downs et al., 2004; Gilbert et al., 2008; Kiene & Barta, 2006; Lightfoot et al., 2007; Martin et al., 2008; Miller et al., 2010; Rosser et al., 2010). Some interventions, however, were tested as part of a total package of components or as supplements to existing approaches (Appleby et al., 1996; Miller & Read, 2006; Peipert et al., 2008; Read et al., 2006; Redding et al., 2004; Roberto et al., 2007). Finally, most of the virtual interventions we reviewed were compared with no-treatment control groups (Davidovich, 2006; Gilbert et al., 2008; Kiene & Barta, 2006; Lightfoot et al., 2007; Miller et al., 2010; Roberto et al., 2007; Rosser et al., 2010) or standard-of-care controls (Appleby et al., 1996; Bull et al., 2009; Downs et al., 2004; Martin et al., 2008; Peipert et al., 2008; Read et al., 2006; Redding et al., 2004).

Virtual Interactive Narratives and Intelligent Agents: New Enabling Technologies

For the most part, virtual interventions for HIV delivered via computer or over the Web have included separate video clips or two-dimensional images. Until recently, with few exceptions (e.g., SOLVE), they have excluded extensive rich embedded sequential interactive video narratives or complex three-dimensional environments simulating the risk-taking or risk-promotion narrative. However, over the past five years, technological developments have rapidly changed the virtual interactive intervention landscape. For example, we have been funded by the California HIV/AIDS Research Program (CHRP) to use the Internet to reach MSM and test the effectiveness of SOLVE interactive videos (Appleby, Miller, et al., 2010; Miller et al., 2010; Miller & Read, 2006; Read et al., 2006) delivered over the Web. The approach involves converting existing interactive videos from our DVD intervention into a virtual interactive intervention for Web delivery using Flash and Actionscript technology that affords playback on a variety of operating systems and browsers.

Another development involves simulating and delivering rich interpersonal narratives for promoting behavior change, using one of a number of available game engines or integrated environments for simplifying the development of a game. Game engines include an engine for rendering two- or three-dimensional graphics and can include a physics engine (for detecting and responding to objects colliding) and other engines for developing and incorporating other key elements of the game (e.g., sound, scripting, animation, artificial intelligence of the agents). Some game engines (e.g., UNITY) can be used across a variety of platforms (e.g., Windows, Mac, iPhone, iPad, Wii, Android smartphones), enhancing the potential for dissemination.

Within such games, users can choose or design an avatar to represent themselves (see Fox, this volume). Recent work (e.g., Yee, Bailenson, & Ducheneaut, 2009) suggests that users given more attractive avatars may feel more desirable and comfortable seeking intimacy within a virtual environment and this effect may carry over into real life. Research also suggests that participants allowed to choose their own avatar (Lim & Reeves, 2006), especially customizable attractive ones (Yee & Bailenson, 2007), might be more engaged. That was also our approach in developing a SOLVE game using intelligent technologies (SOLVE-IT). In some interpersonal interventions, users can interact with other avatars (who may represent real or virtual others). The actions of other avatars can be driven by (1) a human operating online (e.g., in a multiplayer game), (2) rules (e.g., if x does this, this character does y), or (3) virtual realistic intelligent avatars (agents) whose decisions are autonomously driven by the agent's (avatar's) underlying AI/computational model (e.g., specification of the agent's motives and representations of self and others and how these will drive decisions).

One of the most extensively used multi-agent-based simulation environments with intelligent agents is PsychSim (Marsella, Pynadath, & Read, 2004; Pynadath & Marsella, 2004, 2005). Using this environment and adaptations to it, a researcher can construct scenarios wherein a diverse set of entities interact and communicate among themselves. Each entity has its own goals and policies of achievement, relationships with other entities (e.g., liking, distrust), private beliefs, and recursive mental models, or "theory of mind," about self and other. Researchers can manually perturb the simulation by changing the models or specifying actions and messages for any entity to perform. A human user can be substituted for an agent. This creates a highly adaptive test bed for readily personalizing the game to a given user and, with a sufficient animation budget, potentially providing an almost infinite number of interpersonal challenges from other virtual MSM. The simulation can also be readily modified (e.g., by adding new interventions, agents, props) to improve that game or develop new games.

Virtual Interactive Narrative Game Applications

These interactive stories with realistic intelligent agents are designed to scaffold the user in learning how to make better decisions and better cope with real-life situational challenges. For example, Carmen's *Bright IDEAS* (Marsella, Johnson, &

LaBore, 2003) uses interactive stories to teach problem solving skills to mothers of pediatric cancer patients. *FearNot!* (Paiva et al., 2004) provides a virtual environment for children exploring ways to cope with bullying. Mitchell, Parsons, and Leonard (2007) use a virtual café populated with conversational agents to teach social skills to children with autism spectrum disorder. Brosnan, Fitzpatrick, Sharry, and Boyle (2006) train children via story design in virtual environments to better cope with depression or anxiety disorders. Most of these interventions have been found to effectively change desired behavior and/or appear promising, based on pilot work (for more on digital games, see Lieberman, this volume).

SOLVE: Narrative Self-Regulatory Circuitry and Scaffolding

To illustrate the potential of intelligent technologies, let us again consider SOLVE as an example. Currently, we are using UNITY to develop an NIMH-funded HIV/AIDS prevention intervention, SOLVE-IT, using 3-D animated intelligent agents (Miller et al., 2010). This technology enables a more rapid dissemination across platforms over the Web. It also affords risky MSM an opportunity to learn how to make safer choices while enjoying fun dates with their choice of attractive partners. The game starts with the user's choice of and customization of his avatar (e.g., by ethnicity, skin tone, eye color, clothing), followed by that player in his apartment getting ready to meet his friend at a party. The user meets his virtual future self (VFS), his chosen avatar made to appear a few years older. The VFS becomes the user's mentor; its goal is to aid the user in optimizing his self-regulated decisions (because "your decisions affect me").

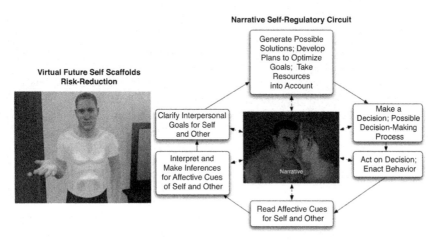

Figure 5.2 Narrative self-regulatory circuitry using a virtual future self in SOLVE-IT

Before going out on his date, the user can take condoms; if he forgets, his VFS reminds him and debunks reasons he might have for not taking them and rewards him when he takes them (this and other choices are recorded and can affect later experiences and feedback).

At the house party the user makes decisions about alcohol (and how much to drink); if the user drinks too much, his VFS may interrupt him with an alcohol intervention message. He stays and starts to make out with the host of the party during which the VFS interrupts to remind him to negotiate safer sex before going to the bedroom. The action proceeds to the bedroom where the realistic three-dimensional animated characters make sexual decisions regarding the type of sex (e.g., oral, mutual masturbation, anal) and whether the sex is protected or not. If and when the user chooses not to use a condom during anal sex, the guides interrupt with an ICAP message. At the end, the VFS recaps the user's choices and responds to them with reward (if the choices were safe) or alternatively describes what he did and why those decisions can lead to negative consequences.

At the second level of the game, the user is at a club in which he seeks out another partner and has new challenges in terms of negotiating safer sex. At the end of the game, if the user made risky choices, he is shown alternative ways he could have responded and how that could have resulted in safer—but still hot—sex. Character choices in negotiating safer sex in the living room and in the bedroom are driven by PsychSim (and the intelligent agents' underlying goal settings). Thus, the action could proceed quite differently if that character's goals were differentially set—providing more and different challenges to the user. With greater funding for the creation of more animation and additional three-dimensional environments, researchers can develop simulations that offer the user more challenges across a broader range of situations, and the user could play multiple versions of the game without repeating similar interactions, thus increasing his exposure to challenging situations and safer ways of handling them.

Another potential advantage of games with intelligent agents is that it may be possible to use PsychSim and related computational models to model the user's own choices throughout the game. That would enable researchers to better predict and anticipate the choices of a given user with different partners and across different situations. With better prediction of how a given user might take risks within a virtual environment, it might be possible to design better interventions within the game for that user. This is important because even in our earlier work using interactive video choices (e.g., Miller et al., 2009, 2010), we found that MSM's virtual interactive choices were predictive of their future similar choices (e.g., regarding alcohol, sex, etc.). If we can increasingly better change more of MSM's virtual behavior, our research suggests we may be better able to increasingly change similar real-life risky choices. That is, emerging intelligent technologies (IT) could afford a cumulative test bed for testing and advancing health communication theory and our interventions' effectiveness. Such a pipeline from IT test bed to rapid dissemination of improved interventions is an exciting possibility for health communication researchers.

Acknowledgments

This work was supported by Grant R01 AI052756 from the National Institute of Allergy and Infectious Diseases (NIAID), Grant R01 MH82671 from the National Institute of Mental Health (NIMH), and Grant R96-USC-160 from the California HIV/AIDS Research Program (CHRP). Its contents are solely the responsibility of the authors and do not necessarily represent the official views of the NIAID, NIMH, or CHRP.

References

Ajzen, I. (1991). The theory of planned behavior. *Organizational Behavior and Human Decision Processes, 50,* 179–211.

Ajzen, I., & Fishbein, M. (1980). *Understanding attitudes and predicting social behavior.* Englewood Cliffs, NJ: Prentice Hall.

Appleby, P. R., Briano, M., Christensen, J. L., Anderson, A. N., Storholm, E. D., Ananias, D. K., et al. (2010). The disparate roles of ethnicity and sexual orientation in predicting methamphetamine use and related beliefs and behaviors among MSM. *Annals of Behavioral Medicine, 39,* s52. Supplemental material retrieved from: http://www.sbm.org/meeting/2010/presentations/Thursday/Paper%20Sessions/Paper%20Session%2002/The%20Disparate%20Roles%20of%20Ethnicity%20and%20Sexual%20Orientation%20in%20Predicting%20Methamphetamine%20Use.pdf.

Appleby, P. R., Godoy, C., Miller, L. C., & Read, S. J. (2008). Reducing risky sex through the use of interactive video technology. In T. Edgar, S. M. Noar, & V. S. Freimuth (Eds.), *Communication perspectives on HIV/AIDS for the 21st century* (pp. 379–384). New York: Lawrence Erlbaum Associates Taylor & Francis Group.

Appleby, P. R., Marks, G., Ayala, A., Miller, L. C., Murphy, S., & Mansergh, G. (2005). Consideration of future consequences and unprotected anal intercourse among men who have sex with men. *Journal of Homosexuality, 50,* 119–133.

Appleby, P. R., Miller, L. C., & Christensen, J. L. (2010, June). *A SOLVE prevention intervention using interactive video: Evidence of immediate enhancement of MSM's condom use and methamphetamine avoidance intentions, beliefs, and self-efficacy.* Paper presented at the 18th annual meeting of the Society for Prevention Research, Denver, CO.

Appleby, P. R., Miller, L. C., & Rothspan, S. (1999). The paradox of trust for male couples: When risking is a part of loving. *Personal Relationships, 6,* 81–93.

Appleby, P. R., Rothspan, S., Read, S. J., Miller, L. C., Marcolina, K., & Adams, D. (1996, March). *Gay men's interactive video.* Poster session presented at the University-wide AIDS Research Program 13th annual Investigators' Meeting, San Francisco, CA.

Balsam, K. F., & Mohr, J. J. (2007). Adaptation to sexual orientation stigma: A comparison of bisexual and lesbian/gay adults. *Journal of Counseling Psychology, 54,* 306–319.

Bandura, A. (1989). Human agency in social cognitive theory. *American Psychologist, 44,* 1175–1184.

Bandura, A. (1994). Social cognitive theory and the exercise of control over HIV infection. In R. J. DiClemente & J. L. Peterson (Eds.), *Preventing AIDS: Theories and methods of behavioral interventions* (pp. 25–29). New York: Plenum.

Bechara, A., Damasio, H., Tranel, D., & Damasio, A. R. (1997). Deciding advantageously before knowing the advantageous strategy. *Science, 275,* 1293–1295.

Beck, A. T. (1970). Cognitive therapy: Nature and relation to behavior therapy. *Behavior Therapy, 1,* 184–200.

Berk, L., & Winsler, A. (1995). *Scaffolding children's learning: Vygotsky and early childhood education.* Washington: National Association for the Education of Young Children.

Bowers, G. H., & Forgas, J. P. (2000). *Affect, memory, and social cognition.* New York: Oxford University Press.

Brosnan, E., Fitzpatrick, C., Sharry, J., & Boyle, R. (2006, April). *An evaluation of the integrated use of a multimedia storytelling system within a psychotherapy intervention for adolescents.* Paper presented at the Conference on Human Factors in Computing Systems (CHI), Montreal, Canada.

Bull, S., Pratte, K., Whitesell, N., Rietmeijer, C., & McFarlane, M. (2009). Effects of an Internet-based intervention for HIV prevention: The Youthnet Trials. *AIDS and Behavior, 13,* 474–487.

Cassell, M. M., Jackson, C., & Cheuvront, B. (1998). Health communication on the Internet: An effective channel for health behavior change? *Journal of Health Communication, 3,* 71–79.

Catania, J., Kegeles, S., & Coates, T. (1990). Towards an understanding of risk behavior: An AIDS risk reduction model (ARRM). *Health Education Quarterly, 17,* 53–72.

Christensen, J. L., Miller, L. C., & Appleby, P. R. (2010, June). *What's to be ashamed? Reducing self-conscious negative affect predicts future decreases in sexual risk-taking.* Paper presented at the 18th annual meeting of the Society for Prevention Research, Denver, CO.

Christensen, J. L., Miller, L. C., Appleby, P. R., Read, S. J., & Corsbie-Massay, C. (2009, November). *Using virtual environments to tailor persuasive appeals: The role of gains and losses given prior decisions to seek or avoid risk.* Poster presented at the annual meeting of the Society for Judgment and Decision-Making, Boston, MA.

Damasio, A. R. (1994). *Descartes' error: Emotion, reason, and the human brain.* New York, NY: Penguin Putnam.

Davidovich, E. (2006). *Liaisons dangereuses.* Amsterdam: Ehud Davidovich.

Downs, J. S., Murray, P. J., de Bruin, W. B., Penrose, J., Palmgren, C., & Fischhoff, B. (2004). Interactive video behavioral intervention to reduce adolescent females' STD risk: A randomized controlled trial. *Social Science and Medicine, 59,* 1561–1572.

Edgar, T., Freimuth, V. S., & Hammond, S. L. (1988). Communicating the AIDS risk to college students: The problem of motivating change. *Health Education Research, 3,* 59–65.

Fishbein, M., & Ajzen, I. (1975). *Belief, attitude, and behavior. An introduction to theory and research.* Reading, MA: Addison-Wesley.

Fisher, J. D., & Fisher, W. A. (1992). Changing AIDS-risk behavior. *Psychological Bulletin, 111,* 455–474.

Fisher, J. D., Fisher, W. A., Bryan, A. D., & Misovich, S. J. (2002). Information-motivation-behavioral skills model-based HIV risk behavior change intervention for inner-city high school youth. *Health Psychology, 21,* 177–186.

Fisher, W. A. & Fisher, J. D. (1998). Understanding and promoting sexual and reproductive health behavior: Theory and method. *Annual Review of Sex Research, 9,* 39–76.

Gilbert, P., Ciccarone, D., Gansky, S. A., Bangsberg, D. R., Clanon, K., McPhee, S. J., et al. (2008). Interactive "Video Doctor" counseling reduces drug and sexual risk behaviors among HIV-positive patients in diverse outpatient settings. *PLoS ONE, 3,* e1988, 1–10.

Herek, G. M. (2002). Heterosexuals' attitudes toward bisexual men and women in the United States. *Journal of Sex Research, 39,* 264–274.

Kiene, S. M., & Barta, W. D. (2006). A brief individualized computer-delivered sexual risk reduction intervention increases HIV/AIDS preventive behavior. *Journal of Adolescent Health, 39,* 404–410.

Kiousis, S. (2002). Interactivity: A concept explication. *New Media & Society, 4,* 355–383.

Lightfoot, M., Comulada, S. W., & Stover, G. (2007). Computerized HIV preventive intervention for adolescents: Indications of efficacy. *American Journal of Public Health, 97,* 1027–1030.

Lim, S., & Reeves, B. (2006, June). *Being in the game: Effects of avatar choice and point of view on arousal responses during play.* Paper presented at the International Communication Association, Dresden, Germany.

Mackenzie, S. L. C., Kurth, A. E., Spielberg, F., Severynen, A., Malotte, C. K., St. Lawrence, J., et al. (2007). Patient and staff perspectives on the use of a computer counseling tool for HIV and sexually transmitted infection risk reduction. *Journal of Adolescent Health, 40,* 572.e9–572.e16.

Marsella, S. C., Johnson, L., & LaBore, C. (2003, July). *Interactive pedagogical drama for health interventions.* Paper presented at the 11th International Conference on Artificial Intelligence in Education, Sydney, Australia.

Marsella, S. C., Pynadath, D. V., & Read, S. J. (2004). PsychSim: Agent-based modeling of social interactions and influence. *Proceedings of the International Conference on Cognitive Modeling, USA,* 243–248.

Martin, S. S., O'Connell, D. J., Inciardi, J. A., Surratt, H. L., & Maiden, K. M. (2008). Integrating an HIV/HCV brief intervention in prisoner reentry: Results of a multisite prospective study. *Journal of Psychoactive Drugs, 40,* 427–436.

Miller, L. C., Appleby, P. R., & Read, S. J. (2011). Virtual sex: Real risk reduction for MSM (NIAID grant # R01 AI052756).Unpublished raw data.

Miller, L. C., Christensen, J., Appleby, P. R., Read, S. J., & Corsbie-Massay, C. (2010, June). *Results of a SOLVE-IAV efficacy trial: Evidence of reduction in insertive and receptive UAI over 3-months for younger (18–24) but not older (25–30) MSM compared to a wait-list control group.* Paper presented at the 18th annual meeting of the Society for Prevention Research, Denver, CO.

Miller, L. C., Christensen, J. L., Godoy, C. G., Appleby, P. R., Corsbie-Massay, C., & Read, S. J. (2009). Reducing risky decision-making in the virtual and in the real-world: Serious games, intelligent agents, and a SOLVE approach. In U. Ritterfeld, M. Cody, & P. Vorderer (Eds.), *Serious Games: Mechanisms and Effects* (pp. 429–447). Routledge/LEA Press.

Miller, L. C., & Murphy, S. T. (1999). A loaf of bread, a jug of wine, and thou: The meaning and impact of alcohol in the sexual sequence [Abstract]. *Annals of Behavioral Medicine, 19:* S006.

Miller, L. C., & Read, S. J. (2006). Virtual sex: Creating environments for reducing risky sex. In S. Cohen, K. Portnoy, D. Rehberger, & C. Thorsen (Eds.), *Virtual decisions: Digital simulations for teaching reasoning in the social sciences and humanities* (pp. 137–160). Mahwah, NJ: Lawrence Erlbaum Associates.

Mitchell, P., Parsons, S., & Leonard, A. (2007). Using virtual environments for teaching social understanding to 6 adolescents with Autistic Spectrum Disorders. *Journal of Autism and Developmental Disorders, 37,* 589–600.

Noar, S. M., Black, H. G., & Pierce, L. B. (2009). Efficacy of computer technology-based HIV prevention interventions: A meta-analysis, *AIDS, 23,* 107–115.

Noar, S. M., Clark, A., Cole, C., & Lustria, M. L. A. (2006). Review of interactive safer sex websites: Practice and potential. *Health Communication, 20,* 233–241.

Noar, S. M., Pierce, L. B., & Black, H. G. (2010). Can computer-mediated interventions change theoretical mediators of safer sex? A meta-analysis. *Human Communication Research, 36,* 261–297.

Paiva, A., Dias, J., Sobral, D., Woods, S., Aylett, R., Sobreperez, P., et al. (2004). Caring for agents and agents that care: Building empathic relations with synthetic agents. *Proceedings of the Third International Joint Conference on Autonomous Agents and Multi Agent Systems, USA, 3,* 194–201.

Peipert, J. F., Redding, C. A., Blume, J. D., Allsworth, J. E., Matteson, K. A., Lozowski, F., et al. (2008). Tailored intervention to increase dual-contraceptive method use: A randomized trial to reduce unintended pregnancies and sexually transmitted infections. *American Journal of Obstetrics & Gynecology, 198,* 630.e1–630.e8.

Peterson J. L., & DiClemente R. J. (Eds.) (2000). *Handbook of HIV prevention.* New York: Kluwer/Plenum Publishing Corporation.

Pos or Not (2009). MTV Networks On Campus Inc. [Digital game]. Retrieved February 23, 2011, from http://blog.aids.gov/2008/05/using-games-in.html.

Prochaska, J. O., & DiClemente, C. C. (1984). *The transtheoretical approach: Crossing the traditional boundaries of therapy.* Homewood, IL: Dow Jones-Irwin.

Pynadath, D. V., & Marsella, S. C. (2004). Fitting and compilation of multiagent models through piecewise linear functions. *Proceedings of the International Conference on Autonomous Agents and Multi Agent Systems, USA, 4,* 243–248.

Pynadath, D. V., & Marsella, S. C. (2005). Psychsim: Modeling theory of mind with decision-theoretic agents. *Proceedings of the International Joint Conference on Artificial Intelligence, UK, 5,* 1181–1186.

Read, S. J., Miller, L. C., Appleby, P. R., Nwosu, M. E., Reynaldo, S., Lauren, A., et al. (2006). Socially optimized learning in a virtual environment: Reducing risky sexual behavior among men who have sex with men. *Human Communication Research, 32,* 1–34.

Redding, C. A., Morokoff, P. J., Rossi, J. S., Meier, K. S., Hoeppner, B. B. Mayer, K., et al. (2004). Effectiveness of a computer-delivered TTM-tailored intervention at increasing condom use in at-risk heterosexual adults: RI Project Respect [Abstract]. *Annals of Behavioral Medicine, 27:* S113.

Roberto, A. J., Zimmerman, R. S., Carlyle, K. E., & Abner, E. L. (2007). A computer-based approach to preventing pregnancy, STD, and HIV in rural adolescents. *Journal of Health Communication, 12,* 53–76.

Rosser, B. R. S., Oakes, J. M., Konstan, J., Hooper, S., Horvath, K. J., Danilenko, G. P., et al. (2010). Reducing HIV risk behavior of men who have sex with men through persuasive computing: Results of the men's INTernet study-II. *AIDS, 24,* 2099–2107.

Salovey, P. (2005). Promoting prevention and detection: Psychologically tailoring and framing messages about health. In R. Bibace, J. D. Laird, K. L. Noller, & J. Valsiner (Eds.), *Science and medicine in dialogue: Thinking through particulars and universals* (pp. 17–42). Westport, CT: Praeger.

Scholes, D., McBride, C. M., Grothaus, L., Civic, D., Ichikawa, L. E., Fish, L. J., et al. (2003). A tailored minimal self-help intervention to promote condom use in young women: Results from a randomized trial. *AIDS, 17,* 1547–1556.

Shagland. (2011). London: Rubberductions [Digital game]. Retrieved February 28, 2011, from http://www.hypegames.com/adventure/867/super-shag-land.html.

Tangney, J. P., & Dearing, R. L. (2002). *Shame and guilt.* New York: Guilford.

Webb, T. L., Joseph, J., Yardley, L., & Michie, S. (2010). Using the Internet to promote health behavior change: A systematic review and meta-analysis of the impact of theoretical basis, use of behavioral change techniques, and mode of delivery on efficacy. *Journal of Medical Internet Research, 12,* e4.

Woolf-King, S. E., Maisto, S., Carey, M., & Vanable, P. (2009). Selection of film clips and development of a video for the investigation of sexual decision making among men who have sex with men. *Journal of Sex Research, 47,* 589–597.

Yee, N., & Bailenson, J. (2007). The proteus effect: The effect of transformed self-representation on behavior. *Human Communication Research, 33,* 271–290.

Yee, N., Bailenson, J., & Ducheneaut, N. (2009). The proteus effect: Implications of transformed digital self-presentation on online and offline behavior. *Communication Research, 36,* 285–312.

Zhang, D., Zhou, L., Briggs, R. O., & Nunamaker, Jr., J. F. (2006). Instructional video in e-learning: Assessing the impact of interactive video on learning effectiveness. *Information & Management, 43,* 15–27.

6

AVATARS FOR HEALTH BEHAVIOR CHANGE

Jesse Fox

You enter a virtual room. Standing before you is you—well, the virtual you. You walk around the representation and find that virtual you looks exactly like you do, from the crooked smile to the scar on your knee to the raised mole on the back of your neck. You hear the voice of your health care provider, Dr. Jones: "If you keep your tanning habit, this is what you can expect." You watch as the crow's feet form around your eyes and the skin on your hands gets leathery. A dark growth becomes apparent at your hairline. *Is that…?* Dr. Jones notices your gaze. "Yes, given your family history, sun exposure, and lack of sun safety practices, I anticipate that at some point in the future you will develop melanoma." Yikes. "If you change now, however…" Suddenly, the virtual you transforms into an older, healthier you with no melanoma growth in sight. Relief. "We've already noticed some change here," Dr. Jones says, as an arrow directs your attention to your neck mole. A calendar pops up and you see how the mole has changed in the last two years. "But as long as it doesn't evolve into this"—the mole grows larger, with an uneven border and color—"you shouldn't worry."

Virtual scenes like this one have transformed from a science fiction fantasy to a laboratory reality, one that may be an everyday exchange in our future. Already, computer-mediated communication is a daily activity for many people via social networking sites, online gaming, chat, commercial websites, and virtual worlds. Commonly, users interact with friends, company representatives, coworkers, opponents, and bots (i.e., preprogrammed computer applications that automatically perform tasks such as data gathering), which are often symbolized using a *virtual representation,* or digital image or figure. Those representations that closely resemble the human form are called *virtual humans.*

Virtual representations can be categorized as either *avatars* or *agents.* The word *avatar* is adapted from the Sanskrit for "descent," used to describe a Hindu god emerging from the heavens and bodily manifesting itself in order to intervene in human affairs (Bailenson & Blascovich, 2004). Generically, the term *avatar* can refer to any representation of a person. Names, online profiles, and playable video game characters can all be considered types of avatars by this broad definition (Bailenson, Yee, Blascovich, & Guadagno, 2008). Neal Stephenson (1992), in his science fiction novel *Snow Crash,* popularized the use of the word as it is commonly understood today to describe a digital representation in a virtual environment. Avatars are distinguished from *agents,* another form of digital representation, by the element of control. Avatars are controlled by human users, whereas agents are controlled by computer algorithms (Bailenson & Blascovich, 2004). For example, in single-player video games, the player at the controls is represented by an avatar, whereas the other characters on the screen are agents controlled by the computer.

Commonly, avatars are used to represent people in Internet chat (Kang & Yang, 2006), video games (Smith, 2006), social virtual worlds (Castronova, 2005), massively multiplayer online role-playing games (MMORPGs; Yee, 2006), social networking sites (Walther, Van Der Heide, Kim, Westerman, & Tong, 2008), and other mediated contexts. With such broad applications, avatars serve many purposes and are often multifunctional within a given context (Fox, Arena, & Bailenson, 2009).

One function of avatars is to help the user parallel the virtual world with the familiar physical world. For example, a user may have a photographic avatar attached to a chat interface to approximate a face-to-face interaction or use an avatar with a human form to navigate virtual space or engage virtual objects, agents, or other avatars. Avatars may also be used to facilitate communication. Whether through a simple smiley face icon or a highly realistic virtual human, avatars may help virtual communication more closely resemble the richness of face-to-face communication by allowing users to convey nonverbal as well as verbal messages. When selecting an avatar for a virtual world, users can often demonstrate group affiliation, social identity, interests, goals, or personality traits through their choice of representation and nonverbal cues. Additionally, avatars may be manipulated to express and convey emotions.

All of these traits indicate how users can adopt avatars to interact in virtual health contexts. Perhaps the most compelling reason to implement avatars, however, is their persuasive abilities. Virtual representations have been used to affect health monitoring (Skalski & Tamborini, 2007), helping behavior (Eastwick & Gardner, 2009), and brand preference (Ahn & Bailenson, 2011). As Bandura (1997) noted, persuasive messages from interpersonal sources can have a direct impact on self-efficacy; using avatars to convey these messages may maximize the impact of mediated messages because they evoke many of the same feelings as interpersonal interactions. A recent meta-analysis further determined that people were more influenced by representations they perceived to be human-controlled avatars than those they perceived to be computer-controlled agents (Fox et al., 2010). Thus, it is likely that in many health contexts, avatars will have a persuasive advantage over agents.

Advantages of Avatars for Health Communication

Given their vast and various purposes, avatars present many advantages to health communication. On a basic level, they provide a way for users to interact virtually with the potential to resolve many issues or inconveniences of remote communication. For example, communicating via phone, email, or text chat can strip out some nonverbal aspects. Although webcams can be useful, they are limited in that they can only portray a current physical state. Avatars can approximate face-to-face communication yet also give interactants the opportunity to project more information than just their current state. Using avatars, patients could graphically portray occurrences of a symptom to show its evolution over time to provide a doctor with more specific information. A doctor could map a patient's previous complaints onto the patient's avatar to get a holistic, head-to-toe view of medical issues. Having all of this information visible might facilitate diagnoses. This visibility might also be useful for doctors to explain the interrelatedness of a patient's complaints (e.g., how a person's weight is causing back and knee pain) and show how these conditions might change the entire body over time.

Avatars also present users the opportunity for an experience beyond mere exposure to mediated imagery. Users embody avatars, controlling the movements and interactions of the representation; thus, the avatar becomes a proxy for the physical self in the virtual world. As Biocca (1997) noted, during avatar embodiment "the mental model of the user's body (body schema or body image) may be influenced by the mapping of the physical body to the geometry and topology of the virtual body." Due to these processes, embodiment may create a realistic and particularly potent experience for the user, and health messages delivered in this setting may have a greater impact than other mediated messages.

Another advantage of avatars is the ability to customize them to tailor a message specifically for the user. Health scholars have long touted the advantages of tailoring messages to audiences (see chapter 8 of this volume); Bandura (2004) suggests that interactive tailoring is the greatest strength of new media. Developments in many virtual worlds have enabled advanced customization of avatars, including body type, age, and race or ethnicity as well as smaller details like hairstyle and eye color. Additionally, worlds could be designed to add medical conditions and symptoms that could be applied to an avatar. For example, a patient could demonstrate to a doctor exactly where and how quickly a rash spread leading up to the time the patient contacted the doctor. A doctor could then illustrate possible future symptoms or warning signs specifically on the patient's avatar so that the patient would know when he or she needed to contact the doctor. Rather than generic descriptions or illustrations from other cases that may or may not look like the patient's manifestation, avatars enable specific, personalized representations that can be customized to each patient's precise needs.

Customization presents two distinct advantages. First, customized avatars can be used for the transmission of specifically tailored messages. Typically, doctors only interact with patients face to face during office visits, limiting their opportunities to convey health-related information. If the patient rarely visits the doctor, the doctor may not have the opportunity to monitor recurring or imminent health issues. Imagine a virtual world in which users' avatars were customized to reflect their physical selves. Researchers or health care providers could monitor these avatars to target specific health messages to them. For example, aging avatars could be targeted for messages about osteoporosis or overweight avatars could be targeted for messages about diabetes or weight loss. Rather than merely sending a message about a health condition, the provider could demonstrate future consequences on the patient's avatar.

A second advantage of customization is that avatars have been shown to increase participants' *identification,* or feelings of being similar to another (Bandura, 1977, 2001). Users become more invested in their avatars and their virtual setting when users have a part in choosing and developing avatars (Lim & Reeves, 2009). Thus, participants might be more receptive to a computer-delivered health message conducted via an avatar rather than, for example, an email.

Virtual Representations of the Self

Another way to bolster identification with another is through apparent similarity (Bandura, 2001). For example, an adolescent girl is more likely to identify with another female in her age group than an adult man. Thus, identification may be greater when the model closely resembles the self.

Recent technological developments enable researchers to use photographs of an individual to create virtual representations that appear highly similar to the self (Bailenson, Blascovich, & Guadagno, 2008). Through the use of digital photographs and head-modeling software, an individual's visage may be replicated in the virtual world. Although this transference is not flawless, it creates relatively accurate models of the human form, and the striking similarity gives these virtual representations of the self (VRSs) great potential as stimuli in virtual realms. These VRSs can then be used as avatars that the user can control or as agents that are controlled by a computer.

The use of a VRS to deliver a health message has many advantages. First, the VRS is maximally similar to the self, so it is very likely that a user will identify with the representation. This similarity will be greater than what is typically accomplished with mediated health campaigns, which can often only match the target audience on a few demographic characteristics such as age or race (although see chapter 8 of this volume). Second, the VRS can be used to accurately portray past, current, and potential future health conditions. Rather than having to exert cognitive effort to imagine oneself in a specific state (and facing the likelihood that this image will not be accurate or comprehensive), a user can experience and observe conditions on his or her own virtual body. Third, traditional media are often limited to portraying only "before" and "after" scenarios, whereas the VRS can be used to depict incremental levels of change or alternate realities depending on what health choices are made. In sum, virtual representations of the self have unique affordances that may make them more potent and effective models than those used in traditional health behavior change efforts.

Target Populations

Because these emergent technologies are still being tested in the lab, many studies have targeted the accessible collegiate population. Although this population might be criticized for being a convenience sample, given college students' technological savvy and high media use, these users are an optimal target audience for such treatments. The college years are also a crucial time for health interventions because young adults are often making decisions without the direct influence of their parents for the first time. Living away from home means making one's own dietary choices and being able to engage more freely in behaviors such as smoking, alcohol and drug use, and sex. Being able to observe the immediate and future consequences of their decisions might help emerging adults make more healthful choices.

Developing interventions are also investigating the utility of these technologies with younger populations. Several health video games have been developed in which users have an avatar that faces various health obstacles, helping the user develop skills regarding the treatment of diabetes, leukemia, and other diseases (see Lieberman, this volume). Another current project by Mette Torp Høybye and her collaborators (2011) is exploring the utility of VRSs for use with young cancer patients. Høybye is exploring how patients may modify their VRSs to express their feelings or current health state at various stages of treatment. Additionally, these avatars may be used to interact with other patients, both local and remote, to seek social support from other children with similar conditions. Indeed, because of the interactivity of customizing an avatar, the potential for social interaction, as well as entertainment value, avatars have great potential for engaging youth and conveying health-related information in a socially oriented virtual setting.

Theories Applied to Avatars and VRSs

Because avatars and VRSs rest at the intersection between mediated messages and interpersonal communication, any number of theories may be applied to studying avatar-based communication. Given that avatars have frequently been used as models for health behavior change, social cognitive theory (SCT) is particularly relevant.

Originally known as social learning theory, SCT posits that humans can learn behaviors through the observation of models (Bandura, 1977, 2001). The subsequent imitation of these learned behaviors is contingent on four factors. *Vicarious reinforcement* suggests that individuals need not experience rewards or punishments themselves in order to learn behaviors; rather, they can observe and interpret the consequences experienced by a model and make inferences as to the likelihood of incurring those outcomes themselves. Observing this reinforcement helps the observer develop *outcome expectancies,* or beliefs in the likelihood of the behavior yielding particular outcomes. *Identification* refers to the extent to which an individual relates to a model and feels that he or she is similar to the model. Another essential component of SCT is *self-efficacy,* the individual's perceived ability to enact a behavior and attain anticipated outcomes. The belief that one is capable of fulfilling one's goals (i.e., successful imitation) is crucial in determining whether or not one will attempt to mimic the behavior. Two of these variables, vicarious reinforcement and identification, are particularly relevant to the development of avatars for use in health messages.

Vicarious reinforcement has been used to demonstrate the benefits and risks associated with health-related behaviors. For example, showing negative consequences in public health campaigns is expected to discourage observers from smoking or drug abuse by showing models punished with appalling physical symptoms or harmed social relationships (Witte & Allen, 2000). Users can be responsible for the health of their avatars and thus observe the rewards and punishments associated with their health-related decisions. Time progression can be used to speed up or slow down the depiction of these consequences so that users can best understand how the consequences develop. Showing rewards and punishments may be particularly potent on a VRS because users can directly observe the effects on their own bodies. Rather than seeing another person become out of shape, they can see the consequences of a sedentary lifestyle on themselves.

Identification refers to the extent to which an individual relates to a model and feels that he or she is similar to the model. Identification has been shown to increase the likelihood of performing learned behaviors (Bandura, 2001; Bandura & Huston, 1961). Observers must feel that the model is similar enough to them that they are able to experience the same outcomes. Similarity may be based on physical traits, personality variables, or shared beliefs and attitudes (Stotland, 1969). Indeed, the likelihood of learning increases when models are of the same sex (Andsager, Bemker, Choi, & Torwel, 2006), race (Ito, Kalyanaraman, Brown, & Miller, 2008), or skill level (Meichenbaum, 1971), as well as when models demonstrate similar opinions (Hilmert, Kulik, & Christenfeld, 2006) or previous behaviors (Andsager et al., 2006).

Avatars allow researchers to present their audience with a choice of representations. Ito et al. (2008) created an interactive CD-ROM that offered its female adolescent participants their choice of avatars to guide them through information about sexually transmitted infections; over 60% of participants chose avatars of the same race/ethnicity. It is likely the participants identified more highly with these guides. With some platforms and technologies (e.g., VRSs), avatars can be tailored very closely to the appearance of the user, which means users can create a representation that they will identify with to a great degree. Thus, following social cognitive theory, we would anticipate that greater identification with these avatar models would lead to a greater likelihood of imitating the avatar's behavior.

Current research is further investigating the depth of an individual's experience with his or her avatar. Avatars are often the method by which users can extend the self into a virtual environment. Users may be embodied in these avatars for days, weeks, or even years in digital environments. Thus, it is unsurprising that people report having strong feelings toward or experiences with their avatars (Lewis, Weber, & Bowman, 2008). Indeed, some studies have found a link between identification with violent game characters and aggression (Konijn, Bijvank, & Bushman, 2007) and identification with characters leading to stereotyping and hostility (Eastin, Appiah, & Cicchirllo, 2009).

Klimmt, Hefner, and Vorderer (2009) distinguish avatars (specifically those in video games) from other media characters because of the interactivity and control that the user has over an avatar that is not possible with a literary role or television character. Klimmt et al. (2009) argue that due to their interactivity and the user's control over the character, video games create a *monadic* relationship wherein "players do not perceive the game (main) character as a social entity distinct from themselves, but experience a merging of their own self and the game protagonist" (p. 354). They also argue that because of the active and responsive nature of this form of identification, it is most similar in concept to role playing. As research in this area continues, it is likely that further theoretical explanations for experiences with avatars will emerge.

Effects of VRSs

We have been examining the use of VRSs for health behavior change. (See Lieberman and Miller et al., this volume, for more on the role of video games and virtual agents, respectively.) One series of studies examined the effectiveness of VRSs in encouraging exercise behavior (Fox & Bailenson, 2009). These studies were conducted in an immersive virtual environment (IVE) in which participants' physical movements around the room were tracked and a virtual world was appropriately rendered in a lightweight helmet, or head-mounted display (HMD), that they wore (see Figure 6.1).

In the first study, participants were instructed that they would be participating in three phases in the virtual environment. In the first phase, they would be asked to exercise. In the second phase, they would be asked to remain inactive. The third phase was voluntary: participants could remain in the virtual environment or they could terminate the experiment. While inside the virtual environment, participants saw one of three treatments: an empty room, a VRS, or a vicariously reinforced VRS that lost weight as the user exercised or gained weight as the user remained inactive. Participants who saw their VRS rewarded and punished chose to stay in the virtual environment and continue exercising, while those who saw an unchanging VRS or an empty room did not exercise in the voluntary phase. Thus, it was determined that observing vicarious reinforcement of the virtual self avatar encouraged people to engage in voluntary exercise.

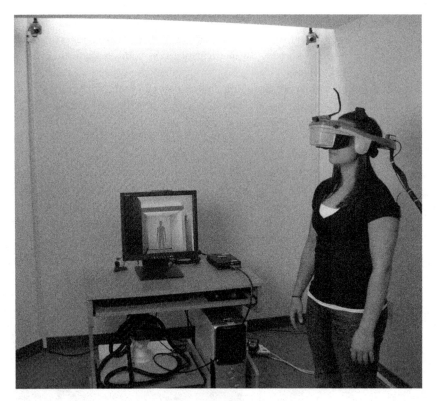

Figure 6.1 An immersive virtual environment (cameras at the corners of the room track the participant's movements to render the virtual environment appropriately in the head-mounted display she is wearing)

The second study aimed to determine whether it was the reward or punishment of their avatars that motivated participants to exercise. This time, the VRS was also contrasted with a same sex, similar age virtual representation of another, unknown person (VRO), yielding four conditions (self-reward, self-punishment, other reward, other punishment). The same three phases as the first experiment were used, except that only one consequence was illustrated (for example, in the reward conditions, participants only saw the avatar lose weight as they exercised, but when they were inactive, no weight gain was shown). The results indicated that it did not matter if the avatar experienced rewards or punishments—both were equally effective in motivating exercise—but the changes were much more effective when depicted on a virtual self. Participants in the Self conditions exercised significantly more than those in the Other conditions.

In a third study, we investigated whether the effects of a VRS would extend outside the laboratory and again compared virtual selves and others to test the role of identification. Participants observed one of three treatments: a VRS running on a treadmill, a VRS loitering, or a VRO running on a treadmill. During the five minutes of exposure, they were told the goal was to memorize numbers flashing on the avatar's chest. The next day, participants were contacted and their levels of activity in the 24 hours following the experiment were assessed. Participants who had seen the virtual self exercising reported over an hour more exercise than participants in the other two conditions. In sum, VRSs have been shown to be effective in persuading individuals to engage in exercise.

Another study we conducted examined the use of VRSs to influence dietary behaviors (Fox, Bailenson, & Binney, 2009). Participants were exposed to a VRS eating (see Figure 6.2). Afterward, they were told to respond to some questionnaire items and were seated at a computer with a bowl of chocolate candy nearby. For participants who experienced *presence* (i.e., they felt the environment was realistic and involving), social facilitation of eating behaviors occurred wherein men ate more and women ate less in the presence of another person (Harrison, Taylor, & Marske, 2006; Herman, Roth, & Polivy, 2003). That is, the same social eating patterns that are observed in the real world were replicated when participants

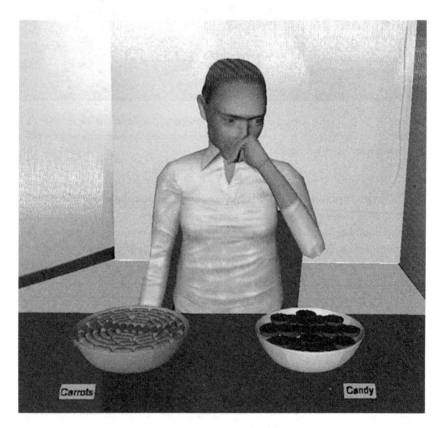

Figure 6.2 A virtual self demonstrates an eating behavior

encountered a virtual person: high-presence men ate more candy, whereas high-presence women suppressed their appetites. Future studies should investigate the use of dietary stimuli to help encourage healthful eating.

Another domain in which avatars have been useful is the examination of body disturbances and eating disorders. Researchers have been investigating the utility of avatars for helping women develop a more accurate and healthful perspective on their own bodies (Alcañiz et al., 2000; Gaggioli, Mantovani, Castelnuovo, Wiederhold, & Riva, 2003; Perpiña et al., 1999). A woman suffering from eating disorders and body dysmorphia might be embodied in an avatar to help her accept a healthy body shape. In the future, it may be possible to incorporate avatars as a form of treatment to help women develop a healthy self-image.

Dissemination Potential

Avatars are prevalent in video games, MMORPGs, online social worlds, and social networking sites. Future efforts may incorporate existing avatars in treatments and campaigns or create new platforms in which users may build an avatar for a specific health application.

Virtual interactions via avatars may be optimal for patients who feel uncomfortable explaining health conditions face to face or who wish to maintain anonymity. Doctors and patients could arrange virtual visits, using avatars to provide verbal and nonverbal feedback throughout the discussion. It may be difficult for a patient to indicate via email, text chat, or phone what "here" means when describing a pain, but an avatar would make it easier to portray that "*this* is what hurts." Patients who are embarrassed to discuss a sexually transmitted disease, for example, may feel more comfortable initially divulging this information to a provider virtually before making a face-to-face appointment. Patients might not feel comfortable discussing the number of sexual partners or particular sexual practices, but delivering this information via an avatar may be easier. Having a relatively anonymous environment at first may prevent them from shying away or being less forthright when seeking treatment in person.

Using photographs and high-end body mapping and modeling technologies, doctors could help patients create three-dimensional virtual models of themselves. Patients who cannot come into the office due to having a debilitating condition or living in a remote location could arrange for a virtual visit with the doctor. Patients could customize their avatars to reflect symptoms or incorporate webcam technologies to map their symptoms to their avatars. Doctors could then examine the avatar, consult the patient's charts and medical history, and come up with a tentative diagnosis. Although these interactions cannot completely replicate a face-to-face experience, they might be optimal for doctors working with familiar patients who have consistent, long-term health care needs.

Another area for dissemination is mobile technologies (see Abroms, Padmanabhan, & Evans, and Fjeldsoe, Miller, & Marshall, this volume). Extensive research has been conducted regarding the use of computer-generated, phone-delivered health interventions to promote healthful behaviors (e.g., Atienza, King, Oliveira, Ahn, & Gardner, 2008; King et al., 2007, 2008). Avatars could be incorporated into these mobile health messages to promote identification and more investment. For example, one could maintain a virtual representation of the self on a mobile phone and use it to give reminders to go to the gym or stick with a diet. Users could input their caloric intake or exercise exertion and watch their virtual selves slim or fatten in response, which may keep them continually motivated to make healthy decisions.

Limitations and Future Directions

Although at this stage the potential for avatars seems limitless, there are many qualifications to our current understanding. First, long-term studies are needed to see how people continue to interact with their avatars. It could be that people become less susceptible to avatar-mediated messages over time. Alternatively, it could be that more time spent with the avatar leads to greater investment and interest, and thus messages become more potent. Second, future research should be oriented toward older populations. New technologies tend to be explored with younger, presumably more technologically savvy populations, but computer literacy is increasing among seniors (Pew Internet & American Life Project, 2010), and they could benefit from avatar treatments as well. Third, more desktop and mobile platforms need to be explored. Second Life, for example, is a completely free, online avatar-based virtual world with millions of users that has been used for medical interventions. Practitioners have used online worlds to treat individuals suffering from social anxiety and agoraphobia, as well as to administer cue exposure therapy to people who suffer from various addictions (Gorini, Gaggioli, Vigna, & Riva, 2008).

Online avatar-based interactions have their drawbacks. First, a health care provider must rely on patients to depict themselves truthfully. Although this is an issue with any patient-provider interaction, an avatar is relatively easy to manipulate or idealize. Wireless biomonitors such as heart rate monitors, scales, or insulin devices that automatically convey information and integrate with the avatar interface may help minimize these issues. Second, privacy may be an issue. There is a risk with the transmission of any Internet data, and a detailed avatar has the potential to be a walking health record. Security and the anonymization of records and representations should be considered with any remote administration. Finally, it is important for researchers of new technologies such as avatars to examine the downside of encouraging people to spend more time in front of screens, which is presumably less time spent outdoors or engaging in vigorous activity.

Currently, the biggest disadvantage to this technology is affordability. The more realistic and immersive a virtual environment, the more expensive it tends to be. Custom creation of avatars requires skilled technicians spending significant time programming and artistically rendering each one. New advancements are making these avatars and their environments more accessible every day, however. Video games such as *Tony Hawk's Underground* enable participants to upload photos to create a highly similar avatar. Recently, Microsoft launched the Kinect, a new video gaming system for the X-Box 360 console that allows players to move in a natural fashion as a camera tracks their motions and renders the game accordingly. Microsoft also announced that it would release a kit for researchers and other interested parties to develop their own ideas, providing great potential for interactive, avatar-based health interventions. Still, these technologies, although widely available, cost hundreds of dollars, which may put them out of reach for many patients and individuals.

As we continue to spend more and more time in the presence of new media technologies, the opportunities for us to reach out and use them for health promotions grows. Avatars are one potent way for humans to bridge the physical and the virtual in health communication.

References

Ahn, S. J., & Bailenson, J. N. (2011). Self-endorsing versus other-endorsing in virtual environments: The effect on brand preference. *Journal of Advertising, 40*(2), 93–106.

Alcañiz, M., Perpiña, C., Baños, R. M., Lozano, J. A., Montesa, J., Botella, C., et al. (2000). A new realistic 3-D body representation in virtual environments for the treatment of disturbed body image in eating disorders. *CyberPsychology & Behavior, 3,* 433–439.

Andsager, J. L., Bemker, V., Choi, H-L., & Torwel, V. (2006). Perceived similarity of exemplar traits and behavior: Effects on message evaluation. *Communication Research, 33,* 3–18.

Atienza, A. A., King, A. C., Oliveira, B. M., Ahn, D. K., & Gardner, C. D. (2008). Using hand-held computer technologies to improve dietary intake. *American Journal of Preventive Medicine, 34,* 514–518.

Bailenson, J. N., & Blascovich, J. (2004). Avatars. In W. S. Bainbridge (Ed.), *Berkshire encyclopedia of human-computer interaction* (pp. 64–68). Great Barrington, MA: Berkshire Publishing Group.

Bailenson, J. N., Blascovich, J., & Guadagno, R. E. (2008). Self representations in immersive virtual environments. *Journal of Applied Social Psychology, 38,* 2673–2690.

Bailenson, J. N., Yee, N., Blascovich, J., & Guadagno, R. E. (2008). Transformed social interaction in mediated interpersonal communication. In E. A. Konijn, S. Utz, M. Tanis, & S. B. Barnes (Eds.), *Mediated interpersonal communication* (pp. 77–99). Mahwah, NJ: Lawrence Erlbaum Associates.

Bandura, A. (1977). *Social learning theory.* Englewood Cliffs, NJ: Prentice-Hall.

Bandura, A. (1997). *Self-efficacy: The exercise of control.* New York: Freeman.

Bandura, A. (2001). Social cognitive theory of mass communication. *Media Psychology, 3,* 265–299.

Bandura, A. (2004). Health promotion by social cognitive means. *Health Education & Behavior, 31,* 143–164.

Bandura, A., & Huston, A. C. (1961). Identification as a process of incidental learning. *Journal of Abnormal & Social Psychology, 63,* 311–318.

Biocca, F. (1997). The cyborg's dilemma: Progressive embodiment in virtual environments. *Journal of Computer-Mediated Communication, 3*(2). Retrieved May 25, 2011, from: http://jcmc.indiana.edu/vol3/issue2/biocca2.html.

Castronova, E. (2005). *Synthetic worlds: The business and culture of online games.* Chicago: University of Chicago Press.

Eastin, M. S., Appiah, O., & Cicchirllo, V. (2009). Identification and the influence of cultural stereotyping on postvideogame play hostility. *Human Communication Research, 35,* 337–356.

Eastwick, P. W., & Gardner, W. L. (2009). Is it a game? Evidence for social influence in the virtual world. *Social Influence, 4,* 18–32.

Fox, J., Ahn, S. J., Janssen, J., Yeykelis, L., Segovia, K. Y., & Bailenson, J. N. (2010, November). *A meta-analysis quantifying the effects of avatars and agents on social influence.* Paper presented at the 96th Annual Conference of the National Communication Association, San Francisco, CA.

Fox, J., Arena, D., & Bailenson, J. N. (2009). Virtual reality: A survival guide for the social scientist. *Journal of Media Psychology, 21,* 95–113.

Fox, J., & Bailenson, J. N. (2009). Virtual self-modeling: The effects of vicarious reinforcement and identification on exercise behaviors. *Media Psychology, 12,* 1–25.

Fox, J., Bailenson, J. N., & Binney, J. (2009). Virtual experiences, physical behaviors: The effect of presence on imitation of an eating avatar. *Presence: Teleoperators & Virtual Environments, 18,* 294–303.

Gaggioli, A., Mantovani, F., Castelnuovo, G., Wiederhold, B., & Riva, G. (2003). Avatars in clinical psychology: A framework for the clinical use of virtual humans. *CyberPsychology & Behavior, 6,* 117–125.

Gorini, A., Gaggioli, A., Vigna, C., & Riva, G. (2008). A second life for eHealth: Prospects for the use of 3-D virtual worlds in clinical psychology. *Journal of Medical Internet Research, 10,* e21.

Harrison, K., Taylor, L. D., & Marske, A. L. (2006). Women's and men's eating behavior following exposure to ideal-body images and text. *Communication Research, 33,* 507–529.

Herman, C. P., Roth, D. A., & Polivy, J. (2003). Effects of the presence of others on food intake: A normative interpretation. *Psychological Bulletin, 129,* 873–886.

Hilmert, C. J., Kulik, J. A., & Christenfeld, N. J. S. (2006). Positive and negative opinion modeling: The influence of another's similarity and dissimilarity. *Journal of Personality & Social Psychology, 90,* 440–452.

Høybye, M. T. (2011, May). *BE Community: Bridging social isolation for teenagers and young adults with cancer.* Paper presented at the 7th Annual Games for Health Conference, Boston, MA.

Ito, K. E., Kalyanaraman, S., Brown, J. D., & Miller, W. C. (2008). Factors affecting avatar use in a STI prevention CD-ROM. *Journal of Adolescent Health, 42,* S19.

Kang, H-S., & Yang, H-D. (2006). The visual characteristics of avatars in computer-mediated communication: Comparison of Internet Relay Chat and Instant Messenger as of 2003. *International Journal of Human-Computer Studies, 64,* 1173–1183.

King, A. C., Ahn, D. K., Oliveira, B. M., Atienza, A. A., Castro, C. M., & Gardner, C. D. (2008). Promoting physical activity through hand-held computer technology. *American Journal of Preventive Medicine, 34,* 138–142.

King, A. C., Friedman, R., Marcus, B., Castro, C., Napolitano, M., Ahn, D., et al. (2007). Ongoing physical activity advice by humans versus computers: The Community Health Advice by Telephone (CHAT) trial. *Health Psychology, 26,* 718–727.

Klimmt, C., Hefner, D., & Vorderer, P. (2009). The video game experience as "true" identification: A theory of enjoyable alterations of players' self-perception. *Communication Theory, 19,* 351–373.

Konijn, E. A., Bijvank, M. N., & Bushman, B. J. (2007). I wish I were a warrior: The role of wishful identification in the effects of violent video games on aggression in adolescent boys. *Developmental Psychology, 43,* 1038–1044.

Lewis, M. L., Weber, R., & Bowman, N. D. (2008). "They may be pixels, but they're MY pixels." Developing a metric of character attachment in role-playing video games. *CyberPsychology & Behavior, 11,* 515–518.

Lim, S., & Reeves, B. (2009). Computer agents versus avatars: Responses to interactive game characters controlled by a computer or other player. *International Journal of Human-Computer Studies, 68,* 57–68.

Meichenbaum, D. H. (1971). Examination of model characteristics in reducing avoidance behavior. *Journal of Personality & Social Psychology, 17,* 298–307.

Perpiña, C., Botella, C., Baños, R. M., Marco, H., Alcañiz, M., & Quero, S. (1999). Body image and virtual reality in eating disorders: Is exposure to virtual reality more effective than the classical body treatment? *CyberPsychology & Behavior, 2,* 149–155.

Pew Internet & American Life Project. (2010). *Generations 2010.* Washington, DC: Author.

Skalski, P., & Tamborini, R. (2007). The role of social presence in interactive agent-based persuasion. *Media Psychology, 10,* 385–413.

Smith, B. P. (2006). The (computer) games people play. In P. Vorderer & J. Bryant (Eds.), *Playing video games: Motives, responses, and consequences* (pp. 43–56). Mahwah, NJ: Lawrence Erlbaum Associates.

Stephenson, N. (1992). *Snow crash.* New York: Bantam Books.

Stotland, E. (1969). Exploratory investigations of empathy. In L. Berkowitz (Ed.), *Advances in experimental social psychology* (Vol. 4, pp. 274–314). New York: Academic Press.

Walther, J. B., Van Der Heide, B., Kim, S-Y., Westerman, D., & Tong, S. T. (2008). The role of friends' appearance and behavior on evaluations of individuals on Facebook: Are we known by the company we keep? *Human Communication Research, 34,* 28–49.

Witte, K., & Allen, M. (2000). A meta-analysis of fear appeals: Implications for effective public health campaigns. *Health Education & Behavior, 27,* 591–615.

Yee, N. (2006). The psychology of massively multi-user online role-playing games: Motivations, emotional investment, relationships and problematic usage. In R. Schroeder & A. S. Axelsson (Eds.), *Avatars at work and play: Collaboration and interaction in shared virtual environments* (pp. 187–207). New York: Springer.

7

DIGITAL GAMES FOR HEALTH BEHAVIOR CHANGE

Research, Design, and Future Directions

Debra A. Lieberman

Digital interactive games deliver powerful and engaging experiences that can motivate and support behavior change. When well designed, they can influence players' attitudes, emotions, self-concepts, self-confidence, social interactions, risk perceptions, knowledge, and development and rehearsal of skills, all of which can contribute to changes in behavior (see Ritterfeld, Cody, & Vorderer, 2009; Vorderer & Bryant, 2006).

This chapter discusses current trends in the research and design of digital games aimed at improving players' health behaviors and the delivery of health care. It includes examples of health games and related research findings and points to advances in technology and game design that show great promise for motivating health behavior change.

Health games can be especially effective when they are designed on the basis of well-established theory and research evidence and then rigorously researched and tested with the target population to improve game design during the early stages of development. After development is done, health games can be evaluated in laboratory and field studies to identify players' processes of behavior change and the health outcomes they experience as a result over the short and long term. Research can lead to the design of more engaging and impactful games that use story lines, game challenges, and game dynamics to motivate behavior change related to specific health topics and to serve targeted groups most effectively.

What Is a Digital Game?

Fundamentally, a game is a rule-based activity that involves challenge to reach a goal and that provides feedback on progress made toward that goal. These three essential components of games—rules, goals, and feedback—are found in a wide range of digital games, from massively multiplayer online role-playing games

(MMORPGs) that involve hundreds of thousands of players participating in an almost limitless number of cooperative and competitive activities over extensive periods of time, to the simplest casual quiz or puzzle game that may take a moment for one person to play. Well-designed games are experiential and compelling. They are goal-driven, challenging, and immersive, and they often involve the player in dramatic narratives and interactions. All of these features can be designed to enhance the attitude change, emotions, self-concepts, learning, and skill development known to improve prevention behaviors, self-care, and delivery of care.

Digital games use interactive technology to support game play in at least one of two ways. First, a game can be technology-*based:* the game is in the technology. The player interacts with the technology, which displays, enacts, or in some other way transmits the results of the player's actions. One example is screen-based games delivered via console, computer, or mobile phone. The player may use various input devices to interact with the game, and the game software could be delivered via a network such as the Internet or reside locally on the player's game device, but in all cases the screen displays the game. Other types of displays are possible, too. A technology-based game could be displayed and transmitted to the player, for example, with the sounds and motions of a robot or with the signals emitted from a toy, medical device, or weight machine in a gym. In technology-based games the player interacts directly with the technology, no matter how the technology displays or delivers the game.

Second, a game can be technology-*supported:* the technology is in the game. In this case technology supports a player who is engaged in activities in the physical world. For example, a geolocation game such as Geocaching involves the player in a quest to arrive at a certain geographic destination and provides clues to help the player figure out where it is located or how to get there; other games involve collecting digital items that can only be obtained by physically going to the location to "get" them so that they will appear on the screen. The mobile phone or other portable device displays the clues, and its GPS system provides feedback about the player's location relative to the target location. However, the player is hiking around in the physical world and looking for the places and the physical or virtual objects mentioned in the clues. The player relies on the digital technology for information and real-time feedback needed to play the game, but the game play itself is located in the physical world and is analog, not digital. Other types of technology-supported games include alternate reality games (ARGs) that add game goals and fictional stories to the player's daily life and, when the goal is health promotion, integrate health-related challenges into the game play and story line; health tracking games that use accelerometers and other sensor-based devices to monitor the player's physical states and daily activities (exercise, calories burned, nutrition, stress, sleep, etc.), and then deliver tools and feedback to help the player monitor and understand his or her progress (for more about personal data tracking and the Quantified Self movement, see Institute for the Future, 2009); and games that use techniques of "gamification" to integrate game dynamics such as incentives, rewards, and social recognition and support into tasks of daily life to increase engagement and participation, as used in customer loyalty reward programs and, for health, in wellness programs for employees or health plan members.

Some games are a combination of technology-based and technology-supported, such as technology-based games that involve teamwork and communication (face to face or online) so that the player is interacting directly with the technology in order to play the game, but there is also game play taking place interpersonally as players strategize together or coach each other. A technology-supported game may also include access to online technology-based mini-games played to reinforce key concepts or specific behaviors that the player is tracking in the physical world.

Game challenges often involve competition between individuals or teams, which can be very motivating, but there are also many other ways to challenge and engage the player. Working alone or in collaboration with others, players could be required to solve a mystery, make a decision that leads to desired outcomes, or use a skill or strategy that must be perfected to achieve the game goal, to name a few examples. In so doing they could be challenged to use creativity, knowledge, logic, memory, cooperation, social skills, persuasive skills, visual or auditory acuity, eye-hand coordination, balance, physical strength, and/or physical endurance. Some games use sensors and challenge players to control their stress level in order to progress in the game, control their brain waves with biofeedback, or move their arms and legs a certain way when using a camera-based movement sensing interface with game technologies such as the Kinect.

Most players of a well-designed game will be intensely motivated to win it (Brown et al., 1997; Vorderer & Bryant, 2006). They will learn and rehearse anything the game demands of them, if they are capable enough to do so, because it will help them win. Games designed so that players avidly learn and rehearse specific content and skills in order to win the game are potentially highly impactful because players gain new levels of experience, insight, and capability.

A variety of technology platforms can deliver interactive digital games, and now games reach almost every demographic group in the United States. Games are available on computers, video game consoles, handheld game devices, mobile phones, arcade machines, electronic toys (such as toy robots, dolls, and other digital devices with sounds, displays, and/or actions that deliver interactive games), electronic learning systems (such as LeapFrog and VTech), and gym equipment (such as stationary bikes with video screens and sport walls that sense when and where they are hit by a ball and provide feedback on the player's success in a variety of sport game challenges).

Sensors (such as video and still cameras, GPS, physiological monitoring devices, accelerometers, software that detects emotional state based on facial movements, and many others) are components of games in which the game state is determined not only by the player's choices and actions but also by the player's context and physical state. A context-aware game uses sensor readings about the player, and these readings come from sources including the environment (location of the player and locations of items in the environment that may contain radio frequency identification [RFID] tags or other forms of transmission to indicate their position and send other signals and data); the player's physical activity (movement of the body, such as reaching or tossing, or movement from one geographical location to another); the player's physiological state (brain waves, stress level, breathing rate, blood oxygen level, heart rate, galvanic skin response, emotional expressions); and other people (their comments about the player and their votes, recommendations, interpretations, and descriptions).

Health Games

The features of digital games discussed above, including technology-based and technology-supported games, social aspects of playing, game challenges, player motivations, platform capabilities, and sensor inputs, are some of the building blocks that game designers use to create compelling game play experiences. These features can be used effectively in health games, which are digital games intended to improve players' health or the delivery of health care. There are thousands of health games available today and the number is growing (find health games and related resources, organizations, and research publications in the Health Games Research online searchable database at http://www.healthgamesresearch.org/database).

A health game could be designed especially for health or it could be an entertainment game that is later repurposed for health. Two examples of games designed for health, and evaluated in clinical trials that found significant improvements, are the cancer education game *Re-Mission,* aimed at increasing cancer patients' adherence to their cancer-related treatment plan (Kato, Cole, Bradlyn, & Pollock, 2008), and the school-based game *Squire's Quest,* intended to instill new attitudes and skills so that elementary school students will increase their daily servings of fruit and vegetables (Baranowski et al., 2003). These games, in addition to being entertaining and engaging, used theory- and research-based behavioral health strategies to improve players' health behaviors and were evaluated in well-designed clinical trials.

Health games made for the delivery of health care have been used by clinicians to diagnose and treat patients' medical and neurological conditions, such as attention deficit disorder (Pope & Bogart, 1996), autism (Griffiths, 2003), mental health problems (Griffiths; Wilkinson, Ang, & Goh, 2008), and deficiencies in the strength, coordination, and balance of people needing physical therapy and rehabilitation (Fritz, Rivers, Merlo, & Duncan, 2009).

Social networks and virtual worlds have presented health games in innovative ways. For instance, in the virtual world Whyville, with content provided by the Centers for Disease Control and Prevention (CDC), children have learned how epidemics can spread and how to respond to them by seeing their own or others' avatar characters catch the "whypox," discovering how to prevent catching the disease or avoid transmitting it, and learning where to receive proper care

(Kafai, Quintero, & Feldon, 2010). Also, in medical training games available in virtual worlds such as Second Life, clinicians have learned how to administer treatments for a wide range of medical problems (Hansen, 2008) and have learned how to deliver emergency care (Barrera, 2008). Crowdsourcing, also called community-based design or participatory design, has been used in social games to gather ideas from the general public to discover new ways to address health problems. Two examples are the game *FoldIt*, in which scientists invite players to come up with original ways to fold proteins so that this information can be used to combat diseases such as cancer and HIV/AIDS, and the game *Breakthroughs to Cures*, in which players imagine and share new ways to accelerate medical research, knowing that scientists are interested and could potentially implement the best ideas that emerge from the game.

Games such as *Dance Dance Revolution* and *Wii Sports* are popular entertainment games that have been repurposed by players, families, schools, community organizations, and clinics to engage people in activities that improve weight management, physical activity, and physical therapy. The health benefits of these repurposed entertainment games have been documented in a growing number of studies (Biddis & Irwin, 2010; Lieberman et al., 2011; Murphy et al., 2009). Car chase games like *Crazy Taxi* have been repurposed to help older adults improve their ability to focus attention and avoid distraction (Belchior, Marsiske, & Mann, 2010). Entertainment games involving car driving have also been used to help therapy patients overcome their fear of driving (Walshe, Lewis, Kim, O'Sullivan, & Wiederhold, 2003).

Health games and entertainment games repurposed for health are available not only on well-known game technologies such as consoles, computers, and hand-held game systems but also on some unexpected technologies including medical devices such as inhalers and spirometers (Bingham, Bates, Thompson-Figueroa, & Lahiri, 2010) and blood glucose meters (e.g., digital meter from Bayer, available at http://www.bayerdidget.co.uk/Home); robots (Fasola & Mataric, 2010); and print and electronic media that deliver game challenges and plot twists in alternate reality games that immerse players in a fictional story that takes place in their everyday surroundings (Johnston, Sheldon, & Massey, 2010). A new smoking cessation game, *Lit to Quit*, is a breath-driven game that smokers play by blowing into the microphone of a mobile phone to move objects around the screen, in either "rush" mode using frequent bursts of breath or "relaxation" mode using slow sustained breaths. The game is designed to help reduce cigarette cravings as players experience the rush and relaxation of the two modes of breathing (Mezei et al., 2010).

Advantages of Games in Health Communication

Games are a popular leisure activity and people in almost every demographic group play digital games enthusiastically and often. Increasingly, even those who do not play digital games during leisure time play health games when teachers, health educators, or physical therapists assign a game as part of an educational or therapeutic program (Murphy et al., 2009; Papastergiou, 2009). But for most people in the United States, digital games have the appeal, availability, and "cool" factor that combine to make them a favorite voluntary pastime and, therefore, a natural way to deliver health messages and health experiences—in the digital worlds where people already live.

Games can reach people in at-risk populations who are unlikely to seek information or help from professional caregivers. For people who obtain health information and care from other sources, digital games can supplement these forms of education and intervention because they can be played during leisure time.

Playing and talking about games can be a springboard for discussion about health concerns, and some games intentionally use collaborative game play and teamwork to foster discussion and social support (e.g., Brown et al., 1997). It is well established that social support is strongly associated with better prevention behaviors, treatment adherence, and health outcomes (Lieberman, 1997; Peterson & Stunkard, 1989). The diabetes self-management game *Packy & Marlon,* a side-scrolling Super Nintendo adventure game that challenges players to keep their character's blood glucose in the normal range through blood glucose testing, nutrition, and insulin—so that the character will be strong enough to achieve other game challenges—uses collaborative play to increase players' discussion, learning, and social support (Brown et al., 1997; Lieberman, 2001).

Digital games can change players' self-concepts, another factor that influences health behaviors. One of the aims of the diabetes game *Packy & Marlon* is to reduce the perceived stigma of having diabetes by providing a way for diabetic players to share and discuss with their friends a game that they are proud to say is about their own medical condition. The game succeeds at reducing stigma because it enables a diabetic young person to broach the topic of diabetes with friends and to discover that friends do not think worse of them for having diabetes. Furthermore, friends often admire their diabetic friend for being able to play the game so expertly, especially an appealing and challenging game that is well produced and clearly targeted to smart, creative, game-savvy young people. *Packy & Marlon* looks like any other Super Nintendo game of its mid-1990s era because it includes characters that are full of personality; a compelling story line; a variety of game challenges in 24 game levels that take place in the playing fields, lakes, mountains, and haunted cabins at a diabetes summer camp; plenty of player control over the character's actions, movements, and choices as Packy or Marlon makes his way forward in the game environment; sophisticated forms of performance feedback including displays of food exchanges each character has eaten in various food groups and a cumulative log of the character's blood glucose readings; new artwork and game play dynamics in each game level; and its own unique sound effects and original music sound track.

In an NIH-funded clinical trial, 59 young people with type 1 diabetes, ages 8 to 16, who were outpatients at Stanford Medical Center and a Kaiser Permanente clinic in San Jose, California were randomized to receive the *Packy & Marlon* game (treatment group) or an entertainment game with no health content (control group) to play at home as little or as much as they wished, as long as they followed their parents' rules about when and for how long they were allowed to play video games. After six months, those in the treatment group, but not in the control group, significantly increased their discussions with parents about diabetes and improved their daily diabetes self-care behaviors. The clinical trial also found that the treatment group experienced a 77% drop in diabetes-related emergency and urgent care visits, moving from 2.5 visits per person per year at the start of the clinical trial down to 0.5 visits per person per year six months later, whereas the control group remained at 2.5 visits per person per year when the trial was completed (Brown et al., 1997; Lieberman, 2001).

Social interactions and networking are used to promote health in a growing number of healthy lifestyle support games on Internet-connected mobile phones (see Abroms, Padmanabhan, & Evans, this volume; Pollock et al., 2010). These games help people track and share their own data and then use the data for self-reflection, course correction, and coaching of friends (Institute for the Future, 2009). The games make healthy behaviors and better health outcomes the focus and purpose of the game challenge. Social connections are an essential component; friends and family members are enlisted to provide encouragement and support, and they have access to the player's tracked data and health outcomes so they can provide motivation and acknowledgment. The games enable players to monitor their physical activity and food intake, calculate calories consumed and expended, and track other lifestyle habits and physiological measures such as stress, sleep, blood pressure, and heart rate. Since the games are on a network, it is easy to share the data with friends and family and with one's doctors and clinical case managers.

Digital games can address a wide variety of health issues and have been used to motivate and support players' healthy lifestyle habits, prevention behaviors, self-care, diagnosis and treatment, adherence to treatment plans, and chronic disease self-management. They have focused on safe sex, HIV prevention, smoking prevention, smoking cessation, alcohol and drug prevention and relapse prevention, weight management, nutrition, exercise, asthma, stress management, diabetes, cystic fibrosis, heart disease, cognitive and problem-solving skills, cancer, stroke rehabilitation, and much more (see Biddis & Irwin, 2010; Hansen, 2008; Lieberman, 1997, 1999, 2009; Lieberman et al., 2011; Papastergiou, 2009). Games have also been used to train clinicians and to help them diagnose and treat patients (e.g., Dev, Heinrichs, & Youngblood, 2011; Pope & Bogart, 1996). Furthermore, at the institutional level, games have helped hospitals, first responders, and the military rehearse how they would handle many types of epidemics and disasters, working in realistic game-based scenarios that are constrained by the actual resources available and the nature of the crisis (e.g., Barrera, 2008). Simulations like these that provide scenario-based learning allow caregivers to rehearse situations that have not yet happened and to try and fail repeatedly in a safe environment that lets them learn by doing and see the positive and negative consequences of their decisions (see Miller et al., this volume).

In addition to their many advantages as dynamic environments for learning and behavior change, digital games have limitations that health communicators should keep in mind. While games do reach all demographic groups, there is still a digital divide in game genre preferences by age and gender, and as a result some groups may be underserved in the health games field. Careful targeting of game genres, story lines, characters, entertainment and health content, technologies, and skill levels can attract the groups that are generally less likely to play digital games yet, in the case of health games, would benefit from playing them. There are many instances where underserved groups have embraced health games that matched their personal interests, needs, and abilities. For example, note the popularity of *Wii Sports* games among seniors, who enjoy this system's intuitive interface and easy-to-learn games, while other game interfaces and genres are not as appealing for the seniors who have problems with vision and manual dexterity.

Another serious issue is the overuse of digital media, for some people, to the point where it displaces and interferes with the time that should be spent in other activities related to work, family, community, and a healthy lifestyle. Also, media users should understand how the media they use could affect and influence them in desirable or undesirable ways. As digital technology becomes ubiquitous in many people's daily lives, with games and other media content always readily available, it is especially important that all people become media literate and able to use media wisely and prudently, with keener awareness of its potential benefits and drawbacks in society and in their own lives.

Reaching Specific Target Populations

Health games targeted to specific populations can focus on serving their unique sets of needs and interests and can offer the game challenges and rewards that are most likely to engage them to increase the chance that the game will improve their health. To learn more about the target population, health game designers can conduct formative research such as focus groups, individual interviews, play testing, and user testing early in the design process (Isbister & Schaffer, 2008). Formative research helps the designers gain deeper insight into the capabilities, interests, and beliefs of the target population; their level of health literacy and their skills related to health behaviors, technology, and games; the perceived and actual obstacles that prevent them from carrying out good health behaviors; how they like to spend their time; the game technologies and genres they like to play; and what is most gratifying to them about playing digital games. Formative research is also useful to find out whether target population members tend to play with others or alone, with whom they play, and what kinds of social interactions result. Answers to these questions will enable game designers to optimize the appeal and effectiveness of the health game for the targeted group. An ongoing cycle of iterative game testing and design can further fine-tune the game and help assure it will be impactful and beneficial.

When a game is completely developed, summative research, also called outcome research or evaluation research, can test whether the game significantly changed target group members' health behaviors and health status, how that group in particular responded to the game play experience, and how those responses contributed to improved health-related knowledge, skills, attitudes, social interactions, behaviors, and outcomes. For games that health care providers will use to diagnose or treat patients, summative research can also investigate whether and how the game helped improve the delivery of care.

Contexts: Where Games Are Played and Why That Matters

The context of game play is important to consider because it can drive developers' decisions about the content and format of a game and how it should be implemented. In informal settings during leisure time, a game competes with all other available activities, including other games, so it must be appealing and engaging in order to be played. No matter how well the game is designed as a health behavior change intervention, the game will have no impact if people do not play it. On the other hand, in formal settings such as school classrooms, worksite wellness meetings, and clinic-based health education classes, games are an assigned activity so they do not need to compete with other leisure-time entertainment options, and instead there is more pressure for these games to be demonstrably effective in achieving health behavior change or in improving the delivery of care. In informal settings, games must be highly appealing or people will not play them, and in formal settings games must be highly effective or teachers will not assign them. Ideally, all health games must be as entertaining, engaging, challenging, and effective as possible regardless of context, but if resources are limited, then there is a natural tendency for producers to cut corners where the least harm will be done.

Location can determine the context of a game. While mobile phones now bring health games and apps to any location (see Abroms, Padmanabhan, & Evans and Fjeldsoe, Miller, & Marshall, this volume), more stationary or nonportable systems exist in new contexts for playing health games in locations such as gyms and health clubs, hotels and cruise ships, schools, after-school programs, clinic waiting rooms, hospital rooms and hospital lounges, museums, zoos, libraries, shopping malls, amusement parks, and other public places. Each of these contexts offers unique challenges and opportunities to health game designers. In addition to the context of location or institution, the social environment is a context to consider in the design of a health game. For example, a game designed for the family to play together should not look and feel the same as a game made for adolescents to play with their peers.

Integrating Behavioral Health Theories into the Design of Digital Games

Many health games aimed at motivating and supporting learning, skill development, or behavior change are not designed on the basis of well-established theory or research, and so they do not take advantage of the rich body of well-tested message design strategies known to work. Among the few health games that are theory-based, it is rare to see published studies that demonstrate their effectiveness and even rarer to see tests of how and why they were effective with the target population. There are innumerable theories and models that could inform, and in some cases are beginning to inform, the research and design of health games in areas such as social comparison, social networking, risk perception, motivation, persuasion, message tailoring, message framing, health beliefs, stages of health behavior change, and much more. Following are just a few examples out of the large number of theories and models that game developers and researchers could use from the fields of communication, psychology, health promotion, education, and human-computer interaction to design effective digital interactive health games.

Social cognitive theory provides a strong foundation for the design of game-delivered behavioral health interventions, with its emphasis on role modeling, vicarious experience, and self-efficacy, all of which can be used to improve learning and behavior change (Bandura, 1986, 1997). People often learn, change their attitudes, and develop skills simply by observing others in action, and this includes observing characters in media and games. Observational learning, in real life or via media, is especially impactful when observers see appealing role model characters demonstrating appropriate behaviors and experiencing personal rewards for engaging in those behaviors. They also learn what not to do when they see role model characters engaging in inappropriate behaviors and suffering negative consequences as a result. A third way to use role models is to portray transitional characters who begin by engaging in inappropriate behaviors and suffering negative consequences, and who later change their attitudes, go through a process of behavior change, and begin to experience rewards, such as having better health, income, quality of life, or social relationships (Singhal & Rogers, 2001).

Digital games are experiential, with many offering opportunities for players to interact with other characters and to take care of their own character, and then to see the immediate consequences. Games provide a form of hands-on experience that combines vicarious observation with realistic direct interaction, two fundamental elements of social cognitive theory. In addition to learning by observing role model characters vicariously, players develop skills in games by interacting directly with characters and events, rehearsing and applying skills, and receiving immediate useful feedback.

Game experiences can also increase players' self-efficacy, which is their level of self-confidence that they are capable of carrying out a particular behavior or task in their own life (Bandura, 1997; Brown et al., 1997; Kato et al., 2008). Behavior change is more likely to occur when self-efficacy for carrying out the behavior has increased. In other words, people must feel confident that they can carry out a behavior or task successfully before they are likely to give it a try.

Another useful tool for the design of health games is the extended parallel process model (Witte, Meyer, & Martell, 2001), which focuses on messages that convey health risks. The model shows that the likelihood of health behavior change increases when individuals realize that they are susceptible to a health problem and that the problem is potentially severe, and they will be more likely to take action against the threat if they also have a strong sense of efficacy for dealing with it effectively. There are two types of efficacy in the model: self-efficacy involves one's level of self-confidence to carry out the health behavior successfully, and response efficacy involves the strength of one's belief that the health behavior itself will be effective enough to reduce the threat. For example, the model would predict that people will become more physically active (behavior change) if they believe that inactivity would harm their own cardiovascular health (susceptibility), the harm would be seriously debilitating or would significantly shorten their life span (severity), they are capable of increasing their physical activity (self-efficacy), and if they did increase their physical activity their cardiovascular health would indeed improve (response efficacy). Health games can be designed to help players improve any of these four factors that are known to motivate behavior change. Studies are now under way, funded by HopeLab (2011), to explore how health games can be designed to strengthen perceptions of susceptibility, severity, self-efficacy, and response efficacy, and thereby influence health behavior change.

Another approach that is well grounded in theory and research is constructivist learning, a pedagogical method that situates learning in an experiential and applied environment, where learners take an active role and personally construct their own knowledge in authentic situations that allow them to build on what they already know (Honebein, Duffy, & Fishman, 1993; Prawat & Flowden, 1994). By building on students' prior knowledge in constructivist learning environments and giving them choice and autonomy, this instructional strategy makes learning more relevant and engaging. Health games can deliver and support constructivist learning by providing compelling challenges that require the player to learn new content, engage in higher-order thinking and problem solving, make decisions, interact with others collaboratively and in leadership roles, and try out new experiences that would be difficult or impossible in the physical world. Constructivist games could be technology-based, where the player interacts entirely with digital screen displays or with robots or toys or other devices, or the games could be technology-supported, where the player is engaged in activities in the physical world and interacts with other people to play the game, while using the technology for computation, measurement, information seeking, communication with distant teammates, recording, sensing, feedback, coaching, co-learning, or many other functions.

Immersiveness and perceived reality are also characteristics of digital interactive games that help make them effective environments for learning and behavior change. Games, like many other media formats, elicit feelings of presence—that is, of really being there (Lee, 2004; Lombard & Ditton, 1997). This authentic mediated experience can elicit the same kinds of arousal, physiological responses, and empathy that real experiences do (Picard, 1997; Reeves & Nass, 1996), and the extent to which a health game delivers immersive and realistic experiences can influence depth of attention, involvement, learning, and behavior change.

Immersion and perceived reality can influence learning and behavior change when a player controls the actions of their own character, or avatar, which is the player's representation of self within a digital virtual environment or game. Research is discovering how avatars affect game player behavior, not only within the game but also in the player's real life (see Fox, this volume). For example, when players are represented by attractive avatars or tall avatars, their perceptions of their own attractiveness, power, or leadership qualities carry over from the virtual world of the game into their real life and there are marked changes in their interpersonal interactions, almost as if they really had the characteristics of their avatar (Yee, Bailenson, & Ducheneaut, 2009).

Processes and Effects of Health Games

There is a growing body of research on the way people process health games and on the health behaviors and outcomes that emerge as a result. Following are a few areas that have been researched.

Studies have been done on the uses, gratifications, and effects of active games that use interfaces involving dance pads, balance boards, gym and sports equipment, and sensors such as accelerometers, GPS, physiological monitors, and cameras. In general, research finds that active games motivate physical activity and increase energy expenditure beyond the energy expended during sedentary activity (Biddis & Irwin, 2010; Papastergiou, 2009). Games that require players to move their bodies vigorously as the interface to the game, such as *Dance Dance Revolution* and certain games on the Wii console and the Wii Fit balance board, require enough exertion so that players experience a moderate to vigorous cardiovascular workout (Graf, Pratt, Hester, & Short, 2009; Leatherdale, Woodruff, & Manske, 2010; Unnithan, Houser, & Fernhall, 2005). In some cases, these games can also improve players' arterial and coronary functioning and weight management (Carson, Murphy, Vosloo, Donley, & Richison, 2006; Murphy et al., 2009). Studies of active games have found mental health benefits, as well. For example, older adults experienced reductions in their subsyndromal depression after participating regularly in exergaming, and they improved their depressive symptoms, mental health-related quality of life (QoL), and cognitive performance (Rosenberg et al., 2010).

In addition to active games, digital games in many genres delivered on a variety of video game technologies have improved players' health behaviors and outcomes. For example, digital games on consoles, computers, and the Internet have increased players' self-efficacy for safer sex negotiation (Thomas, Cahill, & Santilli, 1997), strengthened preadolescents' antismoking attitudes and intentions not to smoke (Tingen, Grimling, Bennett, Gibson, & Renew, 1997), improved children's nutrition habits (Baranowski et al., 2003), reduced phobic patients' fear of driving (Walshe et al., 2003), reduced children's and teens' asthma-related emergencies and reduced their missed school days and parents' missed work days due to their child's asthma (Lieberman, 2001), and improved cancer patients' adherence to their treatment plan (Kato et al., 2008).

These studies found that the games influenced mediating factors, such as self-concepts, self-efficacy, empathy, skill development, and communication and social support, which in turn influenced health behaviors. The games were tested in outcome studies to measure and discover the contributing effects of the mediating factors, many of which were carefully planned and designed into each health game. This approach to game design and outcome testing is costly and requires a team of experts in behavioral health, the health topic, the target population, game design, and games research, yet it is an effective way to design and evaluate health games that aim to change health behavior or the delivery of care. More games are needed that bring together (1) game design principles based on prior theory and research, (2) the expertise of a multidisciplinary design team, and (3) well-designed clinical trials and outcome studies. This approach not only will improve the design and effectiveness of the game being developed by the team but also will generate research findings on processes and effects of health games that will improve future game designs.

Dissemination of Health Games

With the Wii Fit, the Xbox Kinect camera-based game platform, dance pad games, and brain training games leading the way as successes in the marketplace, investors and game developers are beginning to see a market for health games. New start-up companies are being formed, especially for mobile phone health games, social network games, crowd sourced games that bring people together online to engage in mass collaboration and discussion to solve local and global health problems, and incentivized support and reward programs in an approach called the "gamification" of health. Health games for other platforms and contexts are also on the verge of explosive growth.

More funding is needed to support the research and dissemination of health games in areas that may not have a large market but can potentially make important contributions to improving health and health care. In one notable exception, the Robert Wood Johnson Foundation's Pioneer Portfolio has recognized the value and potential of health games, and in 2007 the foundation began to fund research and dissemination through a new national program called Health Games Research, headquartered at the University of California, Santa Barbara (see http://www.

healthgamesresearch.org). Since then, the national program has funded 21 research projects across the nation and has provided scientific leadership to the field. The 21 grantee projects are investigating processes and effects of a wide range of health games played on a variety of game platforms, and Health Games Research gives these grantees technical assistance as they conduct their research and help with promotion and dissemination of their findings.

The projects are focusing on games that motivate and support physical activity and/or self-care. The physical activity games they are studying support rehabilitation for stroke patients, cybercycling for older adults, exercising for older adults who play a game with a "robot motivator," school-based physical activity for teens, and physical activity for overweight youth and their families. The projects investigating self-care games are conducting studies of games for smoking cessation, diabetes-related nutrition, cystic fibrosis self-management, relapse prevention for recovered alcoholics, social skills for children with autism, rehabilitation for people with Parkinson's disease, and improvement of healthy lifestyle habits for people of all ages.

Health Games Research works with health care professionals, game developers, researchers, federal agencies, and the press to get the word out about high-quality health games and the research evidence that demonstrates their design strategies and effectiveness. By focusing its research funding on the mediating factors that lead to effective processing of game play experiences, Health Games Research aims to develop a robust set of well-tested principles of health game design that can guide the design of health games in the future. There is a great deal to be learned about what works, and for whom, with health games. To support this work in addition to funding and assisting grantees, Health Games Research conducts research, develops resources to help people create health games, and provides an online searchable database containing links to health games, research publications, organizations, and resources in the field (http://www.healthgamesresearch.org/database).

Looking toward the Future

Digital games are rich with potential as environments for health-related learning, skill development, and behavior change. They are interactive, engaging, social, and immersive, and when designed by experts in the art and science of game design, they can be very motivating and effective.

To improve our ability to create impactful health games, the field needs more research and funding. Some newcomers to the field are developing games that are neither engaging as entertainment nor effective as health interventions, and so a new norm is needed in which it is understood that health games should be theory- and evidence-based in their design and well researched both during and after game design and development. Also, the decision makers who fund, recommend, purchase, or implement health games must embrace this norm so that they will make good choices and hold the game publishers to a high standard. While more studies are examining the processing of games, the mediating factors that lead to this processing, and how and why certain games are effective for certain target populations, much more work is needed, especially as new technologies, genres, players, and health topics are emerging.

New research tools and methods are addressing new questions about game environments and their effects on health behavior change. Now researchers can gather survey responses from players online around the world and can collect in-game data about game play usage and progress, as well as any sensor data used in the game. Social interactions online can also be captured and analyzed to assess the amount of contact between group members and the purposes of the contacts.

The health games field can make important contributions to health education, health promotion, clinical diagnosis and treatment, and clinical training, but first game development projects must recruit the expert teams that can make compelling and effective health games and can use state-of-the-art research methods to understand how and why people respond to games with passion, empathy, motivation, engagement, and enjoyment. Equipped with this knowledge, health game design teams can make more effective games in the future and integrate them optimally into other forms of health promotion and clinical care.

Acknowledgment

Preparation of this chapter was supported by a grant from the Pioneer Portfolio of the Robert Wood Johnson Foundation.

References

Bandura, A. (1986). *Social foundations for thought and action: A social cognitive theory.* Englewood Cliffs, NJ: Prentice Hall.

Bandura, A. (1997). *Self-efficacy: The exercise of control.* New York: W. H. Freeman.

Baranowski, T., Baranowski, J., Cullen, K. W., Marsh, T., Islam, N., Zakeri, I., et al. (2003). *Squire's Quest!* Dietary outcome evaluation of a multimedia game. *American Journal of Preventive Medicine, 24,* 52–61.

Barrera, M. (2008). Virtual world emergency training. *Occupational Health & Safety, 77,* 10.

Belchior, P., Marsiske, M., & Mann, W. (2010). *Cognitive training with video games to improve selective visual attention in older adults.* Paper presented at the annual meeting of the American Occupational Therapy Association, Orlando, FL.

Biddis, E., & Irwin, J. (2010). Active video games to promote physical activity in children and youth. *Archives of Pediatric and Adolescent Medicine, 164,* 664–672.

Bingham, P. M., Bates, H. T., Thompson-Figueroa, J., & Lahiri, T. (2010). A breath biofeedback computer game for children with cystic fibrosis. *Clinical Pediatrics, 49,* 337–342.

Brown, S. J., Lieberman, D. A., Gemeny, B. A., Fan, Y. C., Wilson, D. M., & Pasta, D. J. (1997). Educational video game for juvenile diabetes: Results of a controlled trial. *Medical Informatics 22,* 77–89.

Carson, L. Murphy, E. S., Vosloo, J., Donley, D., & Richison, K. (2006). *The effects of video games to promote physical activity in obese children.* Paper presented to the National Prevention Summit: Prevention, Preparedness, and Promotion, Washington, DC.

Dev, P., Heinrichs, W. L., & Youngblood, P. (2011). CliniSpace. *Studies of Health Technology and Informatics, 163,* 173–179.

Fasola, J., & Mataric, M. (2010). *Robot motivator: Increasing user enjoyment and performance on a physical/cognitive task.* Paper presented at the International Conference on Development and Learning, Ann Arbor, MI.

Fritz, S. L, Rivers, E. D., Merlo, A. R., & Duncan, B. M. (2009). Examining the effects of commercially available video game systems, the Nintendo Wii and Sony Playstation 2, on balance and mobility in individuals with chronic stroke. *Journal of Neurologic Physical Therapy Abstracts, 33,* 224–232.

Graf, D. L., Pratt, L. V., Hester, C. N., & Short, K. R. (2009). Playing active video games increases energy expenditure in children. *Pediatrics, 124,* 534–540.

Griffiths, M. (2003). The therapeutic use of videogames in childhood and adolescence. *Clinical Child Psychology & Psychiatry, 8,* 547–554.

Hansen, M. M. (2008). Versatile, immersive, creative and dynamic virtual 3-D healthcare learning environments: A review of the literature. *Journal of Medical Internet Research, 10,* e26.

Honebein, P., Duffy, T., & Fishman, B. (1993). Constructivism and the design of learning environments: Context and authentic activities for learning. In T. M. Duffy, J. Lowyck, & D. H. Jonassen (Eds.), *Designing environments for constructive learning* (pp. 87–108). New York: Springer-Verlag.

HopeLab (2011). *Narrative and empathy in Re-Mission. Description of forthcoming research.* Retrieved February 15, 2011, from: http://www.hopelab.org/our-research/narrative-empathy-remission/.

Institute for the Future (2009). *Quantified self: Your body and health as a data system.* Unpublished report, Technology Horizons Program, Institute for the Future, Palo Alto, CA.

Isbister, K., & Schaffer, N. (2008). *Game usability: Advancing the player experience.* San Francisco: Morgan Kaufmann.

Johnston, J., Sheldon, L., & Massey, A. P. (2010). Influencing physical activity and healthy behaviors in college students: Lessons from an alternate reality game. In J. Cannon-Bowers and C. Bowers, *Serious game design and development: Technologies for training and learning* (pp. 270–289). Hershey, PA: IGI Global.

Kafai, Y. B., Quintero, M., & Feldon, D. (2010). Investigating the "Why" in *Whypox*: Casual and systematic explorations of a virtual epidemic. *Games and Culture, 5,* 116–135.

Kato, P. M., Cole, S. W., Bradlyn, A. S., & Pollock, B. H. (2008). A video game improves behavioral outcomes in adolescents and young adults with cancer: A randomized trial. *Pediatrics, 122,* e305–e317.

Leatherdale, S. T., Woodruff, S. J., & Manske, S. R. (2010). Energy expenditure while playing active and inactive video games. *American Journal of Health Behavior, 34,* 31–35.

Lee, K. M. (2004). Presence, explicated. *Communication Theory, 14,* 27–50.

Lieberman, D. A. (1997). Interactive video games for health promotion: Effects on knowledge, self-efficacy, social support, and health. In R. L. Street, W. R. Gold, & T. Manning (Eds.), *Health promotion and interactive technology: Theoretical applications and future directions* (pp. 103–120). Mahwah, NJ: Lawrence Erlbaum Associates.

Lieberman, D. A. (1999). The researcher's role in the design of children's media and technology. In A. Druin (Ed.), *The design of children's technology* (pp. 73–97). San Francisco: Morgan Kaufmann Publishers.

Lieberman, D. A. (2001). Management of chronic pediatric diseases with interactive health games: Theory and research findings. *Journal of Ambulatory Care Management, 24,* 26–38.

Lieberman, D. A. (2009). Designing serious games for learning and health in informal and formal settings. In U. Ritterfeld, M. Cody, & P. Vorderer (Eds.), *Serious games: Mechanisms and effects* (pp. 117–130). New York: Routledge, Taylor and Francis.

Lieberman, D. A., Chamberlin, B., Medina, E., Jr., Franklin, B. A., Sanner, B. M., & Vafiadis, D. K. (2011). The Power of Play: Innovations in Getting Active Summit 2011: A science panel proceedings report from the American Heart Association. *Circulation, 123,* 2507–2516.

Lombard, M., & Ditton, T. (1997). At the heart of it all: The concept of presence. *Journal of Computer-Mediated Communication, 3.* Retrieved from: http://jcmc.indiana.edu/vol3/issue2/lombard.html.

Mezei, J., Alex, N., Jamalian, A., Levitan, P., Hammer, J., & Kinzer, C. (2010). *Lit to Quit: A game intervention for nicotine smokers.* Paper presented at the American Education Research Association, Denver, CO.

Murphy, E. C., Carson, L., Neal, W., Baylis, C., Donley, D., & Yeater, R. (2009). Effects of an exercise intervention using *Dance Dance Revolution* on endothelial function and other risk factors in overweight children. *International Journal of Pediatric Obesity, 4,* 205–214.

Papastergiou, M. (2009). Exploring the potential of computer and video games for health and physical education: A literature review. *Computers & Education, 53,* 603–622.

Peterson, C. & Stunkard, A. J. (1989). Personal control and health promotion. *Social Science and Medicine, 28,* 819–828.

Picard, R. W. (1997). *Affective computing.* Cambridge, MA: MIT Press.

Pollock, J. P., Gay, G., Byrne, S., Wagner, E., Retelny, D., & Humphreys, L. (2010). It's time to eat! Using mobile games to promote healthy eating. *IEEE Pervasive Computing, 9,* 21–27.

Pope, A. T., & Bogart, E. H. (1996). Extended attention span training system: Video game neurotherapy for attention deficit disorder. *Child Study Journal, 26,* 39–50.

Prawat, R. S., & Flowden, R. E. (1994). Philosophical perspectives on constructivist views of learning. *Educational Psychologist, 29,* 37–48.

Reeves, B., & Nass, C. (1996). *The media equation: How people treat computers, television, and new media like real people and places.* New York: Cambridge University Press.

Ritterfeld, U., Cody, M., & Vorderer, P. (Eds.) (2009). *Serious games: Mechanisms and effects.* New York: Routledge, Taylor and Francis.

Rosenberg, D., Depp, C. A., Bahia, I. V., Reichstadt, J., Palmer, B. W., Kerr, J., et al. (2010). Exergames for subsyndromal depression in older adults: A pilot study of a novel intervention. *American Journal of Geriatric Psychiatry, 18,* 221–226.

Singhal, A., & Rogers, E. M. (2001). The entertainment-education strategy in communication campaigns. In R. E. Rice & C. K. Atkin (Eds.), *Public Communication Campaigns* (3rd. ed., pp. 343–356). Thousand Oaks, CA: Sage.

Thomas, R., Cahill, J., & Santilli, L. (1997). Using an interactive computer game to increase skill and self-efficacy regarding safer sex negotiation: Field test results. *Health Education & Behavior, 24,* 71–86.

Tingen, M. S., Grimling, L. F., Bennett, G., Gibson, E. M., & Renew, M. M. (1997). A pilot study of preadolescents to evaluate a video game-based smoking prevention strategy. *Journal of Addictions Nursing, 9,* 118–124.

Unnithan, V. B., Houser, W., & Fernhall, B. (2005). Evaluation of the energy cost of playing a dance simulation video game in overweight and non-overweight children and adolescents. *International Journal of Sports Medicine, 26,* 1–11.

Vorderer, P., & Bryant, J. (Eds.) (2006). *Playing video games: motives, responses, and consequences.* Mahwah, NJ: Lawrence Erlbaum Associates.

Walshe, D. G., Lewis, E. J., Kim, S. I., O'Sullivan, K., & Wiederhold, B. K. (2003). Exploring the use of computer games and virtual reality in exposure therapy for fear of driving following a motor vehicle accident. *CyberPsychology & Behavior, 6,* 329–334.

Wilkinson, N., Ang, R. P., & Goh, D. H. (2008). Online video game therapy for mental health concerns: A review. *International Journal of Social Psychiatry, 54,* 370–382.

Witte, K., Meyer, G., & Martell, D. (2001). *Effective health risk messages.* Thousand Oaks, CA: Sage.

Yee, N., Bailenson, J., & Ducheneaut, N. (2009). The Proteus Effect: Implications of transformed digital self-representation on online and offline behavior. *Communication Research, 36,* 285–312.

8

COMPUTER-TAILORED INTERVENTIONS FOR IMPROVING HEALTH BEHAVIORS

Seth M. Noar and Nancy Grant Harrington

Tailoring has been defined as "any combination of strategies and information intended to reach one specific person, based on characteristics that are unique to that person, related to the outcome of interest, and derived from an individual assessment" (Kreuter, Strecher, & Glassman, 1999). Contrast this approach with traditional health communications (e.g., brochures) that are developed with a broad audience in mind, may or may not be viewed as relevant to a particular individual, and do not involve individual assessment in their creation. The basic premise behind tailored health communication is that information that is customized to an individual (rather than a group) will be viewed as more personally relevant, will be more likely to be read and cognitively processed, and ultimately will have a better chance of stimulating behavioral change (Kreuter & Wray, 2003; Noar, Harrington, & Aldrich, 2009; Skinner, Campbell, Rimer, Curry, & Prochaska, 1999).

The world we live in is changing rapidly, with changes in technology being perhaps the best example. While the concept of using technology to assess an individual before providing health messaging/advice was out of reach decades ago, today this strategy is eminently possible, in some cases with great ease. Indeed, online polls, Web surveys, "voting" via text message, and other forms of assessment using technology are quickly becoming ubiquitous in our society. In the case of tailoring, many early studies relied on telephone interviews or mail surveys for assessment, but increasingly computer technologies such as kiosks and Web surveys are used for assessment. In some applications of tailoring, feedback is presented in the form of tailored print materials. In other cases, technologies such as websites and mobile devices are used for both assessment and feedback, with messaging delivered onscreen immediately following assessment. The term *computer-tailored interventions* (CTIs) can be used to describe these and other applications of tailoring on a variety of computerized platforms (see Table 8.1), and this term will be used in the current chapter.

Table 8.1 Comparison of five delivery channels for computer-tailored interventions (CTIs)

Attributes		Delivery Channels			
	Print	Telephone (automated)	Local computer/kiosk	Internet (website, email)	Mobile device
Low cost	X	X			
Broad reach	X	X		X	
Ease of updates		X		X	
Ease of access		X			X
Ease of multiple assessments/exposures				X	X
No Internet connection necessary	X	X	X		X
No technical support necessary					X
No training/supervision necessary	X	X	X	X	X
No computer skills necessary	X	X			
High intervention fidelity	X	X	X	X	X
Durability	X	X	X	X	
Portability of report	X				X
Interactivity			X	X	X
Multimedia			X	X	X
Visuals	X		X	X	X

Note: Each X indicates a positive attribute of the particular channel.

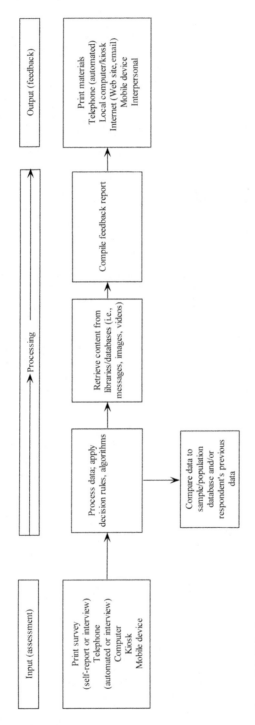

Figure 8.1 Tailoring process

The CTI literature began with the development and testing of tailored print materials (Kreuter, Farrell, Olevitch, & Brennan, 2000; Skinner et al., 1999). Since that beginning, tailoring has been widely applied to a variety of technological platforms. Indeed, as the Internet began to flourish, tailoring was increasingly applied in Internet-based programs (Lustria, Cortese, Noar, & Glueckauf, 2009; Noar et al., 2009; Strecher, 2007). Most recently, tailoring is being applied in the mobile device context, including text messaging (Cole-Lewis & Kershaw, 2010; Fjeldsoe, Marshall, & Miller, 2009; Patrick et al., 2009; Woolford, Clark, Strecher, & Resnicow, 2010) and more sophisticated mobile programs (Abroms, Padmanabhan, Thaweethai, & Phillips, 2011; Arsand, Tatara, Ostengen, & Hartvigsen, 2010; Estrin & Sim, 2010; Whittaker et al., 2011).

Figure 8.1 provides a graphic of how the tailoring process works. Briefly, a participant is first assessed on a variety of characteristics (e.g., demographic, behavioral, psychosocial) that are relevant to the behavior under study. Computer algorithms are then used to drive decision rules that have been developed and programmed to create a feedback report for participants. The core content that is pieced together by the computer into a feedback report comes from a *message library* consisting of hundreds or thousands of messages that have been created by the researchers expressly for this purpose. Other libraries can also exist in tailoring, such as photo or video libraries. The feedback report is then compiled and presented to the participant.

Tailoring Example

Consider the following CTI example. In the HIV/AIDS area, scores of efficacious prevention programs exist (Noar, 2008), and yet disseminating such programs has been a major challenge (Solomon, Card, & Malow, 2006). CTIs may be able to overcome many common barriers to effective dissemination, including fidelity to intervention protocols and cost to consistently deliver interventions. For these reasons, Noar and colleagues developed and are currently testing a CTI in the HIV/AIDS prevention area.

The program that we have developed is called the Tailored Information Program for Safer Sex, or TIPSS. TIPSS is an individually tailored, computer-delivered program designed to increase correct and consistent condom use among 18- to 29-year-old heterosexually active African Americans visiting a sexually transmitted infection (STI) clinic (Noar, Webb, et al., 2011). The program is based on the attitude-social influence-efficacy model (De Vries & Mudde, 1998) and skills training principles (Segrin & Givertz, 2003) and was developed through a two-year process of formative research activities (Noar, Crosby, Benac, Snow, & Troutman, 2011; Noar, Webb, et al., 2011). TIPSS assesses individuals on a host of psychosocial constructs related to condom use and provides individually tailored messages based on individuals' scores on those constructs. The program also delivers two interactive exercises—one focused on correct condom use and another on condom use negotiation. All of these exercises and feedback vary based on whether one has main and/or casual sexual partners. Figure 8.2 presents TIPSS's design; the TIPSS home screen, assessment screen, and feedback screen can be seen in Figures 8.3–8.5, respectively.

The TIPSS program acts in many ways like a human counselor, asking questions and providing feedback to the participant. It also uses interactive exercises to foster skills training in key areas related to safer sexual behavior. The program is currently being tested in a randomized controlled trial examining its ability to increase correct and consistent condom use in the target population (Noar, Webb, et al., 2011). The ultimate potential of such a program is dissemination as a waiting room intervention that all STI clients could access while waiting for care.

Advantages of CTIs

CTIs offer several advantages. While some attributes and advantages are specific to particular platforms (see Table 8.1), there are also cross-platform advantages, which we describe here. First, while there are certainly initial costs involved in the development of a CTI, once developed CTIs are likely to be cost-effective to

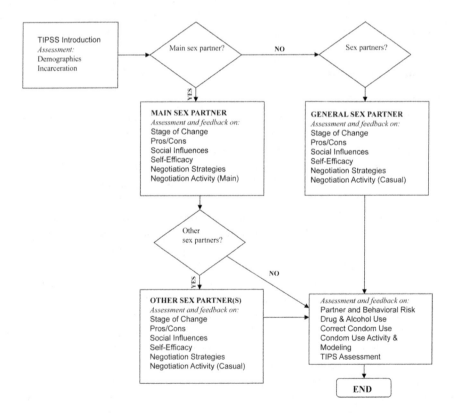

Figure 8.2 TIPSS design

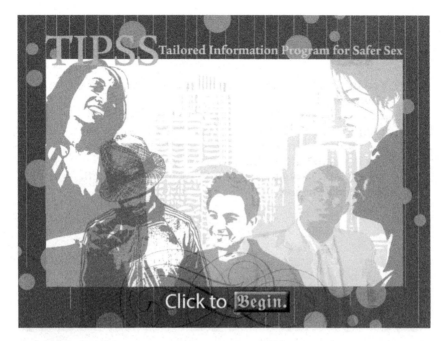

Figure 8.3 TIPSS home screen

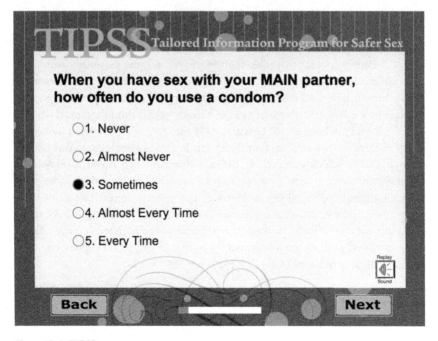

Figure 8.4 TIPSS assessment screen

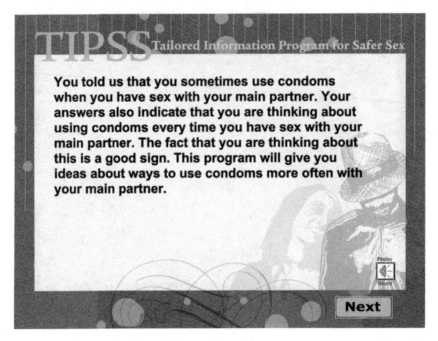

Figure 8.5 TIPSS feedback screen

implement (Lynch, Whitlock, Valanis, & Smith, 2004), especially when compared to the cost of human counseling interventions (Saywell, Champion, Skinner, Menon, & Daggy, 2004). Second, using computer algorithms and interactivity, CTIs can deliver content that is likely to be viewed as more personally relevant to the individual than more generic content (Kreuter & Wray, 2003; Skinner et al., 1999). Indeed, perceived relevance is thought to play a major role in engagement, message processing, and ultimately in the efficacy of eHealth programs (Hawkins, Kreuter, Resnicow, Fishbein, & Dijkstra, 2008; Strecher et al., 2008a). Third, CTIs are very flexible in terms of delivery channels (Noar, Harrington, Van Stee, & Aldrich, 2011), which can include Internet programs (see Buller & Floyd, this volume), mobile apps (see Abroms, Padmanabhan, & Evans, this volume), text messaging (see Fjeldsoe, Miller, & Marshall, this volume), interactive voice technology (see Piette & Beard, this volume), and even social media (see Taubenheim et al., this volume). Finally, through the combination of high reach, high efficacy, and low cost, CTIs have great potential for having an impact on large segments of at-risk audiences (Abrams et al., 1996; Strecher, 2007).

Contexts and Target Populations

CTIs have been applied to an enormous number of health problems, behaviors, and target populations. Our reviews of the tailoring literature have found that the majority of interventions have been focused on smoking, diet, physical activity, multiple behavior change, and, to a lesser extent, mammography screening (Lustria et al., 2009; Noar, Benac, & Harris, 2007; Noar et al., 2009; Noar, Harrington, et al., 2011). Other reviews have found similar results regarding the distribution of behavioral areas in tailoring studies (Krebs, Prochaska, & Rossi, 2010; Richards et al., 2007; Sohl & Moyer, 2007).

In addition, reviews indicate that CTIs have been tested on at least 20 distinct health problems/behaviors, including alcohol use, sun safety, drug use, hypertension, immunization, seatbelt use, safer sex, injury prevention, medical appointments, and cervical and colorectal cancer screening (Noar et al., 2007, 2009; Richards et al., 2007). Not surprisingly, target populations run the gamut from adolescents, college students, parents, and older adults to more specialized populations such as adult cancer survivors and callers to the Cancer Information Service. These and other populations have been accessed at clinics, worksites, schools, and churches; from health maintenance organization insurer lists; through newspaper advertising and random digit dial calling; and through other methods. While many studies in this literature have been conducted in the United States, a significant minority of studies are international studies (Krebs et al., 2010; Noar et al., 2007, 2009).

Theoretical Bases for Interventions

A host of behavioral theories have been used to inform tailored interventions. Constructs from such theories are often used in the tailoring process itself, a strategy referred to as *behavioral construct tailoring* (Kreuter et al., 2000). Theory can also be used in other ways, however, such as providing detailed message design guidance in intervention development (Harrington & Noar, in press).

Reviews of the tailoring literature indicate that the transtheoretical model and stages of change may be the most dominant theoretical perspective in this literature (Noar et al., 2007; Richards et al., 2007). This finding is not surprising, given the influential role that this model played early in the tailoring literature (Noar et al., 2007). In fact, many of the first tailored interventions applied stages of change (Campbell et al., 1994; Skinner, Strecher, & Hospers, 1994) or the full transtheoretical model (Prochaska, DiClemente, Velicer, & Rossi, 1993). Many other widely used theories appear in this literature, however, including social cognitive theory, the health belief model, and the theory of planned behavior (Lustria et al., 2009; Noar et al., 2007; Noar, Harrington, et al., 2011; Richards et al., 2007; Sohl & Moyer, 2007).

It is important to note that tailored interventions often apply multiple theories to inform a single tailored intervention (Noar et al., 2009; Richards et al., 2007). Also, it cannot be assumed that because a particular intervention is "based on" a theory that the intervention tailors messages on the basis of all of that theory's core constructs (Noar et al., 2007; also see Painter, Borba, Hynes, Mays, & Glanz, 2008).

Instead, theory has been used in a very eclectic and utilitarian manner in this literature, with select constructs from a variety of theories often informing one intervention. While theoretical purists may object to this manner of using theory, others defend the use of theoretical constructs for interventions on the basis of their empirical usefulness (Bartholomew, Parcel, Kok, & Gottlieb, 2006; Kreuter et al., 2000) or suggest that the use of multiple theories (with complementary contributions) can actually strengthen interventions (Glanz & Bishop, 2010).

Effects of CTIs

Almost two decades of literature provides a strong empirical basis on which to judge the efficacy of CTIs. Early in the literature, a number of seminal studies demonstrated efficacy and thus provided reasons for optimism (Campbell et al., 1994; Prochaska et al., 1993; Skinner et al., 1994). Subsequently, narrative reviews of the literature asserted that CTIs generally were successful in affecting health behavior change in diverse areas (Skinner et al., 1999), including smoking cessation (Strecher, 1999), nutrition (Brug, Campbell, & Van Assema, 1999) and cancer prevention (Rimer & Glassman, 1999). There have also been more recent systematic reviews that have concluded that CTIs are generally efficacious (Kroeze, Werkman, & Brug, 2006; Neville, O'Hara, & Milat, 2009; Richards et al., 2007). Perhaps most important, three recent meta-analytic projects have examined the literature and provided a more fine-grained analysis of CTI efficacy. We describe these meta-analyses in greater detail next.

Noar et al. (2007) conducted a meta-analysis of 57 studies that tested the ability of tailored print materials to affect health behavior change. The studies primarily consisted of smoking cessation (26%), diet (23%), and mammography screening (21%) interventions. The overall effect size in this study was $r = .074$ (for tailored interventions compared with no-treatment control and alternative interventions), which converts to $d = .15$. Perhaps most important, an analysis that excluded studies that contained only no-treatment control comparison conditions revealed that tailored interventions still outperformed generic or targeted interventions ($r = .058$ or $d = .12$).

Across behaviors, smoking and diet had the largest effect sizes, followed by mammography screening and then exercise. Also, a variety of intervention characteristics moderated intervention efficacy. For example, studies that generated tailored reports in the form of pamphlets/leaflets and newsletters/magazines had significantly larger effect sizes than those generating letters or manuals. In addition, those interventions with more than one contact with participants had significantly larger effects than those with just one contact. Finally, studies tailoring on particular theoretical (e.g., attitudes, self-efficacy, stage of change) and other (e.g., demographic) factors had larger effect sizes than those not tailoring on these variables (Noar et al., 2007).

That same year, Sohl and Moyer (2007) published a meta-analysis of 28 tailored intervention studies focused on increasing mammography screening within print, telephone, and in-person interventions. Results indicated a statistically significant overall effect of the tailored interventions (compared with no-treatment control and alternative interventions) with an odds ratio (OR) equal to 1.42 (which converts to $d = .21$). Telephone, in-person, and print-tailored interventions all had similar impact. In addition, studies that tailored on variables from the health belief model had significantly greater impact than those that did not, and interventions were significantly more effective when a physician recommendation was part of the intervention. Also, studies that measured *recent* mammography as opposed to *regular* mammography tended to have larger effect sizes.

Most recently, Krebs et al. (2010) conducted a meta-analysis of 88 studies testing CTIs delivered using print (75%), computer (22%), and automated telephone (3%) channels. Behaviors examined in this review were diet, smoking, physical activity, and mammography screening, and some studies intervened on more than one behavior at a time. Overall, there was a statistically significant effect of tailored interventions on health behavior change ($d = .17$), and this effect did not vary significantly across tailoring channels. Effects were similar across behaviors, with interventions focused on dietary fat reduction being most efficacious ($d = .22$). In addition, interventions that focused on multiple behaviors did *not* have smaller effects than those focusing on a single behavior.

Krebs et al.'s (2010) meta-analysis also examined tailoring effects over time. Results revealed that effects tended to peak between 4 and 12 months and then gradually decline over time. Interestingly, there was also evidence that dynamically tailored interventions (those reassessing individuals before providing new tailored feedback) had significantly larger effects at most timepoints (including 13–24 month follow-up) than statically tailored interventions (those providing new tailored feedback based on the same baseline assessment). Indeed, only dynamically tailored interventions demonstrated statically significant effects at long-term follow-up.

Overall, these meta-analyses suggest that CTIs have often been successful in stimulating behavior change, and they each contribute to our knowledge about what may make efficacious CTIs. The evidence to date suggests that messages that are more customized to an individual are more successful in influencing health behavior change (Noar et al., 2007) and that carefully constructed interventions can maintain changes over the longer term (Krebs et al., 2010). Effect sizes across all of these meta-analyses were similar ($d = .15–.21$), giving us some indication of what the "typical" effect of a CTI may be. Other important findings from these meta-analyses indicate that tailoring channel does not in and of itself appear to make a difference, but how tailoring is carried out (e.g., choice of theoretical constructs, dynamic versus static tailoring, design of print materials) does appear to have a measurable impact on the efficacy of a CTI.

Dissemination Potential

For tailored interventions to have a real impact on health-related behaviors, their reach needs to be broadened well beyond the participants in the research trials conducted to date. While there is much *potential* in CTIs for dissemination, a central problem is the familiar research-practice gap that exists in much of health promotion and disease prevention research (Glasgow, Lichtenstein, & Marcus, 2003). That is, it is one thing to demonstrate that a particular intervention approach is efficacious within the context of a research trial. It is quite another to find a delivery system for that intervention and see it successfully integrated into practice. This translation is especially challenging considering that there is not an obvious delivery channel for health behavior change interventions in the same way that there is for other health products, such as pharmaceutical medications.

In order to attempt to speed dissemination progress, the National Cancer Institute convened a workgroup to discuss the barriers to dissemination of computer-tailored interventions and to propose some potential solutions (National Cancer Institute, 2008). Some of the key barriers were the following: (1) many agencies want an intervention that covers many behaviors, while most tailored interventions focus on a single behavior; (2) disseminating interventions in a manner that will make individuals aware of them and take the time to interact with them is challenging; (3) many of the computer platforms on which tailored interventions were developed are now out of date; (4) ongoing technical assistance is needed for such interventions, but who will supply such support is not clear; and (5) intellectual property issues arise in the case of some interventions. Many of these barriers come from the fact that many tailored interventions were *not* developed with dissemination in mind. Future studies will benefit from a more careful consideration of how such interventions can be developed in a way that maximizes dissemination potential.

The workgroup proposed several solutions: (1) funding studies to research the best manner in which to disseminate interventions; (2) developing tailored interventions with more flexible software that allows for adaptations to be made when reaching the dissemination stage; (3) partnering with nonprofit and private sector agencies that have an interest in disseminating such interventions; and (4) increasing the dialogue among technical developers as to the best ways to create sustainable interventions and provide technical support over the long term. Also, an article that grew out of this workshop provides a discussion on possible adaptation of existing evidence-based CTIs, focusing on several issues related to appropriate target population(s), amending CTI content for dissemination (e.g., adding, removing content), implementation in the practice setting, data collection and intervention evaluation, intervention management, and legal and regulatory considerations (Vinson et al., 2011).

While reaching many of the above goals will take time, we should note that there has been some substantive movement toward dissemination. Dr. Victor Strecher and his colleagues in the Center for Health Communications Research at the University of Michigan have developed open source software for the creation of CTIs (Center for Health Communications Research, 2011). The software, called the Michigan Tailoring System, is free to use and is open source, making modifications to it possible by any technical developer. Also, Dr. Marci Campbell and her colleagues in the Communications for Health Applications and Interventions (CHAI) core at the University of North Carolina at Chapel Hill have developed *Tailortool,* an open source software toolkit that enables the creation and delivery of CTIs over the Web (Communication for Health Applications and Interventions, 2011). *Tailortool* allows one to develop CTIs that are delivered in a newsletter format on the computer (in PDF format), which can then be printed or saved electronically for later reading. Also in existence are open-source interactive voice response programs that are available for use in developing and delivering CTIs (Vinson et al., 2011).

Finally, while public sector dissemination has so far been a challenge to achieve, companies such as Health Media (founded in 1998; http://www.healthmedia. com/) and Pro-Change Behavior Systems (founded in 1997; http://www. prochange.com/) have for many years been developing and disseminating CTIs in the private sector. In a further step toward broader dissemination, Pro-Change recently announced that it would make its *Lifestyle Management Program,* which focuses on numerous common health risk behaviors, available to the general public for a yearly fee.

Limitations of CTIs and Future Directions for Research

As with any type of intervention, CTIs have their limitations. CTIs require an assessment of the individual, and thus they cannot be used in mass media channels such as television, nor can they be used with individuals who do not wish to be assessed. Also, as CTIs increasingly move into the area of multiple behavior change (Noar, Harrington, et al., 2011), assessment burden will be a greater challenge. Another limitation is the fact that computer technology platforms change so quickly that by the time research trials are over, the technology that was just tested may be nearly out of date (Strecher, 2009). As mentioned above, solutions to this problem will help lead to greater dissemination of CTIs. Finally, a limitation in the field as a whole is that most studies have only addressed the question of "Do CTIs work?" While this research design strategy answers the efficacy question, it does little to advance an understanding of what makes tailoring effective (Abrams, Mills, & Bulger, 1999; Noar et al., 2009; Strecher, 2009). Consequently, developers new to CTIs have been left a bit in the dark regarding best practices for tailoring. Luckily, new studies (briefly discussed below) are beginning to examine the "ingredients" of effective tailoring.

New research on CTIs is critical to advance the field of tailored health communication. The field is clearly shifting from research that addresses *whether* tailoring works to research that addresses *under what conditions* it works. Many of the meta-analyses discussed in this chapter have conducted analyses to explore this question. In addition, recent conceptual work has distinguished among the various types of personalization and feedback strategies that tailored interventions can deliver

Table 8.2 Domains in which tailoring can be achieved and associated theories and variables

Purpose	Theories	Variable types	Specific constructs/variables	Outcomes
Match content to individual's information needs and interests	Transtheoretical model and stages of change health belief model Social cognitive theory Theory of reasoned action Theory of planned behavior	Psychosocial variables, past behavior	Attitudes, beliefs, self-efficacy, social norms, perceived susceptibility, perceived severity, behavioral intentions, stage of change, previous behavior	Argument strength (content was convincing)
Place information in a meaningful context	Audience segmentation Personalization Culturally-oriented theories	Demographic, cultural variables	Gender, age, race Gender norms, cultural norms, ethnic identity, racial pride, religiosity, collectivism	Perceived relevance (intervention was designed for me and reflects my beliefs and values)
Use design, production, and channel elements to capture and keep individual's attention	Activation model Sensation-seeking targeting limited capacity model	Message design variables ("look and feel")	Message sensation value	Attention (intervention kept my attention)
Present information in type and structure preferred by individual	Exemplification theory/narratives Entertainment education Message framing Emotional appeals	Message structure variables (type of appeal)	Narrative vs. statistical Gain vs. loss framing Fear, guilt, warmth, and other appeals	Message processing (thought about information, recalled information later on)

(Dijkstra, 2008; Hawkins et al., 2008). This "new language" will help tailoring researchers better disentangle the various components of tailored messages in order to advance an understanding of how tailoring operates most effectively.

In addition, an important observation about CTIs is the following: to date, tailoring has almost entirely been conceived of as a way to customize intervention *content* to individuals. As a result, nearly all tailoring has focused on what scholars believe to be the key determinants of behavior, which come from the theories of behavior and behavior change described earlier in this chapter (also see Noar & Zimmerman, 2005). Many other factors affect how health content will be received, however, and a number of these communication-oriented factors could also be tailored on. Table 8.2 lists four domains that can be considered in tailoring (Noar et al., 2009; Rimer & Kreuter, 2006). To date, the literature has focused almost entirely on the first row (*content*) and often neglected the other three domains in tailoring. The potential here is enormous: Not only could CTIs ultimately deliver the right *content* to the individual but also they could deliver it in a way that best ensures that content is attended to, cognitively processed, and perceived as personally relevant.

That specific studies are beginning to examine the kinds of questions raised by Hawkins et al. (2008), Noar et al. (2009), Rimer and Kreuter (2006), and others (Dijkstra, 2008; Strecher, 2009) is promising. For example, newer studies are examining novel constructs on which to tailor—especially constructs in the areas of cultural tailoring (Kreuter et al., 2005; Resnicow et al., 2008; Van der Veen, De Zwart, Mackenbach, & Richardus, 2010), environmental tailoring (Van Stralen, De Vries, Bolman, Mudde, & Lechner, 2010; Van Stralen, De Vries, Mudde, Bolman, & Lechner, 2009), and message framing (Latimer et al., 2008; Van't Riet, Ruiter, Werrij, & De Vries, 2010). Research is also examining the effects of different types of tailoring personalization and feedback on intervention efficacy (De Vet, De Nooijer, De Vries, & Brug, 2008; Dijkstra, 2005; Kroeze, Oenema, Dagnelie, & Brug, 2008; Strecher et al., 2008b), mediators and moderators of effective tailoring (Campbell et al., 2008; Ko, Campbell, Lewis, Earp, & DeVellis, 2010; Ko, Campbell, Lewis, Earp, & DeVellis, 2011; Strecher, Shiffman, & West, 2006), different ways of delivering multiple behavior change CTIs (Vandelanotte, Reeves, Brug, & De Bourdeaudhuij, 2008), and even brain responses to tailoring (Chua, Liberzon, Welsh, & Strecher, 2009). Additional studies are needed to help build a cumulative science of best practices in tailoring.

Conclusion

The literature on CTIs is large, diverse, and growing every day. As eHealth becomes an ever more important part of public health and health care (Kreps & Neuhauser, 2010), our ability to develop effective CTIs becomes even more important. New research is thus critical to advance our understanding of what CTI strategies work best with what populations and behaviors using what technological platforms.

The more we learn about what makes effective CTIs, the better able we will be to build more successful CTIs in the future that maximize our ability to positively affect health behavior change and ultimately improve health outcomes.

Acknowledgments

Preparation of this chapter was funded, in part, by grant no. 1-R34-MH077507-01 from the National Institute of Mental Health (principal investigator: Seth M. Noar).

References

Abrams, D. B., Mills, S., & Bulger, D. (1999). Challenges and future directions for tailored communication research. *Annals of Behavioral Medicine, 21,* 299–306.

Abrams, D. B., Orleans, C. T., Niaura, R. S., Goldstein, M. G., Prochaska, J. O., & Velicer, W. F. (1996). Integrating individual and public health perspectives for treatment of tobacco dependence under managed health care: A combined step care and matching model. *Annals of Behavioral Medicine, 18,* 290–304.

Abroms, L. C., Padmanabhan, N., Thaweethai, L., & Phillips, T. (2011). iPhone apps for smoking cessation: A content analysis. *American Journal of Preventive Medicine, 40,* 279–285.

Arsand, E., Tatara, N., Ostengen, G., & Hartvigsen, G. (2010). Mobile phone-based self-management tools for type 2 diabetes: The few touch application. *Journal of Diabetes Science and Technology, 4,* 328–336.

Bartholomew, L. K., Parcel, G. S., Kok, G., & Gottlieb, N. H. (2006). *Planning health promotion programs: An intervention mapping approach* (2nd ed.). San Francisco, CA: Jossey-Bass.

Brug, J., Campbell, M., & Van Assema, P. (1999). The application and impact of computer-generated personalized nutrition education: A review of the literature. *Patient Education & Counseling, 36,* 145–156.

Campbell, M. K., DeVellis, B. M., Strecher, V. J., Ammerman, A. S., DeVellis, R. F., & Sandler, R. S. (1994). Improving dietary behavior: The effectiveness of tailored messages in primary care settings. *American Journal of Public Health, 84,* 783–787.

Campbell, M. K., McLerran, D., Turner-McGrievy, G., Feng, Z., Havas, S., Sorensen, G., et al. (2008). Mediation of adult fruit and vegetable consumption in the national 5 A Day for Better Health community studies. *Annals of Behavioral Medicine, 35,* 49–60.

Center for Health Communications Research (2011). *The Michigan Tailoring System.* Retrieved May 11, 2011, from: http://chcr.umich.edu/mts/.

Chua, H. F., Liberzon, I., Welsh, R. C., & Strecher, V. J. (2009). Neural correlates of message tailoring and self-relatedness in smoking cessation programming. *Biological Psychiatry, 65,* 165–168.

Cole-Lewis, H., & Kershaw, T. (2010). Text messaging as a tool for behavior change in disease prevention and management. *Epidemiologic Reviews, 32,* 56–69.

Communication for Health Applications and Interventions (2011). *The CHAI Core.* Retrieved May 11, 2011, from: http://www.chaicore.com/.

De Vet, E., De Nooijer, J., De Vries, N. K., & Brug, J. (2008). Testing the transtheoretical model for fruit intake: Comparing Web-based tailored stage-matched and stage-mismatched feedback. *Health Education Research, 23,* 218–227.

De Vries, H., & Mudde, A. N. (1998). Predicting stage transitions for smoking cessation applying the attitude-social influence-efficacy model. *Psychology and Health, 13,* 369–385.

Dijkstra, A. (2005). Working mechanisms of computer-tailored health education: Evidence from smoking cessation. *Health Education Research, 20,* 527–539.

Dijkstra, A. (2008). The psychology of tailoring-ingredients in computer-tailored persuasion. *Social and Personality Psychology Compass, 2,* 765–784.

Estrin, D., & Sim, I. (2010). Health care delivery. Open mHealth architecture: An engine for health care innovation. *Science, 330,* 759–760.

Fjeldsoe, B. S., Marshall, A. L., & Miller, Y. D. (2009). Behavior change interventions delivered by mobile telephone short-message service. *American Journal of Preventive Medicine, 36,* 165–173.

Glanz, K., & Bishop, D. B. (2010). The role of behavioral science theory in development and implementation of public health interventions. *Annual Review of Public Health, 31,* 399–418.

Glasgow, R. E., Lichtenstein, E., & Marcus, A. C. (2003). Why don't we see more translation of health promotion research to practice? Rethinking the efficacy-to-effectiveness transition. *American Journal of Public Health, 93,* 1261–1267.

Harrington, N. G., & Noar, S. M. (in press). Reporting standards for studies of tailored interventions. *Health Education Research.*

Hawkins, R. P., Kreuter, M., Resnicow, K., Fishbein, M., & Dijkstra, A. (2008). Understanding tailoring in communicating about health. *Health Education Research, 23,* 454–466.

Ko, L. K., Campbell, M. K., Lewis, M. A., Earp, J., & DeVellis, B. (2010). Mediators of fruit and vegetable consumption among colorectal cancer survivors. *Journal of Cancer Survivorship, 4,* 149–158.

Ko, L. K., Campbell, M. K., Lewis, M. A., Earp, J. A., & DeVellis, B. (2011). Information processes mediate the effect of a health communication intervention on fruit and vegetable consumption. *Journal of Health Communication, 16,* 282–299.

Krebs, P., Prochaska, J. O., & Rossi, J. S. (2010). A meta-analysis of computer-tailored interventions for health behavior change. *Preventive Medicine, 51,* 214–221.

Kreps, G. L., & Neuhauser, L. (2010). New directions in eHealth communication: Opportunities and challenges. *Patient Education & Counseling, 78,* 329–336.

Kreuter, M. W., Farrell, D., Olevitch, L., & Brennan, L. (2000). *Tailoring health messages: Customizing communication with computer technology.* Mahwah, NJ: Lawrence Erlbaum Associates.

Kreuter, M. W., Strecher, V. J., & Glassman, B. (1999). One size does not fit all: The case for tailoring print materials. *Annals of Behavioral Medicine, 21,* 276–283.

Kreuter, M. W., Sugg-Skinner, C., Holt, C. L., Clark, E. M., Haire-Joshu, D., Fu, Q., et al. (2005). Cultural tailoring for mammography and fruit and vegetable intake among low-income African-American women in urban public health centers. *Preventive Medicine, 41,* 53–62.

Kreuter, M. W., & Wray, R. J. (2003). Tailored and targeted health communication: Strategies for enhancing information relevance. *American Journal of Health Behavior, 27,* S227-S232.

Kroeze, W., Oenema, A., Dagnelie, P. C., & Brug, J. (2008). Examining the minimal required elements of a computer-tailored intervention aimed at dietary fat reduction: Results of a randomized controlled dismantling study. *Health Education Research, 23,* 880–891.

Kroeze, W., Werkman, A., & Brug, J. (2006). A systematic review of randomized trials on the effectiveness of computer-tailored education on physical activity and dietary behaviors. *Annals of Behavioral Medicine, 31,* 205–223.

Latimer, A. E., Williams-Piehota, P., Katulak, N. A., Cox, A., Mowad, L., Higgins, E. T., et al. (2008). Promoting fruit and vegetable intake through messages tailored to individual differences in regulatory focus. *Annals of Behavioral Medicine, 35,* 363–369.

Lustria, M. L., Cortese, J., Noar, S. M., & Glueckauf, R. L. (2009). Computer-tailored health interventions delivered over the Web: Review and analysis of key components. *Patient Education & Counseling, 74,* 156–173.

Lynch, F. L., Whitlock, E. P., Valanis, B. G., & Smith, S. K. (2004). Cost-effectiveness of a tailored intervention to increase screening in HMO women overdue for Pap test and mammography services. *Preventive Medicine, 38,* 403.

National Cancer Institute (2008). *Computerized tailored interventions workgroup meeting, executive summary.* Retrieved April 1, 2008, from: http://cancercontrol.cancer.gov/d4d/info_computer_meeting.html. Washington, DC: U.S. Department of Health & Human Services.

Neville, L. M., O'Hara, B., & Milat, A. J. (2009). Computer-tailored dietary behaviour change interventions: A systematic review. *Health Education Research, 24,* 699–720.

Noar, S. M. (2008). Behavioral interventions to reduce HIV-related sexual risk behavior: Review and synthesis of meta-analytic evidence. *AIDS and Behavior, 12,* 335–353.

Noar, S. M., Benac, C. N., & Harris, M. S. (2007). Does tailoring matter? Meta-analytic review of tailored print health behavior change interventions. *Psychological Bulletin, 133,* 673–693.

Noar, S. M., Crosby, R., Benac, C., Snow, G., & Troutman, A. (2011). Application of the attitude-social influence-efficacy (ASE) model to condom use among African-American STD clinic patients: Implications for tailored health communication. *AIDS and Behavior, 15,* 1045–1057.

Noar, S. M., Harrington, N. G., & Aldrich, R. S. (2009). The role of message tailoring in the development of persuasive health communication messages. *Communication Yearbook, 33,* 72–133.

Noar, S. M., Harrington, N. G., Van Stee, S. K., & Aldrich, R. S. (2011). Tailored health communication to change lifestyle behaviors. *American Journal of Lifestyle Medicine, 5,* 112–122.

Noar, S. M., Webb, E. M., Van Stee, S. K., Redding, C. A., Feist-Price, S., Crosby, R., et al. (2011). Using computer technology for HIV prevention among African-Americans: Development of a tailored information program for safer sex (TIPSS). *Health Education Research, 26,* 393–406.

Noar, S. M., & Zimmerman, R. S. (2005). Health behavior theory and cumulative knowledge regarding health behaviors: Are we moving in the right direction? *Health Education Research, 20,* 275–290.

Painter, J. E., Borba, C. P. C., Hynes, M., Mays, D., & Glanz, K. (2008). The use of theory in health behavior research from 2000 to 2005: A systematic review. *Annals of Behavioral Medicine, 35,* 358–362.

Patrick, K., Raab, F., Adams, M. A., Dillon, L., Zabinski, M., Rock, C. L., et al. (2009). A text message-based intervention for weight loss: Randomized controlled trial. *Journal of Medical Internet Research, 11,* e1.

Prochaska, J. O., DiClemente, C. C., Velicer, W. F., & Rossi, J. S. (1993). Standardized, individualized, interactive, and personalized self-help programs for smoking cessation. *Health Psychology, 12,* 399–405.

Resnicow, K., Davis, R. E., Zhang, G., Konkel, J., Strecher, V. J., Shaikh, A. R., et al. (2008). Tailoring a fruit and vegetable intervention on novel motivational constructs: Results of a randomized study. *Annals of Behavioral Medicine, 35,* 159–169.

Richards, K. C., Enderlin, C. A., Beck, C., McSweeney, J. C., Jones, T. C., & Roberson, P. K. (2007). Tailored biobehavioral interventions: A literature review and synthesis. *Research & Theory for Nursing Practice, 21,* 271–285.

Rimer, B. K., & Glassman, B. (1999). Is there a use for tailored print communications in cancer risk communication? *Journal of the National Cancer Institute, 91,* 140.

Rimer, B. K., & Kreuter, M. W. (2006). Advancing tailored health communication: A persuasion and message effects perspective. *Journal of Communication, 56*(S1), S184-S201.

Saywell, R. M., Champion, V. L., Skinner, C. S., Menon, U., & Daggy, J. (2004). A cost-effectiveness comparison of three tailored interventions to increase mammography screening. *Journal of Women's Health, 13,* 909–918.

Segrin, C., & Givertz, M. (2003). Methods of social skills training and development. In J. O. Greene & B. R. Burleson (Eds.), *Handbook of communication and social interaction skills* (pp. 135–176). Mahwah, NJ: Lawrence Erlbaum Associates.

Skinner, C. S., Campbell, M. K., Rimer, B. K., Curry, S., & Prochaska, J. O. (1999). How effective is tailored print communication? *Annals of Behavioral Medicine, 21,* 290–298.

Skinner, C. S., Strecher, V. J., & Hospers, H. (1994). Physicians' recommendations for mammography: Do tailored messages make a difference? *American Journal of Public Health, 84,* 43–49.

Sohl, S. J., & Moyer, A. (2007). Tailored interventions to promote mammography screening: A meta-analytic review. *Preventive Medicine, 45,* 252–261.

Solomon, J., Card, J. J., & Malow, R. M. (2006). Adapting efficacious interventions: Advancing translational research in HIV prevention. *Evaluation & the Health Professions, 29,* 162–194.

Strecher, V. J. (1999). Computer-tailored smoking cessation materials: A review and discussion. *Patient Education & Counseling, 36,* 107–117.

Strecher, V. J. (2007). Internet methods for delivering behavioral and health-related interventions (eHealth). *Annual Review of Clinical Psychology, 3,* 53–76.

Strecher, V. J. (2009). Interactive health communications for cancer prevention and control. In S. M. Miller, D. J. Bowen, R. T. Croyle, & J. H. Rowland (Eds.), *Handbook of cancer control and behavioral science: A resource for researchers, practitioners, and policymakers* (pp. 547–558). Washington, DC: American Psychological Association.

Strecher, V. J., McClure, J. B., Alexander, G. L., Chakraborty, B., Nair, V. N., Konkel, J. M., Couper, M., et al. (2008a). The role of engagement in a tailored Web-based smoking cessation program: Randomized controlled trial. *Journal of Medical Internet Research, 10,* e36.

Strecher, V. J., McClure, J. B., Alexander, G. L., Chakraborty, B., Nair, V. N., Konkel, J. M., Collins, L. M., et al. (2008b). Web-based smoking-cessation programs: Results of a randomized trial. *American Journal of Preventive Medicine, 34,* 373–381.

Strecher, V. J., Shiffman, S., & West, R. (2006). Moderators and mediators of a Web-based computer-tailored smoking cessation program among nicotine patch users. *Nicotine & Tobacco Research, 8,* S95-s101.

Van der Veen, Y. J. J., De Zwart, O., Mackenbach, J., & Richardus, J. H. (2010). Cultural tailoring for the promotion of hepatitis B screening in Turkish Dutch: A protocol for a randomized controlled trial. *BMC Public Health, 10,* 674.

Van Stralen, M. M., De Vries, H., Bolman, C., Mudde, A. N., & Lechner, L. (2010). Exploring the efficacy and moderators of two computer-tailored physical activity interventions for older adults: A randomized controlled trial. *Annals of Behavioral Medicine, 39,* 139–150.

Van Stralen, M. M., De Vries, H., Mudde, A. N., Bolman, C., & Lechner, L. (2009). The working mechanisms of an environmentally tailored physical activity intervention for older adults: A randomized controlled trial. *International Journal of Behavioral Nutrition and Physical Activity, 6,* 83–83.

Van 't Riet, J., Ruiter, R. A. C., Werrij, M. Q., & De Vries, H. (2010). Investigating message-framing effects in the context of a tailored intervention promoting physical activity. *Health Education Research, 25,* 343–354.

Vandelanotte, C., Reeves, M. M., Brug, J., & De Bourdeaudhuij, I. (2008). A randomized trial of sequential and simultaneous multiple behavior change interventions for physical activity and fat intake. *Preventive Medicine, 46,* 232–237.

Vinson, C., Bickmore, T., Farrell, D., Campbell, M., An, L., Saunders, E., et al. (2011). Adapting research-tested computerized tailored interventions for broader dissemination and implementation. *Translational Behavioral Medicine, 1,* 93–102.

Whittaker, R., Dorey, E., Bramley, D., Bullen, C., Denny, S., Elley, C. R., et al. (2011). A theory-based video messaging mobile phone intervention for smoking cessation: Randomized controlled trial. *Journal of Medical Internet Research, 13,* e10.

Woolford, S. J., Clark, S. J., Strecher, V. J., & Resnicow, K. (2010). Tailored mobile phone text messages as an adjunct to obesity treatment for adolescents. *Journal of Telemedicine & Telecare, 16,* 458–461.

9

MOBILE PHONES FOR HEALTH COMMUNICATION TO PROMOTE BEHAVIOR CHANGE

Lorien C. Abroms, Nalini Padmanabhan, and W. Douglas Evans

We have long known that phones can promote health behavior change. Quitlines and other kinds of phone-based counseling services have been shown to be very effective in promoting smoking cessation, weight loss, and physical activity, and in modifying other health behaviors (Anderson & Zhu, 2007; Castro & King, 2002; Eakin, Lawler, Vandelanotte, & Owen, 2007). The advent of mobile phones and more recently smartphones raises the question of what advances these new technologies and their associated features provide beyond landlines and voice capabilities.

A growing body of evidence indicates that mobile phones have promise in helping people modify health behaviors (Cole-Lewis & Kershaw, 2010; Fjeldsoe, Marshall, & Miller, 2009; Whittaker et al., 2009). Most of these interventions have relied upon the text messaging feature of mobile phones and consisted of a series of automated and sometimes interactive text messages that guide a person through the process of behavior change (Cole-Lewis & Kershaw, 2010; also see Fjeldsoe, Miller, & Marshall, this volume).

Yet, despite the widespread use of mobile phones by the public and the growing evidence base that supports their use in health promotion (Kahn, Yang, & Kahn, 2010), there is a limited understanding of the purposes that mobile phones best address. Little is known about how mobile phones can best be used as adjuncts to other existing programs or campaigns. Furthermore, despite their widespread use, little is known about the utility of smartphones for health promotion.

In this chapter, we review the reach and the appeal of mobile phones, the contexts of current use, and the evidence base for mobile phones in health promotion. Some of the evidence reviewed in this chapter is derived from mobile phone applications in health care, such as treatment adherence and disease self-management.

We also consider the theoretical bases that support these contexts and future directions for research using mobile phones for health promotion, including what we need to know about using mobile phones effectively for health promotion.

Reach of Mobile Phones

Mobile phones can be defined as fully functional telephones that do not require a landline connection (Smith, 2010). They run over wireless communication networks through radio waves or satellite transmissions. The vast majority of mobile phones have capabilities for texting via Short Message Service, or SMS. Mobile phones can be differentiated between basic mobile phones, feature phones, and smartphones (Nusca, 2009; see Table 9.1 for a listing of mobile phone features).

The use of mobile phones is widespread both in developed and developing countries. Globally, mobile phones have higher penetration than any other form of information technology, including landlines, PCs, and televisions (Internet World Stats, 2010). Sixty-seven percent of the world's population has a mobile phone. The prevalence is slightly lower in developing countries, with 57% of the population owning a mobile phone; however, in some developed countries such as Finland, the prevalence approaches 100% (International Telecommunication Union, 2010).

In the United States, 82% of American adults have mobile phones (Lenhart, 2010). Among ethnic minorities, 87% of African American and 87% of English-speaking Hispanic adults own a mobile phone, compared to 80% of white adults. Younger adults are more likely to own a mobile phone than older adults, as are adults with college educations and higher annual incomes (Lenhart, 2010).

Two of the main uses of the mobile phone are voice calling and text messaging. *Text messaging* is defined as a short form of communication transmitted between mobile phones, and is usually limited to 160 characters per message. Texting is more prevalent among minority groups than whites; 79% of African Americans and 83% of English-speaking Hispanics text, whereas 68% of whites text (Smith, 2010), making it a communication technology with higher penetration into minority groups. Texting is also more prevalent among younger mobile phone users. Among texters, teens send on average 50 texts per day, whereas adults average 10 (Lenhart, 2010).

Mobile phones are increasingly used as people's primary phones (International Telecommunication Union, 2010). In the United States in 2010, almost one in three households (29.7%) was a mobile phone–only household, a figure which is on the rise (Frommer, 2010). Mobile phone–only households are more prevalent among younger adults and English-speaking Hispanic adults (Smith, 2010). Mobile phones are also being used as a substitute for other devices, such as cameras and computers. Among adults with mobile phones in the United States, 76% have used them to take a picture, 38% have used them to access the Internet, and 11% have used them to purchase a product. In particular, young adults and African American and Hispanic adults are more likely to use their

Table 9.1 Table of technological features by platform

		Platform		
		Mobile phone		
Features	*Landline*	*Basic mobile phone/ feature phone*[*]	*Smartphone*	*Desktop Computer*
Voice	x	x	x	(x)
Text messaging (SMS)		x	x	
Multimedia messaging		(x)	x	
Instant messaging		(x)	x	x
Camera		x	x	(x)
Video		(x)	x	(x)
Web		(x)	x	x
Email			x	x
Games		(x)	x	x
Multimedia			x	x
Runs simple computer programs			x	x
Runs complicated computer programs				x
GPS			x	
Accelerometers			x	
Links to other devices (e.g., glucometer, pedometer)			x	x
Can receive wireless data from other devices			x	x

x = most models; (x) = some models
[*] Basic mobile phones make and receive telephone calls and are generally grouped with feature phones, which have additional features such as text messaging or a camera.

mobile phones for these non-voice functions than are older adults and whites, respectively (Smith, 2010).

Compared with basic or feature mobile phones, smartphones have more powerful operating systems, which allow them to run small computer programs or applications ("apps") in addition to running the standard features of mobile phones (i.e., voice, text messaging, camera, Web). Because of their more sophisticated operating systems, smartphones have some of the functionality of desktop computers and can offer email, games, multimedia (e.g., music, video), access to the Internet (e.g., social networking), and an assortment of other programs. In addition, smartphones can also link to health-related devices (e.g., glucometers, pedometers, air quality sensors) and nonhealth-related devices (e.g., credit card machines, printers), which also increases the potential functionality of the phone (Patrick, Griswold, Raab, & Intille, 2008).

In the United States, smartphones currently comprise about 25% of the mobile market (Nielsen Wire, 2010; Slivka, 2009), and their proportion of the mobile phone market is expected to rise in the near future (Rand Media Group, 2010). Smartphone users are more likely to be younger, wealthier, and male (Sniderman, 2010). However, smartphone purchases are rising most rapidly in the United States among those with lower SES, as consumers opt for a single mobile device in lieu of multiple devices for communications, Internet access, and entertainment (comScore, 2008). Globally, smartphones are beginning to surge in developing countries, especially among younger people who cannot afford computers (Swartz, 2009).

The proliferation of apps for smartphones is noteworthy. Apps, which are generally distributed to the public through an online store, can add various kinds of functionality to the phone and are most commonly used for games, news, and entertainment (Schonfeld, 2010). The iPhone App Store, which houses more than 225,000 apps for the iPhone (Apple Insider, 2010), offers more apps than any other smartphone platform, although Google's Android Market with 83,000 apps is expected to catch up and surpass the iPhone in the near future (Nielsen Wire, 2010). To date, an estimated six billion iPhone apps have been downloaded from the iPhone App Store (Dediu, 2010).

People report being increasingly reliant on their mobile phones (Taylor & Wang, 2010). In an international survey, 75% of survey respondents stated that they never leave home without their mobile phone (Marketing Charts, 2009). Over half of mobile phone owners in the United States report sleeping with their mobile phones beside their bed (Smith, 2010). An increasing number of people rate their mobile phones as a device that they are "not willing to live without." For young adults, mobile phones rank more highly than televisions as essential devices (Taylor & Wang, 2010). In fact, mobile phones are increasingly being used as television substitutes. Video viewing time in the United States is at an all-time high, with much of the increase coming from use of mobile devices (Nielsen Wire, 2010).

Appeal

Much of the appeal to consumers of mobile phones stems from the ability to receive calls or text messages in any place or setting (Fjeldsoe et al., 2009). Text messages generally arrive instantaneously and are asynchronous, which means that they can be read and replied to when convenient. For users of feature phones or smartphones, there are many additional appealing features of mobile phones beyond telephony or texting. These include being able to access the mobile Web, read and send email, take photos and video, read and post on social networking sites, play games, bank, shop, gamble, navigate with GPS, listen to music, watch videos, and read the news. Indeed, mobile users are increasingly relying on mobile phones as their primary mode of searching the Web and taking photos or videos (Arnsdorf, 2010; Smith, 2010). Compared with landlines, the cost of mobile phones, at least basic mobile phones, is generally cheaper. In some parts of developing countries, mobile phones are the only kind of phone service available, as infrastructure for landlines may be nonexistent (International Telecommunication Union, 2010).

For health promotion purposes and to developers of health promotion programs, mobile phones are appealing as a platform for a number of reasons. Most salient is the potential to offer programs that provide help or exchange health information with a user anytime or anywhere. For existing eHealth or Internet-based interventions, mobile phones present the opportunity to offer these same programs, but with increased access by users given that they can be accessed anywhere. Also appealing is the opportunity to offer new kinds of in-the-moment help, which was not feasible for programs that relied on desktop computers or traditional eHealth formats. This type of help might be especially relevant for in-the-moment decision making, such as overcoming cravings to use drugs or making decisions about which foods to eat. Such types of help could be offered via text messaging (e.g., by sending a keyword to a shortcode to get help), mobile-optimized versions of websites, email, or specific health promotion apps on smartphones.

Another appealing aspect of offering health promotion programs through mobile phones is the ability to have or increase contact time with program participants. For text messages and app-based alerts, health promotion programs can make use of computers to send out proactive messages and thereby sustain or increase contact with individuals over time. These messages may provide follow-up check-ins, reminders, and/or support during key points of decision (e.g., a quit date for smoking cessation). Furthermore, these communications may be tailored and interactive, which may provide additional boosts for behavior change.

Both text messaging programs and smartphone apps have great potential for offering programs on a large scale, as the technology facilitates mass distribution. In the case of texts, once a protocol is developed and tested, messages can easily be scaled up and disseminated on a population level. Indeed, many text messaging programs are currently offered to tens of thousands of people (e.g., SEXINFO, text4baby) or in the case of Project Masiluleke in South Africa, to one million people each day (United Nations Foundation, 2009). Additionally, online app stores have made it possible to easily distribute apps globally. Mobile phone users can download an app directly to their phone from anywhere in the world at any time, provided that they have a phone signal. It is noteworthy that the process of downloading apps to a mobile phone is user friendly, even for those with low levels of computer literacy (Sarasohn-Kahn, 2010).

Interventions for mobile phones are also appealing because they are relatively unobtrusive and confidential. This is important in environments where diseases (such as HIV/AIDS or drug addiction) are taboo or not publicly acknowledged. People can engage with a program in public spaces with relative privacy. Additionally, given high rates of mobile phone use in minority populations and reach into areas that may have limited public health infrastructure, such as rural areas in developing countries (Smith, 2010; United Nations Foundation, 2009), mobile phones, particularly through their text messaging capabilities, are valuable for their ability to send messages to groups with the highest need and/or burdens of disease (Cole-Lewis & Kershaw, 2010). This may be important not only for delivering interventions but also evaluating interventions, as sustained contact is often a challenge to evaluating health promotion programs designed to serve low-income communities (Evans, Christoffel, Necheles, & Becker, 2010).

Finally, mobile applications are also promising for health promotion research and program evaluation. Recent studies have documented the challenges of evaluating health promotion programs designed to serve low-income communities facing health disparities (Evans et al., 2010). Mobile contact with such participants has potential to overcome issues such as panel attrition, which is often due to study participants changing addresses or not being easily tracked using public information. Recent studies have pointed out the challenges observed during the course of data collection, including high mobility and low involvement in systems that enable people to be successfully located such as license and/or vehicle registration records, credit history data, and Internet presence (U.S. Census Bureau, 2007). Use of mobile technology for tracking and data collection has been successful in several areas such as tobacco control (Rodgers et al., 2005), diabetes control (Farmer et al., 2005), and vaccination compliance (Vilella et al., 2004). Mobile phones can help to improve tracking and follow-up for health promotion research by retaining mobile phone numbers and sending periodic text messages to stay in contact with participants.

Contexts of Current Use

There are a wide range of uses of mobile phones for health purposes (mHealth) both domestically and internationally. In a comprehensive report on mobile health by the United Nations Foundation (2009), mHealth applications were grouped into six categories, of which health promotion was one. The six categories were (1) education, awareness, and health promotion; (2) diagnostic and treatment support; (3) communication and training for health care workers; (4) disease and epidemic outbreak tracking; (5) remote monitoring; and (6) data collection (United Nations Foundation, 2009). While the current chapter focuses on mobile health promotion—that is, mobile programs aimed at health education, awareness, and health promotion (Bernhardt, 2010)—it is important to recognize that within the health field, the applications of mobile phones can extend to health care, epidemiology, and disease surveillance.

At the population level, at least in the United States where data are available, use of mobile phones for health-related reasons is low but significant, especially among young adults and minorities. According to a recent U.S. survey, 17% of all U.S. mobile phone owners have used their phone to look up health or medical information, and 9% have downloaded a health-related app. Among young adults, these numbers are higher. Twenty-nine percent have looked up health information on their mobile phone, and 15% have downloaded health-related apps. Hispanics are more likely than other groups to have sought out health information with their mobile phones (Fox, 2010).

A variety of mHealth promotion programs and services do exist, both domestically and internationally, and these appear to be offered and subscribed to at increasing rates. Existing mHealth promotion programs have been designed to address a wide range of health issues, including those related to preventing chronic and infectious diseases such as smoking cessation (Haapala, Barengo, Biggs, Surakka, & Manninen, 2009; Rodgers et al., 2005; Whittaker et al., 2009), weight loss and physical activity (Patrick et al., 2009), sex education, and STD and HIV prevention (Levine, McCright, Dobkin, Woodruff, & Klausner, 2008; Lim, Hocking, Hellard, & Aitken, 2008) and those related to disease management and recovery such as diabetes management (Franklin, Waller, Pagliari, & Greene, 2006; Quinn et al., 2008), asthma management (Kramer, 2010), and treating hypertension (Logan et al., 2007). Services primarily target adults, although some notable exceptions have targeted children and adolescents (Franklin et al., 2006).

Text messaging programs exist in many developed countries, such as the United Kingdom, Norway, and New Zealand (Whittaker et al., 2009), and among developing countries, primarily India, South Africa, Uganda, Peru, and Rwanda (United Nations Foundation, 2009). Smartphone apps, which are primarily distributed through online stores based in the United States, are accessible globally. However, there are few data on the geographic distribution of app downloads. Given the low (but growing) levels of smartphone penetration into developing countries (Kang, 2009), we can assume that use of health promotion smartphone apps primarily takes place in developed countries.

The available mHealth programs generally fall into one of two categories: (1) text and multimedia messaging programs and (2) smartphone applications. We discuss each category in the sections that follow.

Text and Multimedia Messaging

Text and multimedia messaging applications for health promotion typically consist of a series of proactive text or multimedia (i.e., photo or video) messages aimed at giving health information, advice, and reminders for behavior change. Proactive applications can be automated and tied to a preplanned schedule. Interactive messages can involve responses directly from an individual, such as a health care provider or public health practitioner. Additionally, some proactive applications can be used to encourage recipients to engage in other forms of two-way interaction, such as prompting them to call a helpline or visit a clinic.

The vast majority of these programs are text only, although some also include video or photos (Free et al., 2009). An example of a prominent text-based program in the United States is text4baby, a mobile messaging service aimed at prenatal and postnatal health. Users self-enroll by sending the keyword BABY to the shortcode 511411. Once enrolled, subscribers are proactively sent messages three times a week that are timed around the baby's due date and are free for the user to receive (Meehan, 2010). While messages are not interactive, they do encourage recipients to call toll-free hotlines for additional help. The ongoing service has an estimated 90,000 subscribers (Meehan, 2010). In a similar service tested in a recent clinical trial in Kenya, WelTel Kenya 1, HIV-infected adults beginning antiretroviral therapy received weekly text message reminders from a clinic nurse; the reminders required a response within 48 hours. The trial reported increased treatment adherence and suppression of plasma HIV-1 RNA load among treatment patients compared to control patients (Lester et al., 2010). Other common formats for text messaging applications include games or quizzes in which users answer questions to learn about a health issue (e.g., about HIV/AIDS in Uganda [United Nations Foundation, 2009]) or to request health information from the service on an as-needed basis and navigate a decision tree via text to get their question answered (e.g., SEXINFO [Levine et al., 2008]).

Besides format, text messaging programs differ on whether the messages are being sent by a real person (e.g., a clinician or health care worker) or whether the messages are being sent automatically by a computer, as in the case of text-4baby. Typically, more clinically oriented programs such as diabetes management involve messages sent by health care practitioners, sometimes in addition to automated messages (e.g., Franklin et al., 2006). Messages additionally vary across programs in the extent to which the messages are tailored. In some cases, the messages are generic and the same messages go out to all users, as is the case for text4baby. In other cases, the messages are tailored and may be made specific to an individual user's characteristics (e.g., gender, age, zip code, behavioral patterns, triggers as in the case of Text2Quit [Abroms, Thaweethai, Sims, Johiri, & Windsor, 2010]).

Finally, programs also differ in the extent to which they encourage interaction. In some cases, the messages are sent one way with no opportunities to reply (e.g., text4baby), while in other cases the messages are interactive and encourage the users to reply (e.g., quizzes or surveys; tracking progress as in the case of Text2Quit [Abroms et al., 2010]). The resolution of these choice points—concerning format, message sender, tailoring, and interaction—is often driven by logistics (e.g., the history of program offerings) and budgets. In general, untailored, automated programs that only involve one-way alerts are cheaper to run.

Smartphones

For smartphones, there are numerous apps in existence that are health related. One study surveyed all health, medical, and fitness-related apps across the major smartphone app stores (e.g., iPhone, Android, Blackberry, Palm) and identified about 6,000 health-related apps (Dolan, 2010a). Of those, 4,200 were identified as intended for use by consumers and patients and 1,800 were intended for use by health care professionals. The vast majority of all apps identified were designed for the iPhone operating system, followed by the Android operating system (Dolan, 2010a). In other studies, 47 iPhone apps were identified for smoking cessation in the iPhone App Store (Abroms, Padmanabhan, Philips, & Thaweethai, 2011) and 207 were identified for weight loss (Breton, Abroms, & Fuemmeler, 2010).

Estimates on reach for particular apps are difficult to find because most app stores do not disclose to the public how many downloads an app receives. One exception is Google's Android Market, which provides categorical information on downloads (e.g., "0–50" downloads; ">250,000" downloads). On the basis of an analysis of the 500 identified health-related apps in Google's Android Market, Android health apps have been downloaded more than three million times (Dolan, 2010a). For the iPhone, which has the highest numbers of health-related apps (Dolan, 2010a), downloads of health-related apps appear to dwarf the estimates for the Android.

For example, one consistently top-ranking free app in the App Store is WebMD Mobile, which can be used for getting information on health symptoms, conditions, drugs, treatments, and first aid (iPhone App Store, 2010). This app currently ranks fourth behind other free apps (iPhone App Store, 2010), and reports indicate that it has been downloaded more than two million times (Dolan, 2010b). Given the many other popular free and paid apps, a conservative estimate for iPhone health-related app downloads is likely to be in the tens of millions.

It is hard to describe a typical app for health promotion since, given the many capabilities of smartphones, apps can be developed around different functionalities of the phone. Apps make use of the phone's camera to scan food labels and provide nutritional information, use the phone's accelerometer and GPS to track running routes, use Bluetooth technology to link to glucometers and track glycemic load over time (Lanzola et al., 2007), and allow the user to post and read posts on social networking websites aimed at weight loss. Many of the popular health-related apps in the iPhone App Store make use of the phone to track and count information over time. For example, some apps keep personal health records and help users share this information with doctors and emergency workers (Fox, 2010).

One study attempted to characterize all iPhone apps aimed at smoking cessation (Abroms et al., 2011). This study reported that most smoking cessation apps could be categorized as, in rank order of incidence (1) calculators (those that calculated the money and health benefits from quitting), (2) calendars/trackers (those that tracked cigarette intake), (3) rationing apps (those that used the clock and alarm features of the phone to limit smoking to particular times of day), and (4) hypnosis apps (those that used the voice and screen of the phone to hypnotize people for quitting smoking). In this study, almost all of the apps were found to be stand-alone apps with no link to existing services or programs (Abroms et al., 2011). It was also noteworthy that none of these apps made use of text messaging or alerts in addition to the previously mentioned smartphone app functions.

Most of the apps included in the review appeared to be developed by technology companies with little or no involvement from public health agencies, although this appears to be changing as more public health groups develop and release apps.

One notable example of a mobile smoking cessation app—not included in the Abroms et al. (2011) study mentioned above—is the LIVESTRONG iPhone app called MyQuit Coach released in November 2010 (see Figure 9.1). This app guides users through the process of creating a personalized quit plan by setting a goal, whether quitting immediately or gradually decreasing their cigarette use. The app allows users to track their cigarette use by date and time in order to better understand their smoking patterns before quitting. After quitting, they can then use personalized tools, such as photos of loved ones, tips, and progress charts to stay motivated. Users also receive awards in the forms of badges as they make progress toward their goal of quitting (LIVESTRONG, 2010). The app offers opportunities for gaining social support by allowing users to use their app to post and view posts on the MyQuit Coach community board, as well as to post progress on Facebook and Twitter (Demand Media, 2010). While the app strives to follow evidence-based recommendations for smoking cessation (Demand Media, 2010), there is no evaluation to date on its efficacy.

In sum, it is clear that smartphones are increasingly being used for health promotion purposes, but very little is known about how, to what extent, and by whom. This will be one of the emerging focal points of future research in mHealth. With smartphones expected to replace feature phones in the near future (Martin, 2008), the opportunities for health promotion uses will continue to grow. Given the fast pace of change, the research agenda to follow these uses will need to develop rapidly.

Evidence

With regard to text messaging, an emerging body of evidence supports its use for health behavior change in the areas of smoking cessation, weight loss, physical activity, and diabetes management (Cole-Lewis & Kershaw, 2010; Fjeldsoe et al., 2009; Whittaker et al., 2009; also see Fjeldsoe, Miller, & Marshall, this volume), and to a lesser extent for STD prevention and treatment (Lim et al., 2008) and in treating hypertension (Logan et al., 2007). Very little is known about the utility of smartphones and their associated applications for health promotion. A review of the literature found no studies that examined the efficacy of smartphone apps for health promotion or disease management, although a few studies have evaluated the quality of apps for smoking cessation (Abroms et al., 2011), weight loss (Breton et al., 2010), and diabetes self-management (Ciemens, Coon, & Sorli, 2010; Rao, Hou, Golnik, Flaherty, & Vu, 2010), as well as their usability for diabetes self-management (Rao et al., 2010).

Effects from randomized trials of text messaging exist among adolescents and adults, among minority and nonminority populations, and across nationalities,

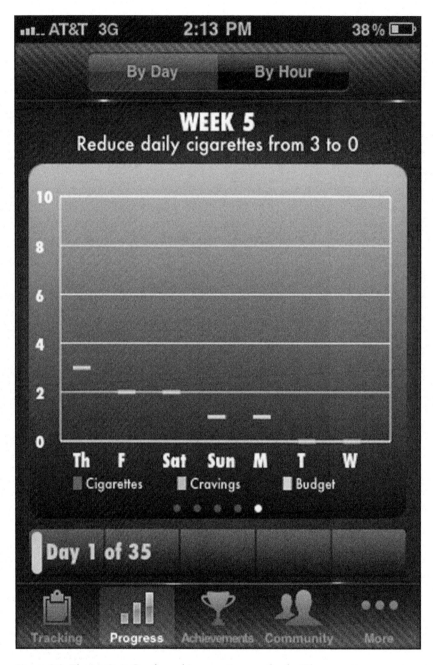

Figure 9.1 The MyQuit Coach smoking cessation app for the iPhone

although none of the studies was conducted in developing countries (Cole-Lewis & Kershaw, 2010). Randomized trials of text messaging with successful outcomes had particular characteristics (see Table 9.2). For example, messages were sent that provided health information, advice, and tips. Users were asked to set goals and track behaviors around these goals and then were given feedback on how they were doing in meeting the goals. Users were also given reminders to do a particular behavior. Some programs used texts to provide social support. For the diabetes management programs that included messages sent by clinicians (Franklin et al., 2006), social support may have simply been getting positive feedback from the clinician.

In other cases, users were offered automated messages from supportive coaches or buddies with whom they could communicate via text (Rodgers et al., 2005). Most programs provided tailored messages, that is, messages that were personalized with the user's name and included personalized reminders and goals (see chapter 8 of this volume). Messages were also tailored on gender, culture, and age. Most programs presented messages that were interactive (see Chung, this volume), and this interactivity varied from asking for feedback on how the user was doing to offering interactive quizzes. The frequency of messages sent ranged from once a week to five or more per day (Cole-Lewis & Kershaw, 2010). Disease prevention studies largely used automated messages while disease management studies included messages from clinicians (Cole-Lewis & Kershaw, 2010).

As noted, studies have evaluated the quality of apps for smoking cessation (Abroms et al., 2011) and weight loss (Breton et al., 2010) as well as the usability of apps for diabetes self-management (Ciemens et al., 2010; Rao et al., 2010). These

Table 9.2 Common approaches in proven health promotion text messaging programs

Approach	Example text message from a hypothetical smoking cessation program
1. Provide health information, advice, and tips that are often tailored around user characteristics	Try using NRT. Smokers who use NRT double their quitrates.
2. Ask users to set goals	How many cigarettes do you hope to cut down to?
3. Provide reinforcement for goals that are met	Congrats! You met your goal.
4. Offer reminders (e.g., to take vitamins, to follow through with goals)	Your quit day is tomorrow.
5. Provide opportunities for tracking progress	Track how many cigarettes you smoked yesterday.
6. Offer social support	Hi! I'm your quitpal. Quitting is tough but if you stick with it, you'll make it through this.

studies have found many of the apps do not follow evidence-based principles, especially in the case of smoking cessation. For example, among 47 smoking cessation apps analyzed, few, if any, apps mentioned, recommended, or linked users to proven treatments and practices based on a list developed from the U.S. Clinical Practice Guidelines (Abroms et al., 2011). This was worrisome, especially since these apps, with the exception of two that linked to a quitline, were independent stand-alone apps. Also worrisome was the fact that while hypnosis apps made up only a fraction of apps available (8%), they dominated what users chose to download (Abroms et al., 2011).

Most of the programs developed using mobile technology for health promotion have been conducted without being guided by behavioral theory, at least based on descriptions in the published literature, which almost exclusively covers text messaging programs (Cole-Lewis & Kershaw, 2010; Fjeldsoe et al., 2009). Some notable exceptions exist, and in these cases the theory used to guide the text messaging program development was social cognitive theory (Rodgers et al., 2005), stages of change theory (Obermayer, Riley, Asif, & Jean-Mary, 2004), or the health belief model (Evans, 2010). In other cases, while no explicit theory was used, some of the practices such as goal setting, cues and reminders, feedback, and reinforcement used in several of the successful projects (e.g., Haapala et al., 2009; Patrick et al., 2009) stem from constructs in traditional behavioral theory (Glanz, Rimer, & Viswanath, 2008).

The text4baby program noted earlier offers one example of a text messaging program that was grounded in theory. First, following the health belief model, text4baby messages serve as a cue to prenatal care action and behavior change for low-income mothers (Glanz, Rimer, & Lewis, 2002). Second, following diffusion theory (Rogers, 1983), text messaging can spread social influence and diffusion of information within a target population. In text4baby, messages diffuse risk information, such as the dangers of alcohol consumption during pregnancy and the benefits of avoiding secondhand smoke both for mother and baby. Third, text4baby uses social cognitive theory to build participants' self-efficacy and provide social models of behavior through text messaging (Bandura, 2004), which helps text4baby develop a brand identity and brand equity (e.g., the brand's market position, consumer loyalty).

In a way, in the mHealth area we find ourselves at the same juncture as in the 1980s, when the personal computer became widespread, or in the 1990s, with the explosion of the Internet. The first impulse was to replicate printed health materials on a computer or on a website. Later insights indicated that programs should make use of the unique capabilities and attributes of computers (Gustafson, Bosworth, Chewning, & Hawkins, 1987) or websites. In a similar vein, we find ourselves with new opportunities with mobile health promotion. Texts and smartphone apps will do best not only guided by behavioral theory but also by an overarching theoretical framework that takes into account in-the-moment cognition of messages and decision making. To date, such theories are lacking.

There is a logical starting point for the development of such a theoretical framework, which is to consider what we have learned from other communication and marketing applications for health. People use mobile devices as one channel for health information in a world filled with other social influences at multiple ecological levels (Maibach, Abroms, & Marosits, 2007). The salience of messages delivered through this channel and audience receptivity must be considered, just as these factors have been staples of health messages delivered through traditional media (Evans, Uhrig, Davis, & McCormack, 2009; Petty & Cacioppo, 1986). Audiences must develop a connection with messages and find them to be credible sources that they can rely on in order to be successful (Evans & Haider, 2008). Health communicators and social marketers have learned that it is critical to build trust and a willingness to participate in programs (Evans, Davis, et al., 2009). Future mHealth programs should build on these lessons to develop health messages that address consumers' quality of life and motivate them to attend to and act upon behavior change promoted through mobile channels. They should aim to make messages and recommended health behaviors fun and reinforcing, thereby providing increased value and benefit for the consumer (Evans, 2010).

Limitations

Despite the appeal of using mobile phones for health promotion, it must be acknowledged that there are a number of limitations of this platform. First and foremost, there is the limitation around access. While access is high overall, especially in the developed world, there remain pockets of the population in the United States with limited access, including the elderly and the poor (Lenhart, 2010). In the case of smartphones, access is overall quite limited, although this is expected to change in the future (Rand Media Group, 2010).

The second limitation revolves around use patterns and usability of mobile phones. While virtually all new mobile phones offer text messaging and access to the Internet, people, for a variety of reasons including cost, may choose not to use these features. People also differ in the extent to which they have their phones near them and therefore are able to receive timely messages from their phone. Another consideration for health promotion program designers is that there is no uniform design for the mobile interface. In some cases, the screen size is very small, limiting the ability to display information, especially textual information.

Perhaps the greatest obstacle in the United States for the widespread dissemination of text messaging programs is the fee structure set by the wireless carriers. While not the case in much of the world outside of the United States, U.S. wireless carriers charge customers to receive (as well as to send) text messages. This makes participating in mobile health promotion programs that involve the receipt of multiple text messages potentially expensive for the end user. Text4baby is notable for having arranged a waiver of fees with the wireless carriers, and in doing so, the program has been able to achieve a high level of dissemination (Meehan, 2010).

However, this arrangement is unprecedented in the health arena, and it remains to be seen whether and to what extent future programs can negotiate a similar fee waiver.

Finally, it is important to note that there may be potential health risks associated with the use of mobile phones. The radiation emitted from mobile phones is considered safe for humans, as most studies have reported no significant association between mobile phone use and disease (e.g. tumors) (Kan, Simonsen, Lyon, & Kestle, 2008; Lahkola, Tokola, & Auvinen, 2006). However, more recent studies indicate that the radiation from mobile phones can lead to alterations in brain activity (Lai & Hardell, 2011; Volkow et al., 2011) and future research is warranted (Volkow et al., 2011). Also, the phenomena of distracted driving, whereby people text on their phones while driving, has been implicated as a prime cause of the recent increase in traffic fatalities in the United States (McCartt, Hellinga, & Bratiman, 2006; Wilson & Stimpson, 2010). Distracted driving represents a serious public health issue worthy of attention and intervention.

Conclusions and Areas for Future Research

In spite of these limitations, and because of widespread penetration, there is a growing sense among health promotion professionals that mobile phones can be effectively used to promote health. By reaching people throughout their day, mobile phones may raise the salience of health behavior change in people's minds and help people track progress, reach goals, obtain social support, and ultimately, change behavior. There is some evidence, in the case of text messaging, to support this excitement because text messaging programs have been shown, at least in the short term, to be effective in promoting smoking cessation, weight loss, and physical activity. The promise of smartphones is to add multimedia and other types of functionality to text messaging-based programs. Although smartphone apps for changing health behaviors abound, there is no evidence to date to support their use. In fact, what little is known suggests that currently available apps, at least for smoking cessation and weight loss, should be approached cautiously, especially as stand-alone programs.

Future research needs to explore how basic mobile phones and smartphones can best be utilized for health promotion, both as stand-alone programs and as adjuncts to existing programs. The existing (and growing) literature on Internet-based interventions can help to inform new programs, but questions remain that are specific to the mobile platform and how to best make use of its capabilities. Specific questions of interest for text messages include identifying the appropriate dose of text messages (e.g., both frequency of sending messages and time period for sending the messages), the appropriate content for text messages (e.g., framing of messages, how to minimize health literacy demands), and how to involve multimedia, as many feature phones now support text messages with photos and videos. With smartphone apps, questions of interest are more basic and center on whether we can design apps that are engaging and result in behavior change. Given the successes of text messaging, it seems that it would be wise to build on these successes of text messaging coupled with the multimedia functionality of smartphones, something that very few apps currently do.

Finally, research is needed to develop and test new theories that can guide the development of mobile-based health promotion programs. Theories are needed that integrate health behavior theory with the types of in-the-moment communication and decision making that are the hallmarks of communication through mobile phones.

References

Abroms, L. C., Padmanabhan, N., Philips, T., & Thaweethai, L. (2011). iPhone apps for smoking cessation: A content analysis. *American Journal of Preventative Medicine, 40,* 279–285.

Abroms, L. C., Thaweethai, L., Sims, J., Johiri, R., & Windsor, R. W. (2010, November). *The Text2Quit Program: Results from a pilot test of an interactive mobile health program designed to help people quit smoking.* Paper presented at the mHealth Summit, Washington, DC.

Anderson, C. M., & Zhu, S-H. (2007). Tobacco quitlines: Looking back and looking ahead. *Tobacco Control, 16,* i81–i86.

Apple Insider. (2010, June 7). *Apple says App Store has made developers over $1 billion.* Retrieved October 2, 2010, from: http://www.appleinsider.com/articles/10/06/07/apple_says_app_store_has_made_developers_over_1_billion.html.

Arnsdorf, I. (2010, June 23). The best shot: Cell or camera? *Wall Street Journal.* Retrieved October 2, 2010, from: http://online.wsj.com/article/SB10001424052748704853404575322794209091082.html.

Bandura, A. (2004). Health promotion by social cognitive means. *Health Education and Behavior, 31,* 143–164.

Bernhardt, J. (2010, November). *mHealth promotion.* Paper presented at the American Public Health Association Annual Meeting, Philadelphia, PA.

Breton, E., Abroms, L. C., & Fuemmeler, B. F. (2010). *Weight loss iPhone applications and their adherence to best practices for weight loss: A content analysis.* Unpublished manuscript.

Castro, C. M., & King, A. C. (2002). Telephone-assisted counseling for physical activity. *Exercise and Sport Sciences Reviews, 30,* 64–68.

Ciemens, E., Coon, P., & Sorli, C. (2010). An analysis of data management tools for diabetes self-management: Can smart phone technology keep up? *Journal of Diabetes Science and Technology, 4,* 958–960.

Cole-Lewis, H., & Kershaw, T. (2010). Text messaging as a tool for behavior change in disease prevention and management. *Epidemiologic Reviews, 32,* 56–69.

comScore. (2008, October 27). *In tough economy, lower income mobile consumers turn to iPhone as Internet & entertainment device* [Press release]. Retrieved December 8, 2009, from: http://www.comscore.com/Press_Events/Press_Releases/2008/10/Lower_Income_Mobile_Consumers_use_Iphone/(language)/eng-US.

Dediu, H. (2010, September 8). iTunes app total downloads to overtake songs this year. *Asymco.* Retrieved October 2, 2010, from: http://www.asymco.com/2010/09/08/itunes-app-total-downloads-to-overtake-songs-this-year/.

Demand Media. (2010, November 17). *Livestrong.com dares you to quit smoking* [Press release]. Retrieved January 19, 2011, from: http://www.demandmedia.com/press-releases/2010/11/17/livestrongcom-dares-you-to-quit-smoking.

Dolan, B. (2010a, March 11). 3 million downloads for Android health apps. *MobiHealthNews*. Retrieved October 12, 2010, from: http://mobihealthnews.com/6908/3-million-downloads-for-android-health-apps.

Dolan, B. (2010b, October 7). WebMD personalizes WebMD Mobile with PHR data. *MobiHealthNews*. Retrieved October 12, 2010, from: http://mobihealthnews.com/9121/webmd-personalizes-webmd-mobile-with-phr-data/.

Eakin, E. G., Lawler, S. P., Vandelanotte, C., & Owen, N. (2007). Telephone interventions for physical activity and dietary behavior change: A systematic review. *American Journal of Preventive Medicine, 32,* 419–434.

Evans, W. D. (2010, August). *Evaluation of mobile health interventions: Case study of text4baby*. Paper presented at the 4th Annual CDC Health Marketing Conference, Atlanta, GA.

Evans, W. D., Christoffel, K. K., Necheles, J. W., & Becker, A. B. (2010). Social marketing as a childhood obesity prevention strategy. *Obesity, 18,* S23–S26.

Evans, W. D., Davis, K. C., Ashley, O. S., Blitstein, J., Koo, H., & Zhang, Y. (2009). Efficacy of abstinence promotion media messages: Findings from an online randomized trial. *Journal of Adolescent Health, 45,* 409–416.

Evans, W. D., & Haider, M. (2008). Public health brands in the developing world. In W. D. Evans and G. Hastings (Eds.), *Public health branding: Applying marketing for social change* (pp. 215–232). London: Oxford University Press.

Evans, W. D., Uhrig, J., Davis, K., & McCormack, L. (2009). Efficacy methods to evaluate health communication and marketing campaigns. *Journal of Health Communication, 14,* 315–330.

Farmer, A. J., Gibson, O. J., Dudley, C., Bryden, K., Hayton, P. M., Tarassenko, T., et al. (2005). A randomized controlled trial of the effect of real-time telemedicine support on glycemic control in young adults with type 1 diabetes. *Diabetes Care, 28,* 2697–2702.

Fjeldsoe, B. S., Marshall, A. L., & Miller, Y. D. (2009). Behavior change interventions delivered by mobile telephone short-message service. *American Journal of Preventive Medicine, 36,* 165–173.

Fox, S. (2010, October 19). Mobile health 2010. *Pew Internet and American Life Project*. Retrieved October 19, 2010, from: http://pewinternet.org/Reports/2010/Mobile-Health-2010.aspx.

Franklin, V. L., Waller, A., Pagliari, C., & Greene, S. A. (2006). A randomized controlled trial of Sweet Talk, a text-messaging system to support young people with diabetes. *Diabetic Medicine, 23,* 1332–1338.

Free, C., Whittaker, R., Knight, R., Abramsky, T., Rodgers, A., & Roberts, I. G. (2009). Txt2stop: A pilot randomised controlled trial of mobile phone-based smoking cessation support. *Tobacco Control, 18,* 88–91.

Frommer, D. (2010, August 18). Chart of the day: Almost a third of U.S. households have cut the landline cord. *Business Insider*. Retrieved October 2, 2010, from: http://www.businessinsider.com/chart-of-the-day-almost-a-third-of-us-households-have-cut-the-landline-cord-2010-8.

Glanz, K., Rimer B. K., & Lewis, F. M. (Eds.). (2002). *Health behavior and health education: Theory, research, and practice* (3rd ed.). San Francisco: Jossey-Bass.

Glanz, K., Rimer, B. K., & Viswanath, K. (Eds.). (2008). *Health behavior: Theory, research, and practice* (4th ed.). San Francisco: Jossey-Bass.

Gustafson, D. H., Bosworth, K., Chewning, B., & Hawkins, R. P. (1987). Computer-based health promotion: Combining technological advances with problem-solving techniques to effect successful health behavior changes. *Annual Reviews of Public Health, 8,* 387–415.

Haapala, I., Barengo, N. C., Biggs, S., Surakka, L., & Manninen, P. (2009). Weight loss by mobile phone: A 1-year effectiveness study. *Public Health Nutrition, 12,* 2382–2391.

International Telecommunication Union. (2010). *Measuring the Information Society 2010* [Report brief]. Retrieved September 29, 2010, from: http://www.itu.int/ITU-D/ict/publications/idi/2010/Material/MIS_2010_Summary_E.pdf.

Internet World Stats. (2010). *Usage and population statistics.* Retrieved October 12, 2010, from: http://www.internetworldstats.com/stats.htm.

iPhone App Store. (2010). Retrieved October 10, 2010, from: http://www.apple.com/iphone/from-the-app-store/.

Kahn, J. G., Yang, J. S., & Kahn, J. S. (2010). "Mobile" health needs and opportunities in developing countries. *Health Affairs, 29,* 252–258.

Kan, P., Simonsen, S. E., Lyon, J. L., & Kestle, J. R. W. (2008). Cellular phone use and brain tumor: A meta-analysis. *Journal of Neurooncology, 86,* 71–78.

Kang, T. (2009, October 8). Smartphone growth in emerging markets. *Strategy Analytics.* Retrieved October 12, 2010, from: http://www.strategyanalytics.com/default.aspx?mod=ReportAbstractViewer&a0=5062.

Kramer, C. (2010, April 22). M-health: Blue Flow mobile sensor would monitor asthma conditions. *Mobile Behavior Blog.* Retrieved October 12, 2010, from: http://www.mobilebehavior.com/2010/04/22/m-health-blue-flow-mobile-sensor-would-monitor-asthma-conditions/.

Lahkola, A., Tokola, K., & Auvinen, A. (2006). Meta-analysis of mobile phone use and intracranial tumors. *Scandinavian Journal of Work, Environment, and Health, 32,* 171–177.

Lai, H., & Hardell, L. (2011). Cell phone radiofrequency radiation exposure and brain glucose metabolism. *Journal of the American Medical Association, 305,* 828–829.

Lanzola, G., Capozzi, D., D'Annunzio, G., Ferrari, P., Bellazzi, R., & Larizza, C. (2007). Going mobile with a multiaccess service for the management of diabetic patients. *Journal of Diabetes Science and Technology, 1,* 730–737.

Lenhart, A. (2010, September 2). Cell phones and American adults. *Pew Internet & American Life Project.* Retrieved October 2, 2010, from: http://pewinternet.org/Reports/2010/Cell-Phones-and-American-Adults/Overview.aspx.

Lester, R. T., Ritvo, P., Mills, E. J., Kariri, A., Karanja, S., Chung, M. H., et al. (2010). Effects of a mobile phone short message service on antiretroviral treatment adherence in Kenya (WelTel Kenya 1): A randomized trial. *Lancet, 376,* 1838–1845.

Levine, D., McCright, J., Dobkin, L., Woodruff, A. J., & Klausner, J. D. (2008). SEXINFO: A sexual health text messaging service for San Francisco youth. *American Journal of Public Health, 98,* 393–395.

Lim, M. S. C., Hocking, J. S., Hellard, M. E., & Aitken, C. K. (2008). SMS STI: A review of the uses of mobile phone text messaging in sexual health. *International Journal of STD & AIDS, 19,* 287–290.

LIVESTRONG. (2010). *MyQuit Coach—Dare to quit smoking mobile app.* Retrieved January 19, 2011, from: http://www.livestrong.com/quit-smoking-app/.

Logan, A. G., McIsaac, W. J., Tisler, A., Irvine, M. J., Saunders, A., Dunai, A., et al. (2007). Mobile phone-based remote patient monitoring system for management of hypertension in diabetic patients. *American Journal of Hypertension, 20,* 942–948.

Maibach, E. W., Abroms, L. C., & Marosits, M. (2007). Communication and marketing as tools to cultivate the public's health: A proposed "people and places" framework. *BMC Public Health, 7,* 88–103.

Marketing Charts. (2009, October 2). *Half of Americans sleep with cellphone.* Retrieved October 12, 2010, from: http://www.marketingcharts.com/interactive/half-of-americans-sleep-with-cellphone-10620/.

Martin, R. (2008, April 1). Cell phones face extinction as smartphones take over. *Information Week.* Retrieved October 12, 2010, from: http://www.informationweek.com/news/mobility/converence/showArticle.jhtml?articleID=207000858.

McCartt, A. T., Hellinga, L. A., & Bratiman, K. A. (2006). Cell phones and driving: Review of research. *Traffic Injury Prevention, 7,* 89–106.

Meehan, J. (2010, August). *Text4baby promotional strategy.* Paper presented at CDC Conference on Health Marketing, Atlanta, GA.

Nielsen Wire. (2010, August 2). *Android soars, but iPhone still most desired as smartphones grab 25% of U.S. mobile market.* Retrieved September 29, 2010, from: http://blog.nielsen.com/nielsenwire/online_mobile/android-soars-but-iphone-still-most-desired-as-smartphones-grab-25-of-u-s-mobile-market/.

Nusca, A. (2009, August 20). Smartphone vs. feature phone arms race heats up; which did you buy? *ZDNet.* Retrieved October 12, 2010, from: http://www.zdnet.com/blog/gadgetreviews/smartphone-vs-feature-phone-arms-race-heats-up-which-did-you-buy/6836.

Obermayer, J. L., Riley, W. T., Asif, O., & Jean-Mary, J. (2004). College smoking-cessation using cell phone text messaging. *Journal of American College Health, 53,* 71–78.

Patrick, K., Griswold, W. G., Raab, F., & Intille, S. S. (2008). Health and the mobile phone. *American Journal of Preventive Medicine, 35,* 177–181.

Patrick, K., Rabb, F., Adams, M. A., Dillon, L., Zabinski, M., Rock, C. L., et al. (2009). A text message-based intervention for weight loss: Randomized controlled trial. *Journal of Medical Internet Research, 11,* e1.

Petty, R. E., & Cacioppo, J. T. (1986). The elaboration likelihood model of persuasion. *Advances in Experimental Social Psychology, 19,* 123–205.

Quinn, C. C., Clough, S. S., Minor, J. M., Lender, D., Okafor, M. C., & Gruber-Baldini, A. (2008). WellDoc mobile diabetes management randomized controlled trial: Change in clinical and behavioral outcomes and patient and physician satisfaction. *Diabetes Technology & Therapeutics, 10,* 160–168.

Rand Media Group. (2010). *Smartphone market set to grow.* Retrieved October 2, 2010, from: http://www.randmediagroup.com/smartphone-market-set-to-grow.

Rao, A., Hou, P., Golnik, T., Flaherty, J., & Vu, S. (2010). Evolution of data management tools for managing self-monitoring of blood glucose results: A survey of iPhone applications. *Journal of Diabetes Science and Technology, 4,* 949–957.

Rodgers, A., Corbett, T., Bramley, D., Riddell, T., Wills, M., Lin, R. B., et al. (2005). Do u smoke after txt? Results of a randomized trial of smoking cessation using mobile phone text messaging. *Tobacco Control, 14,* 255–261.

Rogers, E. M. (1983). *Diffusion of innovations.* New York: Free Press.

Sarasohn-Kahn, J. (2010, April). How smartphones are changing health care for consumers and reporters. *California Health Care Foundation.* Retrieved October 12, 2010, from: http://www.chcf.org/publications/2010/04/how-smartphones-are-changing-health-care-for-consumers-and-providers.

Schonfeld, E. (2010, February 25). When it comes to iPhone games, what sells is action, adventure, and arcade. *TechCrunch.* Retrieved October 12, 2010, from: http://techcrunch.com/2010/02/25/iphone-games-what-sells-distimo/.

Slivka, E. (2009, December 17). iPhone finally surpasses Windows Mobile in U.S. smartphone usage. *MacRumors.* Retrieved January 6, 2009, from: http://www.macrumors.com/2009/12/17/iphone-finally-surpasses-windows-mobile-in-u-s-smartphone-usage/.

Smith, A. (2010, July 7). Mobile access 2010. *Pew Internet & American Life Project*. Retrieved July 8, 2010, from: http://pewinternet.org/Reports/2010/Mobile-Access-2010/Summary-of-Findings.aspx.

Sniderman, Z. (2010, August 26). Why smartphone adoption may not be as big as you think. *Mashable*. Retrieved September 29, 2010, from: http://mashable.com/2010/08/26/smartphone-adoption-trends/.

Swartz, J. (2009, October 21). Marketers salivating over smartphone potential. *USA Today*. Retrieved October 12, 2010, from: http://www.usatoday.com/tech/news/2009-10-20-social-network-smartphone_N.htm.

Taylor, P., & Wang, W. (2010, August 19). The fading glory of the television and telephone. *Pew Research Center Social and Demographic Trends*. Retrieved October 12, 2010, from: http://pewsocialtrends.org/pubs/762/fading-glory-television-telephone-luxury-necessity.

United Nations Foundation. (2009). *mHealth for development: The opportunity of mobile technology for healthcare in the developing world*. Retrieved October 12, 2010, from: http://www.unfoundation.org/press-center/publications/mhealth-for-development-mobile-technology-for-healthcare.html.

U.S. Census Bureau. (2007). *American Community Survey*. Retrieved October 11, 2010, from: http://www.census.gov/acs.

Vilella, A., Bayas, J-M., Diaz, M-T., Guinovart, C., Diez, C., Simó, D., et al. (2004). The role of mobile phones in improving vaccination rates in travelers. *Preventive Medicine, 38*, 503–509.

Volkow, N. D., Tomasi, D., Wang, G-J., Vaska, P., Fowler, J. S., Telang, F., et al. (2011). Effects of cell phone radiofrequency signal and exposure on brain glucose metabolism. *Journal of the American Medical Association, 305*, 808–813.

Whittaker, R., Borland, R., Bullen, C., Lin, R. B., McRobbie, H., & Rodgers, A. (2009). Mobile phone-based interventions for smoking cessation. *Cochrane Database of Systematic Reviews, 4*, 1–22.

Wilson, F. A., & Stimpson, J. P. (2010). Trends in fatalities from distracted driving in the United States, 1999 to 2008. *American Journal of Public Health, 100*, 2213–2219.

10

TEXT MESSAGING INTERVENTIONS FOR CHRONIC DISEASE MANAGEMENT AND HEALTH PROMOTION

Brianna S. Fjeldsoe, Yvette D. Miller,
and Alison L. Marshall

It is hard to imagine a world without the mobile phone: The personal convenience it affords has revolutionized the way people communicate. Mobile phone use is almost ubiquitous in developed countries and is becoming rapidly integrated in developing countries. In 2010, there were an estimated five billion mobile phone subscriptions worldwide, and these subscriptions were increasing at a rate of two million every day (International Telecommunication Union, 2010a). Although the number of subscriptions does not necessarily reflect the number of individuals using mobile phones (one person can have multiple subscriptions, and one subscription may serve multiple users), we are fast approaching a world with one mobile phone subscription per person.

Text messages are the economical way of using a mobile phone to keep in touch, give quick updates, or send reminders. The ability of broadcast programs to create personally tailored text messages and to efficiently communicate them en masse has attracted the attention of health behavior change professionals. Three systematic reviews that appraised the peer-reviewed literature concluded that text-based behavior change interventions can be effectively delivered (Atun & Sittampalam, 2006; Cole-Lewis & Kershaw, 2010; Fjeldsoe, Marshall, & Miller, 2009). In addition to these systematic reviews, a particularly good selection of case study commentaries has been published by the Stanford Persuasive Technology Lab (Fogg & Adler, 2009; Fogg & Eckles, 2008). This chapter aims to provide an understanding of recent evidence about how text messaging is used in behavior change interventions, the limitations of using text messaging to deliver interventions, and future directions of text-based behavior change interventions.

What Is Text Messaging?

A *text message* is a short written message, usually limited to 160 characters, sent from one mobile phone to another or from an operator to a mobile phone via the SMS.[1] Text message services are colloquially referred to as "texts," "SMS," and "TMS," depending on region and culture. Other mobile phone technologies have been used to transmit health information; these include image or video messaging and Web-based applications (see Abroms, Padmanabhan, & Evans, this volume). Of these technologies, text messaging is currently the most widely adopted and least expensive mobile phone technology (Fogg & Adler, 2009). The emerging importance of text messaging is evident in the redesign of mobile phone handsets (e.g., mobile phone keypads that resemble computer keyboards, the development of predictive text functions for faster texting). Popularity has grown to the extent that the term *texting* (a verb meaning the act of sending text messages) has entered the common lexicon and is listed in the Merriam-Webster Dictionary.

Contexts in Which Text Messaging Is Used

Text messages are used for a variety of health-related purposes, including to (1) enhance health service provision (e.g., appointment reminders), (2) distribute mass health education messages (e.g., sexual health education), (3) encourage better disease self-management practices (e.g., medication adherence), and (4) deliver personalized health promotion interventions (e.g., smoking cessation programs).

Text messages are commonly being used to enhance health care service provision. Appointment reminders via text message have improved business efficiency by decreasing the number of missed appointments (Downer, Meara, & Da Costa, 2005; Foley & O'Neill, 2009). Reminder services have also improved patient outcomes by prompting adherence to repeated vaccinations (Kharbanda, Stockwell, Fox, & Rickert, 2009; Vilella et al., 2004), HIV antiretroviral medications (Andrade et al., 2005; Fairley et al., 2003), atopic dermatitis treatments (Pena-Robichaux, Kvedar, & Watson, 2010), and breast self-examinations (Khokhar, 2009). There are examples of sexual health clinics using text messages to deliver test results, trace sexual partners, and monitor contraceptive adherence (Lim, Hocking, Hellard, & Aitken, 2008). These uses of text messaging take advantage of its cost-effectiveness for replacing conventional forms of communication (e.g. telephone calls, mailed print materials) in health care service delivery.

Another use of text messages, facilitated by their one-to-many feature, is mass communication of health education messages. Some countries are exploring the use of text messages to distribute health warnings about communicable disease outbreaks (Atun & Sittampalam, 2006; Kaplan, 2006), although these systems are reliant upon consumers opting in, thus minimizing the potential of a hypothetically efficient system. This mass distribution approach also carries the risk of desensitizing receivers to repeated, impersonal messages.

Text messaging systems are rapidly being adapted to deliver programs that educate, support, and facilitate self-management of chronic disease and behavior change (Cole-Lewis & Kershaw, 2010; Fjeldsoe et al., 2009). Compared with evidence for other mediated approaches such as print, phone, or the Internet, the evidence for text messaging interventions is relatively new. The first evaluation of a text-based health behavior change program appeared in the scientific literature in 2002, when a letter to the editor in the *British Medical Journal* touted, "Mobile phone text messaging can help young people manage asthma" (Neville, Greene, McLeod, Tracy, & Surie, 2002, p. 600). Since then there has been a steady increase in the number of papers appearing in the peer-reviewed literature.

Why Is Text Messaging Appropriate for Behavior Change?

The distinctive features of text messaging adapt perfectly to known characteristics of effective health behavior change interventions: commonly used theories (e.g., self-regulation theory, social cognitive theory), behavior change strategies (e.g., self-monitoring), and principles of effective social marketing (e.g., personally tailored, engaging language, require minimal active retrieval by recipients). Text messaging (1) is accessible by the majority of the population, (2) has relatively low cost and recipient burden, (3) can reach people in a place and at a time that is most meaningful for individual behavior change, (4) allows for efficient individual tailoring, and (5) can develop a virtual relationship that enables interactivity and accountability.

Mass Reach and Accessibility

The rapid integration of text messaging into virtually all aspects of society across the world creates an opportunity for cost-effective delivery of health behavior change messages at the population level. Today text messaging is the most widely used mobile data service. Approximately 80% of all mobile phone subscribers worldwide are active text message users, with particularly high use in Finland, Sweden, and Norway (over 85% of the population [Portio Research, 2010]) and Australia (88% of the population [Australian Communications and Media Authority, 2009]). There are also high rates of text message use in China (the average person sends four texts/day [Zhang & Prybutok, 2005]) and the Philippines (the average person sends 19 texts/day [Evans, 2009]).

Text messaging reaches population groups at higher risk of poor health that are often excluded when using other communication channels (Atun & Sittampalam, 2006; Dutta-Bergman, 2005; Haller, Sanci, Sawyer, Coffey, & Patton, 2006; Leena, Tomi, & Arja, 2005). The digital divide along the socioeconomic gradient is less pronounced for mobile phone use than for other communication technologies, such as the Internet (Forestier, Grace, & Kenny, 2002; Rice & Katz, 2003). The low cost of text messaging and the simple user interface have contributed to the successful adoption of mobile phones with the less economically advantaged and less literate. Almost 80% of adult Americans and more than 97% of young Australians are willing to engage in health programs delivered via text messaging (Cellular Telecommunications Industry Association, 2009; Haller et al., 2006). Numerous studies in specific population groups (described later in this chapter) also demonstrate the high levels of acceptance for interventions delivered via text messaging.

Low Cost

Text messages can be delivered at a cost lower than postal, voice phone, or face-to-face communication (Atun & Sittampalam, 2006). On average, one text message costs less than a quarter of one voice minute for prepaid mobile phone services (International Telecommunication Union, 2010b). Messages can also be automated and preprogrammed, minimizing time and effort in data entry. One of the only studies to investigate the cost-effectiveness of text messaging was a study promoting chlamydia screening among Australian tertiary education students, which found that using traditional promotional approaches (e.g., flyers, events) cost AUD$175.11 per test versus AUD$27.13 per test using text messaging and a AUD$10 cash incentive to get tested (Currie et al., 2010). The low cost of text messaging increases the capacity for longer term intervention contact, which has demonstrated benefits for behavior change maintenance after intensive intervention periods (Fjeldsoe, Neuhaus, Winkler, & Eakin, 2011; Fry & Neff, 2009).

Accessibility in Space and Time

Text messages are sent to handheld devices that are in a person's almost constant possession, providing instantaneous and direct access to individuals. Behavioral cues to action, reinforcement, social support, and other key constructs of effective behavior change can be delivered to people in real time and in their own environment, where the messages received may be most relevant and conducive to encouraging or reinforcing healthy choices. The possibility of linking message delivery with mobile phone global positioning systems also provides an opportunity to prompt about proximal health opportunities in real time. For example, persons could be sent a text message when in close proximity to a walking track to prompt them to use it, or when in proximity to a grocery store, they could be reminded about their dietary goals.

Asynchronous communication such as text messaging (the sender and receiver not necessarily concurrently engaged in conversation) carries low participant burden compared with other communication methods. Text messages can reach people on voice calls at the time of receipt, can be sent and received when it is impractical to have audible conversations, and can be accessed by the recipient when it is convenient and potentially most useful for reinforcing behavior. The capacity to save and store text messages enables individuals to keep messages that they find most useful and to refer to them when and as often as they like.

Personally Tailored Communication

There is substantial evidence supporting the importance of tailoring intervention content to individuals' characteristics for improving the effectiveness of mass-reach behavior change interventions (Kreuter, Strecher, & Glassman, 1999; Noar, Benac, & Harris, 2007; Ryan & Lauver, 2002; also see chapter 8 of this volume). Text messaging programs enable customized messaging via predeveloped systems and automated databases that incorporate personal data from recipients. Text messaging interventions that use individually tailored messages more commonly influence behavioral outcomes than untailored text message interventions (Fjeldsoe et al., 2009). Additionally, the confidentiality and direct communication features of text messaging make it suitable for the transfer of personal information (Atun & Sittampalam, 2006).

Interactivity and Accountability

Text messaging allows for a "virtual personal relationship" to be established between the sender and recipient, without the necessity of voice-to-voice contact (Franklin, Waller, Pagliari, & Greene, 2003; Obermayer, Riley, Asif, & Jean-Mary, 2004). Text messaging can be much more conversational and interactive than email or written materials, as evidenced by the extensive use of question-answer dialogue in many text-based interventions (Fjeldsoe et al., 2009; Katz & Aakhus, 2002). Text message interactivity can also support self-monitoring strategies shown to be important for changing physical activity and dietary behaviors (Michie, Abraham, Whittington, McAteer, & Gupta, 2009) and maintaining weight loss (Butryn, Phelan, Hill, & Wing, 2007; Wing & Phelan, 2005). Frequent text messaging can develop a relationship between recipient and sender that reinforces accountability and emotional support for behavior change. Text messages can be used to unobtrusively remind people to monitor and report on their progress and provide an important opportunity for supportive feedback tailored to recent successes or failures.

Outcomes of Text Messaging Interventions

The last decade has seen a rapid increase in the number of published articles that report on text message interventions for health behavior change (Figure 10.1). A systematic search of PubMed, MEDLINE, Web of Science, and PsycINFO for articles published between 2000 and 2010 including the keywords *mobile phone or cell phone, SMS or text message, health or health intervention, and behavior* resulted

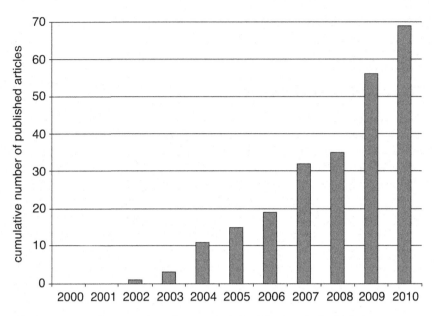

Figure 10.1 Cumulative number of peer-reviewed publications on health behavior change interventions delivered via text message over the past decade

in 69 intervention studies. These interventions cover a variety of chronic disease management strategies related to diabetes ($n = 13$), asthma ($n = 7$), weight loss ($n = 9$), hypertension ($n = 3$), vaccination ($n = 3$), HIV ($n = 5$), or other treatment adherence ($n = 9$). There is also a growing interest in using text message programs to promote healthy behaviors, most commonly physical activity ($n = 8$), smoking cessation ($n = 6$), sexual health behaviors ($n = 4$), regular breast self-examinations ($n = 1$), and regular sunscreen use ($n = 1$). The following section provides an overview of relevant study findings from the most advanced areas of research, highlighting reasons for intervention success and areas requiring further investigation.

Chronic Disease Self-Management Interventions

To date the most common text message interventions have targeted chronic disease self-management among clinically diagnosed populations. Thirteen interventions were found that targeted improved management of type 1 or type 2 diabetes mellitus in children and adolescents (Carroll, Marrero, & Downs, 2007; Franklin, Waller, Pagliari, & Greene, 2006; Gammon et al., 2005; Hanauer, Wentzell, Laffel, & Laffel, 2009; Rami, Popow, Horn, Waldhoer, & Schober, 2006; Wangberg, Arsand, & Andersson, 2006) or adults (Benhamou et al., 2007; Cho, Lee, Lim, Kwon, & Yoon, 2009; Ferrer-Roca, Cardenas, Diaz-Cardama, & Pulido, 2004;

Kim, 2007; Kollmann, Reidl, Kastner, Schreier, & Ludvik, 2007; Kwon et al., 2004; Vahatalo, Virtamo, Viikari, & Ronnemaa, 2004). Seven interventions targeted improved management of asthma in adolescents (Holtz & Whitten, 2009; Ostojic et al., 2005; Pinnock, Slack, Pagliari, & Sheikh, 2007) or adults (Anhoj & Moldrup, 2004; Cleland, Caldow, & Ryan, 2007; Prabhakaran, Chee, Chua, Abisheganaden, & Wong, 2010; Strandbygaard, Thomsen, & Backer, 2010). The primary behaviors targeted in these interventions were regular symptom monitoring (e.g., blood glucose monitoring, asthma symptom monitoring) and medication adherence.

All 20 interventions targeted compliance with regular symptom monitoring. Symptom data were collected using blood glucose monitors or peak expiratory flow meters (to measure lung capacity) that were integrated into mobile phone handsets (e.g., Carroll et al., 2007) and were connected via infrared technologies/ USB cable (e.g., Cleland et al., 2007; Gammon et al., 2005) or relied on participants manually entering their data via text message (e.g., Anhoj & Moldrup, 2004). Two studies required patients to submit symptom data via a separate website (Ferrer-Roca et al., 2004; Kim, 2007). The authors of these studies reported low use of the Web for data entry and participants' preference for text message-delivered components of the intervention. All studies also targeted medication adherence and required health care professionals to survey the symptom monitoring and medication adherence data to tailor the advice provided to participants.

Outcomes reported in these studies are mostly clinical indicators of diabetes or asthma management. Diabetes trials show clinically meaningful decreases in fluctuations of blood glucose levels (HbA1c) ranging from 0.25% (Benhamou et al., 2007) to 1.15% (Kim, 2007). While clinical outcomes used to monitor asthma management varied between trials (e.g., improved lung function [reductions in peak expiratory flow variability] [e.g., Ostojic et al., 2005], reduced number of asthma treatments [nebualizations] [e.g., Prabhakaran et al., 2010]), all of the trials found positive, clinically meaningful outcomes among participants. Some of the diabetes interventions also targeted healthy dietary behaviors and regular physical activity (Franklin et al., 2006; Hanauer et al., 2009; Kim, 2007; Kollmann et al., 2007; Kwon et al., 2004; Rami et al., 2006; Wangberg et al., 2006); however, none reported on behavioral outcomes. Only one study stated that the intervention was developed based on behavioral theory (Franklin et al., 2006).

Importantly, the diabetes and asthma management trials collected qualitative and process evaluation data (Table 10.1). Common themes from these evaluations are that people perceive a greater feeling of control over their diabetes (Franklin et al., 2003) or asthma symptoms (Cleland et al., 2007; Pinnock et al., 2007) while engaging with text-based support. Parents of young children expressed a greater feeling of engagement in their children's diabetes control when they received regular texts (Gammon et al., 2005; Wangberg et al., 2006). However, some participants expressed concern about perceptions of "nagging" or "spying" on children (Gammon et al., 2005) or of increased dependence on health care professionals (Pinnock et al., 2007). A key feature of the chronic disease self-management interventions is that they initiate interventions via clinical referral during face-to-face consultations (Table 10.1), increasing the accountability of the patients to their health care provider. However, relying on this initiation modality limits the reach of interventions to people already engaged in the health care system.

Weight Loss Interventions

Experimental evidence shows that supplementary contact following a weight loss intervention results in less weight regain (Deforche et al., 2005; Svetkey et al., 2008; Wilfley et al., 2007). Due to the low cost and low participant burden of text messaging, it could play a key role in delivering ongoing intervention contact. Nine studies have examined weight loss interventions delivered partly by text messaging to overweight or obese adults (Gerber, Stolley, Thompson, Sharp, & Fitzgibbon, 2009; Haapala, Barengo, Biggs, Surakka, & Manninen, 2009; Park, Kim, & Kim, 2009; Patrick et al., 2009) or adolescents (Bauer, de Niet, Timman, & Kordy, 2010; Shrewsbury et al., 2009; Woolford, Clark, Strecher, & Resnicow, 2010) or promoting weight control in healthy adults (Joo & Kim, 2007; Lombard, Deeks, Jolley, Ball, & Teede, 2010). All nine interventions targeted dietary and physical activity behavior change, and three specified that they were theory-based (all used social cognitive theory: Haapala et al., 2009; Lombard et al., 2010; Shrewsbury et al., 2009). Average participant weight loss ranged from 1.60 kg (3.53 lb.) (Park et al., 2009) to 4.50 kg (9.92 lb.) (Haapala et al., 2009), and all six studies that measured weight outcomes reported significant and clinically mean-ingful decreases. Only two of the nine trials reported on behavioral outcomes, each providing evidence of meaningful improvements in diet quality and physical activity (Haapala et al., 2009; Lombard et al., 2010). All studies reported on pro-cess or acceptability outcomes and reported positive reactions from intervention participants.

Most text-based weight loss interventions were initiated following participa-tion in individual (Joo & Kim, 2007; Park et al., 2009; Woolford et al., 2010) or group-based face-to-face counseling sessions (Bauer et al., 2010; Gerber et al., 2009; Lombard et al., 2010; Shrewsbury et al., 2009). This is good practice in terms of integrating text-based programs with existing practice, but it limits the mass-reach potential of such programs via barriers to attending face-to-face ses-sions (Table 10.1). Future research should explore alternative ways of initiating text-based weight loss interventions that do not require participants to attend face-to-face sessions, especially in light of evidence that text-based interventions can be effective at promoting weight loss on their own (Haapala et al., 2009) or in combination with other mediated (non-face-to-face) modalities such as tele-phone counseling and print materials (Patrick et al., 2009).

Most text message weight loss programs used participant data to tailor text message content and/or frequency. One extreme example asked participants to write their own personal text messages during the counseling sessions on topics on which they felt that they required the most support and then sent the messages at a frequency nominated by participants (Gerber et al., 2009). Other studies allowed participants to select the timing (time of day) and frequency (e.g., two to five texts per day) of the text messages and allowed for participants to change their preferences during the program when experiencing behavioral setbacks or a reduced need for support (Patrick et al., 2009). No studies have examined the level of content tailoring as a predictor of weight loss or collected acceptability data for level of tailoring. However, process data from weight loss studies suggest that participants appreciate the opportunity to tailor frequency and timing of texts (Patrick et al., 2009).

Smoking Cessation Interventions

The field of text-based smoking cessation programs is the most advanced. More than in other fields, smoking cessation has evolved in an iterative way with text-based interventions developed using theories and methods known to be effective from previous smoking cessation evidence. Six studies have examined the impact of text-delivered smoking cessation interventions in young adults (Haug, Meyer, Schorr, Bauer, & John, 2009; Obermayer et al., 2004; Riley, Obermayer, & Jean-Mary, 2008) or adults (Brendryen & Kraft, 2008; Free et al., 2009; Rodgers et al., 2005). Most of these interventions were grounded in the transtheoretical model of behavior change (Haug et al., 2009; Riley et al., 2008; Rodgers et al., 2005) or self-regulation theory (Obermayer et al., 2004; Riley et al., 2008).

All but one study showed significant increases in self-reported quit rates. The New Zealand-based STOMP program (relative risk [RR] of quitting = 2.20 [95% CI 1.79–2.70] [Rodgers et al., 2005]), the UK adaptation of this program, Txt2Stop (RR of quitting = 2.08 [95% CI 1.11–3.89] [Free et al., 2009]), and the Happy Ending program (odds ratio of quitting = 1.91 [95% CI 1.12–3.26] [Brendryen & Kraft, 2008]) all demonstrated meaningful and significant increases in quit rates. One pilot study found no significant between-group effect on quit rates due to parallel quit rates in the control group (Haug et al., 2009).

Key features of smoking cessation interventions include integration of social support, self-monitoring, and craving support strategies (Table 10.1). The Txt2Stop and STOMP interventions use intraprogram quit buddies for support and encourage participants to text their family and friends to request support (Free et al., 2009; Rodgers et al., 2005). Other interventions send emails to participant-nominated family and friends to encourage them to provide support for participants' quit intentions (Obermayer et al., 2004; Riley et al., 2008). These interventions also encourage participants to self-monitor their smoking withdrawal symptoms and quit goals. For example, one intervention texted participants once per day following their quit day to monitor their current quit status

(Obermayer et al., 2004). All six of the smoking cessation interventions include a participant-initiated crave support strategy that triggered either a reply text offering support (e.g., Riley et al., 2008) or an automated interactive voice response (Brendryen & Kraft, 2008). The perceived usefulness of these "crave texts" was not reported, but one study reported that participants preferred instructive feedback over generic encouragement in the reply text (Haug et al., 2009).

Smoking cessation programs use varying modes of program initiation. Two trials used Web-based initiation (Brendryen & Kraft, 2008; Obermayer et al., 2004), two studies used face-to-face meetings (Haug et al., 2009; Riley et al., 2008), and two programs appeared to be initiated via text messaging, although initiation was not clearly described (Free et al., 2009; Rodgers et al., 2005). One study specifically examined the impact of the initiation process by replicating Obermayer and colleagues' intervention with face-to-face initiation instead of having participants independently initiate the program via a website (Riley et al., 2008). Riley and colleagues suggest that the additional support for initiating the program led to better acceptability and quit rates. When Web-based and text message–based strategies are offered within the same intervention, Web-based components are used less frequently than text-based components (Obermayer et al., 2004; Riley et al., 2008).

Compared to other fields, smoking cessation uses the highest frequency of text messages, presumably because of the high frequency of the targeted behavior. Some participants preferred less frequent texts than five per day (over four weeks) (Free et al., 2009), while others wanted more than one to three per day (Riley et al., 2008). Smoking cessation researchers have found no difference in quit rates between groups randomized to receive one versus three texts per week (Haug et al., 2009). The frequency of text messages could be tailored based on participants' expressed need for support at different times during the intervention (Obermayer et al., 2004), but the efficacy of this preference-based system has not been investigated.

Physical Activity Interventions

Eight published studies have used text messages to increase physical activity among healthy adults or adolescents (Fjeldsoe, Miller, & Marshall, 2010; Fukuoka, Vittinghoff, Jong, & Haskell, 2010; Hurling et al., 2007; Prestwich, Perugini, & Hurling, 2010; Shapiro et al., 2008; Sirriyeh, Lawton, & Ward, 2010), adolescents with type 1 diabetes (Newton, Wiltshire, & Elley, 2009), or adults with chronic obstructive pulmonary disease (Nguyen, Gill, Wolpin, Steele, & Benditt, 2009). Most were pilot or feasibility studies that demonstrated some success in changing physical activity, despite inadequate sample sizes or retention rates in some. Increases in physical activity ranged from 18 minutes/week (Fjeldsoe et al., 2010) to 48 minutes/week (Newton et al., 2009), or 609 steps/day (Nguyen et al., 2009) to 800 steps/day (Fukuoka et al., 2010). Most studies report that participants found it easy to engage with the text message interventions and that there was high and ongoing engagement with the programs.

All of the interventions incorporated texts to increase social support and self-monitoring. Social support for physical activity was targeted by sending texts directly to a participant-nominated friend or family member (Fjeldsoe et al., 2010), regularly prompting participants to seek social support (Fukuoka et al., 2010), or offering online discussion forums with other program participants (Hurling et al., 2007). Self-monitoring was encouraged through recording pedometer step counts (Nguyen et al., 2009), Bluetooth connectivity to an accelerometer (Hurling et al., 2007), and text-based questions about meeting weekly goals (Fjeldsoe et al., 2010). Participants' reactions to social support and self-monitoring strategies were positive, although one intervention reported participants' desire for more instrumental social support from their nominated support person (Fjeldsoe et al., 2010), and another reported decreased pedometer use for self-monitoring over the course of the intervention (Nguyen et al., 2009).

Half of the interventions based text message content on behavioral theories, such as social cognitive theory (Fjeldsoe et al., 2010; Nguyen et al., 2009), theory of planned behavior (Sirriyeh et al., 2010), or implementation intentions (Prestwich et al., 2010). Two studies experimentally manipulated text message content to examine the impact of targeting different theoretical mediators (Prestwich et al., 2010; Sirriyeh et al., 2010). Text messages targeting affective beliefs about physical activity (e.g., enjoyment, pleasure, fun) were more successful in changing the behavior of adolescents than messages that targeted instrumental beliefs or a combination of the two (Sirriyeh et al., 2010). Text-based "plan reminders" and "goal reminders" were equally effective for changing physical activity (Prestwich et al., 2010). This research is fundamental to understanding how to adapt the principles of behavior change theories to the limited-character context of text messages.

Limitations of Current Research

Little is known about the maintenance of behavioral changes as a result of text messaging interventions because most trials only assess outcomes immediately following the end of the intervention. Some studies did not assess behavioral outcomes, particularly those reporting clinical markers associated with behavior change (e.g., HbA1c, weight loss). Process outcomes (e.g., number of texts received and sent) are key to informing intervention improvements, yet these are rarely reported. Importantly, researchers need to focus on adapting evidence from interventions that use other delivery modalities to text-based interventions. Similarly, we need to ground the content of text-based programs in the extensive body of literature on behavioral theory and test the success of changing these proposed mediators. As the field matures, it is important to move away from underpowered, prepost design pilot studies to powered, randomized controlled trials and comparative effectiveness trials.

Table 10.1 Strengths and weaknesses of text messaging interventions currently published in the peer-reviewed literature

	Keys to success	*Room for improvement*
Chronic disease self-management interventions	• Fulfills need for ongoing surveillance of patients' symptoms and medication by health care professionals • Easy integration of electronic symptom monitors with mobile phone handsets • High acceptability among young people, who are traditionally hard to engage in disease management • Referral from health care professional increases accountability	• Target behaviors other than symptom monitoring and medication adherence for a holistic approach to disease management • Assess behavioral outcomes as well as clinical outcomes when evaluating the impact of interventions • Reduce barriers to regular symptom monitoring by exploiting the ease of text messaging data entry
Weight loss interventions	• Incorporates text messages into current treatment practice • Tailors text message content and frequency to individual's needs	• Assess behavioral outcomes as well as weight-related outcomes when evaluating the impact of the interventions • Explore modes of initiation other than face-to-face counseling sessions to increase potential reach of programs
Smoking cessation interventions	• Use of interactive text messages for relapse support • Use of text messages to elicit social support from peers • Builds on existing body of evidence on smoking cessation programs	• Ensure that modes of initiation are not a barrier to program participation • Investigate optimal frequency and timing of text messages for behavior change and participant satisfaction
Physical activity interventions	• Use of text messages to elicit social support from peers • Tailors text message content to individual's needs • Starting to manipulate message content to evaluate impact on different theoretical mediators of behavior change	• Investigate different initiation modes to engage participants • Ensure that "other" intervention modalities (e.g., pedometers) are well integrated into text-based programs

Limitations of Text Messaging as an Intervention Delivery Modality

While use of mobile phones is ever-increasing, older generations use them less than younger generations, and when they do use them it is predominantly for voice calls (Atun & Sittampalam, 2006). People in developing countries use mobile phones differently from people in developed countries. For example, while up to 10 million new subscribers are added to mobile phone networks in India each month, these networks record some of the lowest text message usage in the world (Kathuria, Uppal, & Mamta, 2009). Multiple languages, extensive illiteracy, and cheap voice calls all conspire to limit the popularity of text messages in developing countries (Uppal & Kathuria, 2009).

The information delivery capacity of a single text message is limited (typically to 160 characters), challenging interventionists to isolate the key messages they need to transmit to maximize participant attention and message impact. Text messages may not be suitable for delivering interventions that require large amounts of complex information to be communicated or clinically sensitive information that requires explanation. Personal tailoring and mass delivery of text messages requires comprehensive databases and automated delivery software that can be costly to set up but should develop cost-effectiveness over long-term use.

The mobile phone is a device acquired for personal convenience and use. Some users may perceive health-related messages as an invasion of their privacy. This can be overcome by offering opt-in programs and establishing a trusted source. As text messaging is increasingly exploited for mass commercial advertising, behavioral interventionists need to navigate an increasingly difficult legislative environment (Norwell, 2003; Terry, 2008).

Future Directions for Text Messaging Interventions

The concept of delivering behavior change interventions by text message has been endorsed through feasibility and pilot research. The future development of this modality will depend on greater collaboration between behavioral scientists, health professionals, social marketers, software developers, and the telecommunications industry.

To establish text message interventions as a fundable alternative to more established interventions, these interventions need to be tested in comparative effectiveness trials. Only one diabetes management trial so far has attempted this: Hanauer and colleagues (2009) compared text-delivered versus email-delivered programs and found them equally effective, but participants reported a preference for text message delivery. More trials like this are needed to evaluate the effects of combined delivery modalities on behavior change, cost-effectiveness, ongoing use, and satisfaction.

It is important that future text messaging research remains behavior- and population-specific, with cautious transfer of effective strategy components across fields. For example, clinical studies have reported mixed findings on the acceptability of an after-treatment support program delivered by text message to people suffering from bulimia nervosa (Bauer, Percevic, Okon, Meermann, & Kordy, 2003; Robinson et al., 2006). Formative research with a specific population group is crucial for establishing preferences for text-based programs.

An important consideration that underpins the dissemination value of text-based interventions is the optimal process of program initiation (in which information is collected to tailor text message content). Various initiation methods have been tested ranging from face-to-face consultation to depersonalized online registration. The presence of a person during the initiation process (either via face-to-face or telephone) may affect perceptions of text message content and the sincerity of the support offered compared with Web- or text-based initiation processes. While it is acknowledged that most text-based programs will need to deliver some intervention components via other delivery modalities (particularly the initiation process), these modalities should be carefully selected so as not to limit the reach of text-based interventions.

Much research has been conducted using mobile phone technologies other than text messaging (e.g., Klasnja, Consolvo, McDonald, Landay, & Pratt, 2009; also see Abroms, Padmanabhan, & Evans, this volume). From a population health perspective, it is important to utilize technologies accessible across the social divide of populations (Fogg & Adler, 2009). Furthermore, smartphone applications often mimic the behavioral strategies of more traditional Web-based interventions but are delivered on a handheld device, and they may be affected by similar limitations as those of Web-based interventions (e.g., low rates of repeat use of the program).

Conclusion

Text messaging has the potential to bridge the gap between the least and most advantaged audiences for delivery of behavior change programs. The future of this technology for behavior change is exciting and rapidly developing. Our current challenge is to translate the broad and sophisticated evidence we have about successful behavior change via other delivery modalities into this socially absorbed and widely accepted communication channel.

Note

1. Comparable alternative text messaging systems use email messaging technology rather than text messages, including "SkyMail" and "Short Mail" in Japan.

References

Andrade, A. S. A., McGruder, H. F., Wu, A. W., Celano, S. A., Skolasky, R. L., Jr., Selnes, O. A., et al. (2005). A programmable prompting device improves adherence to highly active antiretroviral therapy in HIV-infected subjects with memory impairment. *Clinical Infectious Diseases, 41,* 875–882.

Anhoj, J., & Moldrup, C. (2004). Feasibility of collecting diary data from asthma patients through mobile phones and SMS (Short Message Service): Response rate analysis and focus group evaluation from a pilot study. *Journal of Medical Internet Research, 6,* e42.

Atun, R. A., & Sittampalam, S. R. (2006, March). A review of the characteristics and benefits of SMS in delivering healthcare. *The Role of Mobile Phones in Increasing Accessibility and Efficiency in Healthcare: The Vodafone Policy Paper Series, 4,* 18–28. Retrieved September 2, 2011, from: http://www.enlightenmenteconomics.com/assets/vodafone_policy_paper_4_march06.pdf.

Australian Communications and Media Authority. (2009). *ACMA Communications Report 2008–09.* Retrieved September 2, 2011, from: http://www.acma.gov.au/webwr/_assets/main/lib311252/08–09_comms_report.pdf.

Bauer, S., de Niet, J., Timman, R., & Kordy, H. (2010). Enhancement of care through self-monitoring and tailored feedback via text messaging and their use in the treatment of childhood overweight. *Patient Education & Counseling, 79,* 315–319.

Bauer, S., Percevic, R., Okon, E., Meermann, R., & Kordy, H. (2003). Use of text messaging in the aftercare of patients with bulimia nervosa. *European Eating Disorders Review, 11,* 279–290.

Benhamou, P. Y., Melki, V., Boizel, R., Perreal, F., Quesada, J. L., Bessieres-Lacombe, S., et al. (2007). One-year efficacy and safety of Web-based follow-up using cellular phone in type 1 diabetic patients under insulin pump therapy: The PumpNet study. *Diabetes & Metabolism, 33,* 220–226.

Brendryen, H., & Kraft, P. (2008). Happy ending: A randomized controlled trial of a digital multi-media smoking cessation intervention. *Addiction, 103,* 478–484.

Butryn, M. L., Phelan, S., Hill, J. O., & Wing, R. R. (2007). Consistent self-monitoring of weight: A key component of successful weight loss maintenance. *Obesity, 15,* 3091–3096.

Carroll, A. E., Marrero, D. G., & Downs, S. M. (2007). The HealthPia GlucoPack diabetes phone: A usability study. *Diabetes Technology & Therapeutics, 9,* 158–164.

Cellular Telecommunications Industry Association. (2009, October 8). *National study reveals mHealth has vast appeal in America.* Retrieved September 3, 2011 from: http://www.harrisinteractive.com/vault/Harris_Interactive_CTIA_2009_10_08.pdf.

Cho, J-H., Lee, H-C., Lim, D-J., Kwon, H-S., & Yoon, K-H. (2009). Mobile communication using a mobile phone with a glucometer for glucose control in type 2 patients with diabetes: As effective as an Internet-based glucose monitoring system. *Journal of Telemedicine and Telecare, 15,* 77–82.

Cleland, J., Caldow, J., & Ryan, D. (2007). A qualitative study of the attitudes of patients and staff to the use of mobile phone technology for recording and gathering asthma data. *Journal of Telemedicine and Telecare, 13,* 85–89.

Cole-Lewis, H., & Kershaw, T. (2010). Text messaging as a tool for behavior change in disease prevention and management. *Epidemiologic Reviews, 32,* 56–69.

Currie, M. J., Schmidt, M., Davis, B. K., Baynes, A. M., O'Keefe, E. J., Bavinton, T. P., et al. (2010). "Show me the money": Financial incentives increase chlamydia screening rates among tertiary students: A pilot study. *Sexual Health, 7,* 60–65.

Deforche, B., De Bourdeaudhuij, I., Tanghe, A., Debode, P., Hills, A. P., & Bouckaert, J. (2005). Post-treatment phone contact: A weight maintenance strategy in obese youngsters. *International Journal of Obesity, 29,* 543–546.

Downer, S. R., Meara, J. G., & Da Costa, A. C. (2005). Use of SMS text messaging to improve outpatient attendance. *Medical Journal of Australia, 183,* 366–368.

Dutta-Bergman, M. J. (2005). Theory and practice in health communication campaigns: A critical interrogation. *Health Communication, 18,* 103–122.

Evans, P. (2009). 2009 Philippines—Telecoms, mobile and broadband. *BuddeComm.* Retrieved July 26, 2010, from: http://www.budde.com.au/Research/Philippines-Telecoms-Mobile-and-Broadband.html#overview.

Fairley, C. K., Levy, R., Rayner, C. R., Allardice, K., Costello, K., Thomas, C., et al. (2003). Randomized trial of an adherence programme for clients with HIV. *International Journal of STD & AIDS, 14,* 805–809.

Ferrer-Roca, O., Cardenas, A., Diaz-Cardama, A., & Pulido, P. (2004). Mobile phone text messaging in the management of diabetes. *Journal of Telemedicine and Telecare, 10,* 282–286.

Fjeldsoe, B. S., Marshall, A. L., & Miller, Y. D. (2009). Behavior change interventions delivered by mobile telephone short-message service. *American Journal of Preventive Medicine, 36,* 165–173.

Fjeldsoe, B. S., Miller, Y. D., & Marshall, A. L. (2010). MobileMums: A randomized controlled trial of an SMS-based physical activity intervention. *Annals of Behavioral Medicine, 39,* 101–111.

Fjeldsoe, B. S., Neuhaus, M., Winkler, E., & Eakin, E. (2011). Systematic review of maintenance of behavior change following physical activity and dietary interventions. *Health Psychology, 30,* 99–109.

Fogg, B. J., & Adler, R. (Eds.). (2009). *Texting 4 health: A simple, powerful way to improve lives.* Stanford: Stanford Captology Media.

Fogg, B. J., & Eckles, D. (Eds.). (2008). *Mobile persuasion: 20 perspectives on the future of behavior change.* Stanford: Stanford Captology Media.

Foley, J., & O'Neill, M. (2009). Use of mobile telephone short message service (SMS) as a reminder: The effect on patient attendance. *European Archives of Paediatric Dentistry, 10,* 15–18.

Forestier, E., Grace, J., & Kenny, C. (2002). Can information and communication technologies be pro-poor? *Telecommunications Policy, 26,* 623–646.

Franklin, V. L., Waller, A., Pagliari, C., & Greene, S. A. (2003). "Sweet Talk": Text messaging support for intensive insulin therapy for young people with diabetes. *Diabetes Technology & Therapeutics, 5,* 991–996.

Franklin, V. L., Waller, A., Pagliari, C., & Greene, S. A. (2006). A randomized controlled trial of Sweet Talk, a text-messaging system to support young people with diabetes. *Diabetic Medicine, 23,* 1332–1338.

Free, C., Whittaker, R., Knight, R., Abramsky, T., Rodgers, A., & Roberts, I. G. (2009). Txt2stop: A pilot randomised controlled trial of mobile phone-based smoking cessation support. *Tobacco Control, 18,* 88–91.

Fry, J. P., & Neff, R. A. (2009). Periodic prompts and reminders in health promotion and health behavior interventions: Systematic review. *Journal of Medical Internet Research, 11,* e16.

Fukuoka, Y., Vittinghoff, E., Jong, S. S., & Haskell, W. (2010). Innovation to motivation—pilot study of a mobile phone intervention to increase physical activity among sedentary women. *Preventive Medicine, 51,* 287–289.

Gammon, D., Arsand, E., Walseth, O. A., Andersson, N., Jenssen, M., & Taylor, T. (2005). Parent-child interaction using a mobile and wireless system for blood glucose monitoring. *Journal of Medical Internet Research, 7,* e57.

Gerber, B. S., Stolley, M. R., Thompson, A. L., Sharp, L. K., & Fitzgibbon, M. L. (2009). Mobile phone text messaging to promote healthy behaviors and weight loss maintenance: A feasibility study. *Health Informatics Journal, 15,* 17–25.

Haapala, I., Barengo, N. C., Biggs, S., Surakka, L., & Manninen, P. (2009). Weight loss by mobile phone: A 1-year effectiveness study. *Public Health Nutrition, 12,* 2382–2391.

Haller, D., Sanci, L., Sawyer, S., Coffey, C., & Patton, G. (2006). R U OK 2 TXT 4 RESEARCH? Feasibility of text messaging communication in primary care research. *Australian Family Physician, 35,* 175–176.

Hanauer, D. A., Wentzell, K., Laffel, N., & Laffel, L. M. (2009). Computerized Automated Reminder Diabetes System (CARDS): E-mail and SMS cell phone text messaging reminders to support diabetes management. *Diabetes Technology & Therapeutics, 11,* 99–106.

Haug, S., Meyer, C., Schorr, G., Bauer, S., & John, U. (2009). Continuous individual support of smoking cessation using text messaging: A pilot experimental study. *Nicotine & Tobacco Research, 11,* 915–923.

Holtz, B., & Whitten, P. (2009). Managing asthma with mobile phones: A feasibility study. *Telemedicine Journal and e-health, 15,* 907–909.

Hurling, R., Catt, M., De Boni, M., Fairley, B. W., Hurst, T., Murray, P., et al. (2007). Using Internet and mobile phone technology to deliver an automated physical activity program: Randomized controlled trial. *Journal of Medical Internet Research, 9,* e7.

International Telecommunication Union. (2010a, February 15). *ITU sees 5 billion mobile subscriptions globally in 2010.* Retrieved July 26, 2010, from: http://www.itu.int/newsroom/press_releases/2010/06.html.

International Telecommunication Union. (2010b). *World Telecommunication/ICT Indicators Database 2010* (15th ed.). Retrieved September 3, 2011, from: http://www.itu.int/ITU-D/ict/publications/world/world.html.

Joo, N. S., & Kim, B. T. (2007). Mobile phone short message service messaging for behaviour modification in a community-based weight control programme in Korea. *Journal of Telemedicine and Telecare, 13,* 416–420.

Kaplan, W. A. (2006). Can the ubiquitous power of mobile phones be used to improve health outcomes in developing countries? *Globalization and Health, 2,* 9.

Kathuria, R., Uppal, M., & Mamta. (2009, January). An econometric analysis of the impact of mobile. *India: The Impact of Mobile Phones: The Vodafone Policy Paper Series, 9,* 5–20. Retrieved September 3, 2011, from: http://www.vodafone.com/content/dam/vodafone/about/public_policy/policy_papers/public_policy_series_9.pdf.

Katz, J., & Aakhus, M. (Eds.). (2002). *Perpetual contact: Mobile communication, private talk, public performance.* Cambridge: Cambridge University Press.

Kharbanda, E. O., Stockwell, M. S., Fox, H. W., & Rickert, V. I. (2009). Text4Health: A qualitative evaluation of parental readiness for text message immunization reminders. *American Journal of Public Health, 99,* 2176–2178.

Khokhar, A. (2009). Short text messages (SMS) as a reminder system for making working women from Delhi breast aware. *Asian Pacific Journal of Cancer Prevention, 10,* 319–322.

Kim, H-S. (2007). A randomized controlled trial of a nurse short-message service by cellular phone for people with diabetes. *International Journal of Nursing Studies, 44,* 687–692.

Klasnja, P., Consolvo, S., McDonald, D. W., Landay, J. A., & Pratt, W. (2009). Using mobile & personal sensing technologies to support health behavior change in everyday life: Lessons learned. *Proceedings of the American Medical Informatics Association Annual Symposium, USA,* 338–342. Retrieved September 3, 2011, from: http://dub.washington.edu/djangosite/media/papers/Klasnja_amia2009.pdf.

Kollmann, A., Reidl, M., Kastner, P., Schreier, G., & Ludvik, B. (2007). Feasibility of a mobile phone-based data service for functional insulin treatment of type 1 diabetes mellitus patients. *Journal of Medical Internet Research, 9,* e36.

Kreuter, M. W., Strecher, V. J., & Glassman, B. (1999). One size does not fit all: The case for tailoring print materials. *Annals of Behavioral Medicine, 21,* 276–283.

Kwon, H-S., Cho, J-H., Kim, H-S., Lee, J-H., Song, B-R., Oh, J-A., et al. (2004). Development of Web-based diabetic patient management system using short message service (SMS). *Diabetes Research and Clinical Practice, 66,* s133–s137.

Leena, K., Tomi, L., & Arja, R. (2005). Intensity of mobile phone use and health compromising behaviours—how is information and communication technology connected to health-related lifestyle in adolescence? *Journal of Adolescence, 28,* 35–47.

Lim, M. S. C., Hocking, J. S., Hellard, M. E., & Aitken, C. K. (2008). SMS STI: A review of the uses of mobile phone text messaging in sexual health. *International Journal of STD & AIDS, 19,* 287–290.

Lombard, C., Deeks, A., Jolley, D., Ball, K., & Teede, H. (2010). A low intensity, community based lifestyle programme to prevent weight gain in women with young children: Cluster randomised controlled trial. *British Medical Journal, 341,* c3215.

Michie, S., Abraham, C., Whittington, C., McAteer, J., & Gupta, S. (2009). Effective techniques in healthy eating and physical activity interventions: A meta-regression. *Health Psychology, 28,* 690–701.

Neville, R., Greene, A., McLeod, J., Tracy, A., & Surie, J. (2002). Mobile phone text messaging can help young people manage asthma. *British Medical Journal, 325,* 600.

Newton, K. H., Wiltshire, E. J., & Elley, C. R. (2009). Pedometers and text messaging to increase physical activity: Randomized controlled trial of adolescents with type 1 diabetes. *Diabetes Care, 32,* 813–815.

Nguyen, H. Q., Gill, D. P., Wolpin, S., Steele, B. G., & Benditt, J. O. (2009). Pilot study of a cell phone-based exercise persistence intervention post-rehabilitation for COPD. *International Journal of Chronic Obstructive Pulmonary Disease, 4,* 301–313.

Noar, S. M., Benac, C. N., & Harris, M. S. (2007). Does tailoring matter? Meta-analytic review of tailored print health behavior change interventions. *Psychological Bulletin, 133,* 673–693.

Norwell, N. (2003). Text messaging raises medicolegal issues. *British Medical Journal, 326,* 1148.

Obermayer, J. L., Riley, W. T., Asif, O., & Jean-Mary, J. (2004). College smoking-cessation using cell phone text messaging. *Journal of American College Health, 53,* 71–78.

Ostojic, V., Cvoriscec, B., Ostojic, S. B., Reznikoff, D., Stipic-Markovic, A., & Tudjmam, Z. (2005). Improving asthma control through telemedicine: A study of short-message service. *Telemedicine and e-Health, 11,* 28–35.

Park, M-J., Kim, H-S., & Kim, K-S. (2009). Cellular phone and Internet-based individual intervention on blood pressure and obesity in obese patients with hypertension. *International Journal of Medical Informatics, 78,* 704–710.

Patrick, K., Raab, F., Adams, M. A., Dillon, L., Zabinski, M., Rock, C. L., et al. (2009). A text message-based intervention for weight loss: Randomized controlled trial. *Journal of Medical Internet Research, 11,* e1.

Pena-Robichaux, V., Kvedar, J. C., & Watson, A. J. (2010). Text messages as a reminder aid and educational tool in adolescents and adults with atopic dermatitis: A pilot study. *Dematology Research and Practice, 2010,* 1–6.

Pinnock, H., Slack, R., Pagliari, D., & Sheikh, A. (2007). Understanding the potential role of mobile phone-based monitoring on asthma self-management: Qualitative study. *Clinical and Experimental Allergy, 37,* 794–802.

Portio Research. (2010). *Mobile messaging futures 2010–2014: Analysis and growth forecasts for mobile messaging markets worldwide* (4th ed.). Chippenham, Wilts, UK: Portio Research Limited.

Prabhakaran, L., Chee, W. Y., Chua, K. C., Abisheganaden, J., & Wong, W. M. (2010). The use of text messaging to improve asthma control: A pilot study using the mobile phone short messaging service (SMS). *Journal of Telemedicine and Telecare, 16*, 286–290.

Prestwich, A., Perugini, M., & Hurling, R. (2010). Can implementation intentions and text messages promote brisk walking? A randomized trial. *Health Psychology, 29*, 40–49.

Rami, B., Popow, C., Horn, W. T., Waldhoer, T., & Schober, E. (2006). Telemedical support to improve glycemic control in adolescents with type 1 diabetes mellitus. *European Journal of Pediatrics, 165*, 701–705.

Rice, R. E., & Katz, J. E. (2003). Comparing Internet and mobile phone usage: Digital divides of usage, adoption, and dropouts. *Telecommunications Policy, 27*, 597–623.

Riley, W., Obermayer, J., & Jean-Mary, J. (2008). Internet and mobile phone text messaging intervention for college smokers. *Journal of American College Health, 57*, 245–248.

Robinson, S., Perkins, S., Bauer, S., Hammond, N., Treasure, J., & Schmidt, U. (2006). Aftercare intervention through text messaging in the treatment of bulimia nervosa—feasability pilot. *International Journal of Eating Disorders, 39*, 633–638.

Rodgers, A., Corbett, T., Bramley, D., Riddell, T., Wills, M., Lin, R. B., et al. (2005). Do u smoke after txt? Results of a randomised trial of smoking cessation using mobile phone text messaging. *Tobacco Control, 14*, 255–261.

Ryan, P., & Lauver, D. R. (2002). The efficacy of tailored interventions. *Journal of Nursing Scholarship, 34*, 331–337.

Shapiro, J. R., Bauer, S., Hamer, R. M., Kordy, H., Ward, D., & Bulik, C. M. (2008). Use of text messaging for monitoring sugar-sweetened beverages, physical activity, and screen time in children: A pilot study. *Journal of Nutrition Education and Behavior, 40*, 385–391.

Shrewsbury, V. A., O'Connor, J., Steinbeck, K. S., Stevenson, K., Lee, A., Hill, A. J., et al. (2009). A randomised controlled trial of a community-based healthy lifestyle program for overweight and obese adolescents: The Loozit study protocol. *BMC Public Health, 9*, 119.

Sirriyeh, R., Lawton, R., & Ward, J. (2010). Physical activity and adolescents: An exploratory randomized controlled trial investigating the influence of affective and instrumental text messages. *British Journal of Health Psychology, 15*, 825–840.

Strandbygaard, U., Thomsen, S. F., & Backer, V. (2010). A daily SMS reminder increases adherence to asthma treatment: A three-month follow-up study. *Respiratory Medicine, 104*, 166–171.

Svetkey, L. P., Stevens, V. J., Brantley, P. J., Appel, L. J., Hollis, J. F., Loria, C. M., et al. (2008). Comparison of strategies for sustaining weight loss: The weight loss maintenance randomized controlled trial. *Journal of the American Medical Association, 299*, 1139–1148.

Terry, M. (2008). Text messaging in healthcare: The elephant knocking at the door. *Telemedicine Journal and e-health, 14*, 520–524.

Uppal, M., & Kathuria, R. (2009, January). The impact of mobiles in the SME sector. *India: The Impact of Mobile Phones: The Vodafone Policy Paper Series, 9*, 51–61. Retrieved September 3, 2011, from: http://www.vodafone.com/content/dam/vodafone/about/public_policy/policy_papers/public_policy_series_9.pdf.

Vahatalo, M. A., Virtamo, H. E., Viikari, J. S., & Ronnemaa, T. (2004). Cellular phone transferred self blood glucose monitoring: Prerequisites for positive outcome. *Practical Diabetes International, 21*, 192–194.

Vilella, A., Bayas, J-M., Diaz, M-T., Guinovart, C., Diez, C., Simo, D., et al. (2004). The role of mobile phones in improving vaccination rates in travelers. *Preventive Medicine, 38*, 503–509.

Wangberg, S. C., Arsand, E., & Andersson, N. (2006). Diabetes education via mobile text messaging. *Journal of Telemedicine and Telecare, 12,* 55–56.

Wilfley, D. E., Stein, R. I., Saelens, B. E., Mockus, D. S., Matt, G. E., Hayden-Wade, H. A., et al. (2007). Efficacy of maintenance treatment approaches for childhood overweight: A randomized controlled trial. *Journal of the American Medical Association, 298,* 1661–1673.

Wing, R. R., & Phelan, S. (2005). Long-term weight loss maintenance. *American Journal of Clinical Nutrition, 82,* 222S–225S.

Woolford, S. J., Clark, S. J., Strecher, V. J., & Resnicow, K. (2010). Tailored mobile phone text messages as an adjunct to obesity treatment for adolescents. *Journal of Telemedicine and Telecare, 16,* 458–461.

Zhang, X. N., & Prybutok, V. R. (2005). How the mobile communication markets differ in China, the U.S., and Europe. *Communications of the Association for Computing Machinery, 48,* 111–114.

11

INTERACTIVE VOICE RESPONSE TECHNOLOGY FOR CHRONIC DISEASE MANAGEMENT

John D. Piette and Ashley J. Beard

Interactive voice response, or IVR, is the technology allowing patients to receive information and communicate with others asynchronously using their mobile or landline telephone. Using IVR, patients interact with a structured series of recorded message components and respond to queries using their touch-tone keypad or voice recognition technology. On the basis of their responses, patients receive recorded messages tailored to their individual needs (see chapter 8 of this volume). Others involved in patients' care can receive updates based on the IVR assessment reports, along with structured feedback about what clinicians and informal caregivers can do to improve disease management and outcomes. Those updates can be delivered via IVR, structured emails, faxes, pagers, or Internet summary reports.

This chapter focuses on the role of IVR in self-management support for patients with chronic health problems. We do not present a comprehensive systematic review of IVR, but rather cite key studies and present examples illustrating uses of IVR for improving patients' experience and outcomes.

An Example of IVR in Practice: The CarePartner Model

The CarePartner model is designed to use IVR to improve patient outcomes through the following three mechanisms of action (Figure 11.1): (1) tailored self-care information to patients provided during IVR interactions, (2) feedback about urgent issues to patients' clinical teams, and (3) targeted advice for caregivers about how to address problems and communicate effectively. Patients receive IVR assessment and behavior change calls at times they designate. Call frequency can vary depending on a predefined schedule, clinicians' preferences, or changes in patients' status. The content for the IVR calls has been developed in conjunction with behavior change researchers and experts in the target conditions. Clinicians can specify which urgent problems generate a fax alert, and patients' caregivers can receive feedback via structured emails or a voicemail service.

We pilot tested a version of the CarePartner model among heart failure patients (Piette et al., 2008). Fifty-two patients received weekly calls, using multiple automated calling attempts. The call content was guided by an algorithm-based self-care support protocol. During each call, patients reported information about their health and self-care, including their diet, symptoms, weight, and medication adherence, and they received immediate recorded messages with tailored feedback. Urgent reports such as worsening breathing problems were automatically reported to the patients' clinical team via fax. Email alerts to out-of-home social network members (i.e., "CarePartners") were structured to convey why a problem was important and how to follow up. CarePartners also had access to a Web-based summary with detailed information about heart failure self-care support and information about the patients' status in four domains: overall health, breathing, weight, and medication use.

Only 13% of potential participants identified from medical records were unable to participate because they could not identify someone living outside of their household with email access willing to be their CarePartner. Sixty-seven percent of CarePartners were adult children, 20% were friends, and 13% were other family members. Patients completed assessments during 90% of the weeks in which one was attempted, and there was no drop off in completion rates over the course of patients' participation. Overall, 35% of patients reported running out of medications at least once, 50% reported increased difficulty breathing, and 29% reported problems with their diet. Both patients and CarePartners reported high levels of satisfaction with the service.

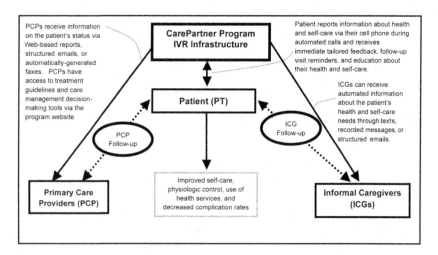

Figure 11.1 CarePartner program infrastructure

In 2009, we launched a randomized trial of the CarePartner program for long-term management of heart failure patients treated in the Veterans Affairs (VA) hospital. To date, more than 200 patient-CarePartner pairs have been enrolled, with half of those CarePartners receiving weekly reports of patients' status over 12 months. Fewer than 2% of patients receiving weekly IVR assessments have dropped out of the study. Clinicians report that they find the fax reports useful and use them to allocate their time to patients with complex needs. Qualitative interview data collected one month into the program yielded feedback such as the following:

> Patient: "This program has helped me keep track of my salt intake and remembering to take my pills."
> CarePartner: "I know more about what's going on with my [patient-partner]—If I just ask him he says he's fine, but now I know what's really happening and we can talk about his health issues."

Advantages of IVR for Health Communication

The Ubiquitous Mobile Phone

Mobile phones have diffused throughout the world more rapidly than any other technology in history. Over 80% of the U.S. population has a mobile phone and, as early as 2002, mobile phones outnumbered landline phones worldwide, with more than one billion subscribers (Castells, Fernandez-Ardevol, Qui, & Sey, 2006).

Latin America provides an illustrative example of the expanding potential for phone-based health care services. Nearly half a billion people in the region have mobile phones, and that number is growing rapidly (International Telecommunications Union, 2007). The number of mobile phone users in Colombia increased from 2 million users in 1999 to 42 million in 2009 (Asociación de la Industria Celular en Colombia, n.d.), and roughly 95% of low-income patients in Santiago, Chile have telephone access (Piette et al., 2006). In 2009, we surveyed 624 chronically ill adults in Honduras, the second poorest country in the hemisphere (Piette, Mendoza-Avelares, Milton, Lange, & Fajardo, 2010). Although more than one in four were illiterate, 78% reported having a mobile phone, and 84% reported having either a mobile or "landline" phone. Patients are particularly accessible via mobile phones because in many Latin American countries calls can be received without a monthly calling plan or paying any "minute" charges.

IVR as a Low-Cost Tool for Improving Patient Care

IVR has cost benefits compared with its alternatives. For example, despite consistent evidence for the effectiveness of "live" telephone care management calls (Inglis et al., 2010), the cost and complexity of this approach have limited implementation in real-world practices. The per-contact cost of IVR, however, is very low, and patients using IVR can receive much more frequent and tailored information about their health and self-care than would be possible in almost any health care system relying on face-to-face encounters or nurse telephone follow-up.

Programs for home telehealth monitoring often require special equipment to measure physiologic indicators, provide tailored advice, or facilitate communication with clinicians. While such monitoring can positively affect patients' health (Inglis et al., 2010), it can be prohibitively expensive and requires an infrastructure for equipment distribution and retrieval, training, and maintenance. While IVR per se lacks the capacity to directly gather objective physiologic measures, it also avoids these complexities that have limited the dissemination of telehealth programs requiring specialized equipment. Web-based disease management services also avoid cost and infrastructure problems and have the added benefits of providing a rich array of tools including video, access to online communities, and advice from clinicians. However, many people still lack Internet access, have inadequate bandwidth, or are not comfortable with Web-based communication (Lober et al., 2006; Piette, 2007). Further, Internet support tools require that patients be motivated enough to log on. Use often declines as enthusiasm wanes, and such systems are more likely to be used by patients with fewer challenges. In contrast, IVR is a "push" technology that proactively contacts patients via phone rather than requiring them to log on to a website. Because it is so accessible, IVR may be more effective at reaching patients who are less able, organized, or motivated to make and maintain changes in their self-management regimen (Glasgow, Bull, Piette, & Steiner, 2004).

Contexts in Which IVR Has Been and Could Be Used

Chronic Disease Self-Management Support

Disease self-management usually requires adherence to multiple and often changing medication schedules, regular follow-up visits with clinicians, efforts to identify potential acute events early, and difficult lifestyle behavior changes such as weight loss or increases in physical activity. Not surprisingly, many patients fall short of self-care goals and experience preventable complications as a result. Some patients with chronic conditions need weekly or even daily support to manage their complex regimens. Comorbid distress, anxiety, and depression are common among patients with chronic conditions and further complicate their self-care (Egede & Ellis, 2010; Fisher et al., 2010).

IVR communication with patients between outpatient visits can promote more effective disease self-management. In one early study, we found that low-income patients with type 2 diabetes completed more than 75% of attempted IVR assessment calls and reported a number of health problems that might otherwise have gone unnoticed by clinicians (Piette & Mah, 1997). Most patients reported that they would like to receive automated monitoring calls as part of their usual care (89%) and that such calls would make them more satisfied with their health services (77%). In a randomized trial, diabetes patients who received weekly IVR calls for one year completed more than 4,000 assessments, representing 71% of all assessment attempts (Piette, McPhee, Weinberger, Mah, & Kraemer, 1999).

Non-English-Speaking Patients

Language minority patients in the United States can and will use IVR as part of their chronic illness care (Brodey, Rosen, Brodey, Sheetz, & Unutzer, 2005; Lorig, Ritter, Villa, & Piette, 2008; Piette, et al., 1999). IVR reminders can reduce return visit failures for tuberculosis patients who speak Spanish, Tagalog (Filipino), or Vietnamese (Tanke & Leirer, 1994; Tanke, Martinez, & Leirer, 1997). In a trial of diabetes patients, we found that Spanish speakers were even more interested than English speakers in accessing information about their self-care using IVR (Piette, 1999). Others have shown that Spanish speakers were interested in telephone support for chronic illness care (Sarkar, Piette, et al., 2008). Spanish- and Cantonese-speaking patients with diabetes have used IVR to report adverse health events (Sarkar, Handley, et al., 2008), and IVR communication can yield higher contact rates than group medical visits for language minority groups (Schillinger et al., 2008).

Enhancing Support from Informal Caregivers

For patients with complex chronic conditions, an informal caregiver can play an important role in supporting efforts to follow self-management plans, identify early warning signs of acute illness, and cope emotionally with the stresses of the disease (Jecker, 1990; Noelker & Whitlatch, 2005; Ward, Sherman, & LaGory, 1984). Unfortunately, many patients have no one living within their household who is able to provide that assistance (Piette, Rosland, Silveira, Kabeto, & Langa, 2010). Although more than 93% of chronically ill older adults in the United States have adult children, and 78% report at least weekly telephone contact (Piette, Rosland, et al., 2010), out-of-home social network members often lack the skills and resources they need to be effective care supporters (Hopp, 2000). IVR can help them play clearly defined support roles in patients' disease self-management.

Follow-Up after Acute Care

One in five hospitalized patients experiences a poor outcome in the first month following discharge (Forster, Murff, Peterson, Gandhi, & Bates, 2003; Jencks, Williams, & Coleman, 2009). Clinicians working at cross-purposes, patients confused by their self-management goals, and inadequate efforts to involve caregivers frequently lead to preventable acute events, emergency department visits, and higher health care costs (Corrigan & Martin, 1992; Weissman et al., 1999). Intensive care management postdischarge can reduce rehospitalization rates and mortality risk (McAlister, Stewart, Ferrua, & McMurray, 2004; Ofman et al., 2004; Phillips et al.,

2004). Unfortunately, telemedicine follow-up is labor intensive, and the resources required to provide these services are often unavailable (Jack et al., 2009; Jones, Clark, Bradford, & Dougherty, 1988).

IVR is a potentially useful technology for improving patient care during transitions from hospital to home. IVR contacts can identify important health concerns arising postdischarge, and studies suggest that some patients may even prefer IVR follow-up to a "live" follow-up call from a clinician (Forster, Boyle, Shojania, Feasby, & Van Walraven, 2009; Forster et al., 2008; Forster & van Walraven, 2007). Other studies have reported high levels of patient responsiveness to IVR monitoring and patient satisfaction (Finkelstein, Khare, & Vora, 2009; Nguyen, Gill, Wolpin, Steele, & Benditt, 2009; Young, Sparrow, Gottlieb, Selim, & Friedman, 2001).

Mental Health

Patients with cognitive impairments, mental health disorders, or substance abuse problems have been among the most studied recipients of IVR monitoring and behavior change support. Studies have consistently shown that IVR is a potential resource for gathering accurate and timely feedback about these patients' needs between in-person encounters and may be an effective strategy for providing assistance with behavior change. Patients with psychiatric problems report reliable information about their symptoms and behaviors using IVR (Kobak et al., 1997a & b; Perrine, Mundt, Searles, & Lester, 1995).

We have found that patients with depression report reliable information about their symptoms using IVR. During weekly IVR assessment and behavior change calls, depressed patients report information about their symptoms using the PHQ-9 (Kroenke, Spitzer, & Williams, 2001). Trend scores are calculated and patients receive advice regarding medication adherence, engaging in pleasurable activities, and seeking follow-up attention from clinicians. Patients who are at risk for self-harm have the option of connecting directly to a suicide hotline. The clinical team for such patients is informed by fax, and informal caregivers enrolled with those patients receive updates on their mobile phone with suggestions on how to help. Results to date indicate that depressed patients may be even more satisfied with IVR-supported disease management than heart failure or diabetes patients.

Managing Chronic Diseases in Underdeveloped Countries

Sixty percent of all deaths worldwide are due to chronic diseases, with 80% of those occurring in low- to middle-income countries (Daar et al., 2007). Diabetes alone represents an international crisis, with estimated global prevalence of 439 million people by 2030 compared to 285 million in 2009 (International Diabetes Federation, 2009). In Latin America, an aging population, migration to urban centers, and the ubiquitous presence of junk food have caused chronic cardiovascular disease rates to skyrocket (International Diabetes Federation, 2009; Pan American Health Organization, 2007).

In a survey of 624 chronically ill Honduran adults, we found that the majority were willing to use IVR as part of a telehealth service designed to improve their chronic illness care (Piette, Mendoza-Avelares, et al., 2010). Eighty-eight percent of respondents reported that they would be willing to receive automated telephone reminders about upcoming appointments, 80% were willing to receive IVR health status monitoring for their symptoms and self-care needs, and 81% were willing to participate in automated self-management education.

Effects of the Approach

The Reliability and Validity of IVR Assessments

IVR monitoring can provide reliable and valid information about patients' status between outpatient visits (Balas et al., 1997; Corkrey & Parkinson, 2002; Krishna, Balas, Spencer, Griffin, & Boren, 1997; Piette, 2000a). In a large randomized trial, we found that English- and Spanish-speaking diabetes patients reported valid and reliable clinical information during IVR calls (Piette et al., 1999). Nurse educators verified 4,400 automated assessment reported problems during follow-up calls. Patients indicated that their automated assessment information was what they had intended to report more than 85% of the time. Overall, 82% reported that they would be more satisfied with their health care if IVR assessment and behavior change calls were available, and 76% reported that they would choose to receive such calls in the future (Piette, 1999, 2000b).

Patients using IVR can report reliably about sensitive issues including alcohol use, alcohol-related problems, and HIV risk behaviors (Andersson, Soderpalm Gordh, & Berglund, 2007; Helzer et al., 2008; Midanik & Greenfield, 2008, 2010; Perrine, et al., 1995; Schroder & Johnson, 2009; Schroder, Johnson, & Wiebe, 2007; Tucker, Foushee, Black, & Roth, 2007). Use of IVR assessments can substantially decrease the staffing time required for low-risk events (Krenzelok & Mrvos, 2009). In one study, older adults with complex neuropsychological deficits completed IVR assessments consistently and with good convergent validity when compared to other measures (Mundt, Kinoshita, Hsu, Yesavage, & Greist, 2007). Depressive symptoms and anxiety also can be assessed accurately using IVR (Kim, Bracha, & Tipnis, 2007; Kobak et al., 1997a & b; Mundt et al., 2006; Turvey, Willyard, Hickman, Klein, & Kukoyi, 2007). Other problems such as back pain (Shaw & Verma, 2007), smoking (Toll, Cooney, McKee, & O'Malley, 2005), addiction severity (Brodey et al., 2004, 2005; Hall & Huber, 2000), and health-related quality of life (Millard & Carver, 1999) have been reliably reported by patients using IVR calls.

Impacts on Patient Outcomes

IVR-supported nursing care can improve patients' self-care and health outcomes (Piette, Weinberger, & McPhee, 2000; Piette, Weinberger, McPhee, &

Mah, 2000). In a trial of underinsured diabetes patients, participants receiving IVR calls reported significantly better self-care than control patients at their 12-month follow-up in the areas of home glucose monitoring, foot care, and weight monitoring. Intervention patients were substantially less likely than controls to report one or more problems with medication adherence at follow-up (44% versus 64%, $p < .01$), and more than twice as many intervention patients had acceptable glycemic control at 12 months (18% versus 8%, $p = .01$). Compared to controls, intervention patients reported fewer symptoms of diabetes and depression (both $p < .001$), were more satisfied with their care, had greater perceived access to care, and had more confidence (i.e., self-efficacy) in managing their self-care (all $p < .05$). Outcomes in a VA trial were similar (Piette, Weinberger, Kraemer, & McPhee, 2001).

Other studies also have shown that IVR services can improve health care and health outcomes of patients with a range of chronic conditions. IVR assessments can be an efficient alternative to "live" assessments for the prevention of cognitive impairment among community dwelling older adults (Sano et al., 2010). IVR assessments have been shown to improve medication adherence in patient groups ranging from asthma to cardiac surgery patients postdischarge (Bender et al., 2010; Sherrard et al., 2009). In a diverse low-income population of diabetes patients served by a safety net health care system, investigators found that an IVR service coupled with nurse care management achieved physical activity objectives at modest cost (Handley, Shumway, & Schillinger, 2008). Other studies have reported important improvements in the body mass index of children participating in a lifestyle change intervention (Estabrooks et al., 2009), smoking cessation rates among heart disease patients (Reid, Pipe, Quinlan, & Oda, 2007), unhealthy drinking among HIV patients (Aharonovich et al., 2006), and mental health symptoms among caregivers of patients with Alzheimer's disease (Mahoney, Tarlow, & Jones, 2003).

Not all trials of IVR-supported disease management have shown positive outcomes. A recent study examined the use of automated calls to health plan members with diabetes to remind them about disease management services such as eye examinations (Simon et al., 2010). Most patients did not respond to the IVR calls sent to their homes and there was no difference in examination rates compared to controls. The null finding may reflect the fact that patients had no prior knowledge about the program and no choice whether to participate. In another study, results showed that IVR calls with educational content and an opportunity to transfer to a scheduling center were not successful in increasing rates of bone mineral density testing among members at risk for osteoporosis (Polinski et al., 2006). Finally, a trial evaluating the marginal benefit of IVR follow-up among Spanish-speaking patients already receiving peer-supported self-care education showed the IVR had no impact (Lorig et al., 2008). This may mean that among patients receiving another evidence-based intervention, the marginal improvement in care associated with IVR is minimal.

Current and Future Dissemination Potential

There is substantial potential for experimentation and dissemination of IVR-based services, including IVR programs linked with other strategies for reaching patients between visits. Here, we describe an area in which our research team is developing new approaches for making available evidenced-based IVR applications.

Delivering IVR Using a Cloud Computing Model

Cloud computing is a new approach in which an end user (e.g., physicians' practice or public clinic) accesses a computing infrastructure remotely over the Internet. With cloud computing, users do not need to maintain the hardware, software, or expertise to manage the technologic infrastructure in the "cloud" that supports them. For IVR programs, a cloud computing model means that clinics can access the core informatics infrastructure from anywhere in the world. Patient information can be entered via a website and IVR calls can be generated from the central server to patients' mobile phones using the low-cost Voice over IP (VoIP) technology that makes Skype, magicJack, and Vonage possible. As such, cloud computing could make IVR-supported disease management available to communities without the technological infrastructure needed for IVR calls.

We recently developed the first cloud computing model for providing IVR support for disease self-management across international boundaries. The system's technologic infrastructure is maintained on a server at the University of Michigan and can be accessed by clinics in other countries via the Web. Clinicians can schedule patients' IVR calls and designate where and how follow-up should be directed to patients' clinical teams and informal caregivers.

In the summer of 2010, 85 diabetes patients were enrolled in an IVR-based disease management program in Honduras (Piette et al., 2011). Despite the country's limited telecommunications infrastructure, patients completed the majority of their weekly IVR assessment calls. Clinicians received urgent alerts about problems such as severe hypoglycemic symptoms and were able to use that information for treatment planning. Patients reported important changes in their diabetes self-care, and mean A1c levels (a measure of glycemic control) decreased from 10.0% at baseline to 8.9% at follow-up ($p < .01$).

We currently are developing the capacity for a larger IVR-supported chronic illness care program that could serve multiple sites in less developed areas of the world. Projects are underway with partners in Monterrey, Mexico; Quito, Ecuador; Bogota, Colombia; and La Paz, Bolivia. The system is being designed so that primary care providers in those areas will be able to access the program via a user-friendly website. Patients will receive IVR calls from the system at a provider-specified frequency, with specified call windows and repeat calls, if necessary. During each IVR call, patients will report information about their health and self-care using their touch-tone telephone and will receive recorded information designed to promote more effective self-care and use of clinical services. Clinicians will auto matically be sent structured faxes when patients report urgent health issues and will be able to review their patients' progress via Web-based reports.

Privacy Concerns

Particularly when IVR services are provided outside of patients' immediate sources of care, the security of data transfer and storage are important concerns. State-of-the-art encryption, firewalls, authentication, and other data security procedures should always be employed. For smaller health centers, cloud computing may be even more secure than onsite data management, since highly specialized professionals can use the most advanced hardware and software to keep patient data safe. Patients should be informed about how the information they provide during IVR calls will be used and stored, using easily understandable, nontechnical language. Research suggests that IVR calls without patient consent are less effective (Simon, et al., 2010), and in our experience, patients are very comfortable with IVR programs including offsite data management when the security of those systems is clearly described. HIPAA regulations allow patients to share their health information with whomever they choose. With appropriately informed patient users, no concerns have been expressed by health care systems, patients, or family caregivers regarding the targeted sharing of self-care support information as part of the CarePartner program.

Limitations and Conclusions

While IVR represents an important part of the portfolio of services improving access to health information, its use does pose challenges. Some potential patient users and health professionals perceive negative connotations of "robo-calls" and see IVR as an attempt to trade off in-person assistance for a cheap and potentially frustrating alternative (Forster et al., 2009). Due to the explosion of mobile communication options (e.g., text messaging, online social networks, and email; see Abroms, Padmanabhan, & Evans, and Fjeldsoe, Miller, & Marshall, this volume), some potential users are unwilling to accept the additional information that IVR can provide (Fava & Guidi, 2007). Some patients may be reticent to share health information with family members, and these new caregiver roles may increase burden or relationship stress. However, our experience with more than 800 patient/caregiver pairs participating in the CarePartner program suggests that a large number of patients and families welcome these new information tools.

In summary, IVR represents an important, evidence-based tool for improving patients' access to health information and providing others involved in their care with accessible data about how to improve patients' management. IVR is low cost and widely accessible without requiring specialized hardware or access to the Internet. IVR has been used successfully with diverse populations, and studies indicate that it can improve patients' self-care behavior and health outcomes. The unsuccessful trials discussed in this chapter suggest that careful consideration must go into the design and dissemination of IVR programs. The technology alone is insufficient to create positive impacts; it is the technology combined with program content that makes a difference. IVR lends itself well to the paradigm of cloud computing and, with Voice over IP, could be used to dramatically improve access to self-care support in some of the most economically challenged areas of the world.

References

Aharonovich, E., Hatzenbuehler, M. L., Johnston, B., O'Leary, A., Morgenstern, J., Wainberg, M. L., et al. (2006). A low-cost, sustainable intervention for drinking reduction in the HIV primary care setting. *AIDS Care, 18,* 561–568.

Andersson, C., Soderpalm Gordh, A. H., & Berglund, M. (2007). Use of real-time interactive voice response in a study of stress and alcohol consumption. *Alcoholism: Clinical and Experimental Research, 31,* 1908–1912.

Asociación de la Industria Celular en Colombia *(n.d.)*. *Densidad celular en Colombia.* Retrieved June 29, 2011, from: http://www.asocel.org.co/pdf/densidad_celular_en_%20 colombia_90.pdf.

Balas, E. A., Jaffrey, F., Kuperman, G. J., Boren, S. A., Brown, G. D., Pinciroli, F., et al. (1997). Electronic communication with patients. Evaluation of distance medicine technology. *Journal of the American Medical Association, 278,* 152–159.

Bender, B. G., Apter, A., Bogen, D. K., Dickinson, P., Fisher, L., Wamboldt, F. S., et al. (2010). Test of an interactive voice response intervention to improve adherence to controller medications in adults with asthma. *Journal of the American Board of Family Medicine, 23,* 159–165.

Brodey, B. B., Rosen, C. S., Brodey, I. S., Sheetz, B. M., & Unutzer, J. (2005). Reliability and acceptability of automated telephone surveys among Spanish- and English-speaking mental health services recipients. *Mental Health Services and Research, 7,* 181–184.

Brodey, B. B., Rosen, C. S., Brodey, I. S., Sheetz, B. M., Steinfeld, R. R., & Gastfriend, D. R. (2004). Validation of the Addiction Severity Index (ASI) for Internet and automated telephone self-report administration. *Journal of Substance Abuse Treatment, 26,* 253–259.

Castells, M., Fernandez-Ardevol, M., Qui, J. L., & Sey, A. (2006). *Mobile communication and society: A global perspective: A project of the Annenberg Research Network on international communication.* Cambridge, MA: MIT Press.

Corkrey, R., & Parkinson, L. (2002). Interactive voice response: Review of studies 1989–2000. *Behavior Research Methods, Instruments, & Computers, 34,* 342–353.

Corrigan, J. M., & Martin, J. B. (1992). Identification of factors associated with hospital readmission and development of a predictive model. *Health Services Research, 27,* 81–101.

Daar, A. S., Singer, P. A., Persad, D. L., Pramming, S. K., Matthews, D. R., Beaglehole, R., et al. (2007). Grand challenges in chronic non-communicable diseases. *Nature, 450,* 494–496.

Egede, L. E., & Ellis, C. (2010). Diabetes and depression: Global perspectives. *Diabetes Research and Clinical Practice, 87,* 302–312.

Estabrooks, P. A., Shoup, J. A., Gattshall, M., Dandamudi, P., Shetterly, S., & Xu, S. (2009). Automated telephone counseling for parents of overweight children: A randomized controlled trial. *American Journal of Preventive Medicine, 36,* 35–42.

Fava, G. A., & Guidi, J. (2007). Information overload, the patient and the clinician. *Psychotherapy and Psychosomatics, 76,* 1–3.

Finkelstein, J., Khare, R., & Vora, D. (2009). Home automated telemanagement (HAT) system to facilitate self-care of patients with chronic diseases. *Systemics, Cybernetics, and Informatics, 1,* 78–82.

Fisher, L., Mullan, J. T., Arean, P., Glasgow, R. E., Hessler, D., & Masharani, U. (2010). Diabetes distress but not clinical depression or depressive symptoms is associated with glycemic control in both cross-sectional and longitudinal analyses. *Diabetes Care, 33,* 23–28.

Forster, A. J., Boyle, L., Shojania, K. G., Feasby, T. E., & van Walraven, C. (2009). Identifying patients with post-discharge care problems using an interactive voice response system. *Journal of General Internal Medicine, 24,* 520–525.

Forster, A. J., LaBranche, R., McKim, R., Faught, J. W., Feasby, T. E., Janes-Kelley, S., et al. (2008). Automated patient assessments after outpatient surgery using an interactive voice response system. *American Journal of Managed Care, 14,* 429–436.

Forster, A. J., Murff, H. J., Peterson, J. F., Gandhi, T. K., & Bates, D. W. (2003). The incidence and severity of adverse events affecting patients after discharge from the hospital. *Annals of Internal Medicine, 138,* 161–167.

Forster, A. J., & van Walraven, C. (2007). Using an interactive voice response system to improve patient safety following hospital discharge. *Journal of Evaluation in Clinical Practice, 13,* 346–351.

Glasgow, R. E., Bull, S. S., Piette, J. D., & Steiner, J. F. (2004). Interactive behavior change technology: A partial solution to the competing demands of primary care. *American Journal of Preventive Medicine, 27*(2 Suppl), 80–87.

Hall, J. A., & Huber, D. L. (2000). Telephone management in substance abuse treatment. *Telemedicine Journal and e-Health, 6,* 401–407.

Handley, M. A., Shumway, M., & Schillinger, D. (2008). Cost-effectiveness of automated telephone self-management support with nurse care management among patients with diabetes. *Annals of Family Medicine, 6,* 512–518.

Helzer, J. E., Rose, G. L., Badger, G. J., Searles, J. S., Thomas, C. S., Lindberg, S. A., et al. (2008). Using interactive voice response to enhance brief alcohol intervention in primary care settings. *Journal of Studies on Alcohol and Drugs, 69,* 251–258.

Hopp, F. P. (2000). Preferences for surrogate decision makers, informal communication, and advance directives among community-dwelling elders: Results from a national study. *Gerontologist, 40,* 449–457.

Inglis, S. C., Clark, R. A., McAlister, F. A., Ball, J., Lewinter, C., Cullington, D., et al. (2010). Structured telephone support or telemonitoring programmes for patients with chronic heart failure. *Cochrane Database of Systematic Reviews,* CD007228.

International Diabetes Federation. (2009). *The diabetes atlas.* Retrieved July 1, 2011, from: http://www.idf.org/Facts_and_Figures.

International Telecommunications Union. (2007, May 16). *World Information Society 2007 Report: Beyond WSIS.* Retrieved July 1, 2011, from: http://www.itu.int/osg/spu/publications/worldinformationsociety/2007/report.html.

Jack, B. W., Chetty, V. K., Anthony, D., Greenwald, J. L., Sanchez, G. M., Johnson, A. E., et al. (2009). A reengineered hospital discharge program to decrease rehospitalization: A randomized trial. *Annals of Internal Medicine, 150,* 178–187.

Jecker, N. S. (1990). The role of intimate others in medical decision making. *Gerontologist, 30*, 65–71.

Jencks, S. F., Williams, M. V., & Coleman, E. A. (2009). Rehospitalizations among patients in the Medicare fee-for-service program. *New England Journal of Medicine, 360*, 1418–1428.

Jones, J., Clark, W., Bradford, J., & Dougherty, J. (1988). Efficacy of a telephone follow-up system in the emergency department. *Journal of Emergency Medicine, 6*, 249–254.

Kim, H., Bracha, Y., & Tipnis, A. (2007). Automated depression screening in disadvantaged pregnant women in an urban obstetric clinic. *Archives of Women's Mental Health, 10*, 163–169.

Kobak, K. A., Taylor, L. H., Dottl, S. L., Greist, J. H., Jefferson, J. W., Burroughs, D., Katzelnick, D. J., et al. (1997a). Computerized screening for psychiatric disorders in an outpatient community mental health clinic. *Psychiatric Services, 48*, 1048–1057.

Kobak, K. A., Taylor, L. H., Dottl, S. L., Greist, J. H., Jefferson, J. W., Burroughs, D., Mantle, J. M., et al. (1997b). A computer-administered telephone interview to identify mental disorders. *Journal of the American Medical Association, 278*, 905–910.

Krenzelok, E. P., & Mrvos, R. (2009). The use of an automated interactive voice response system to manage medication identification calls to a poison center. *Clinical Toxicology, 47*, 425–429.

Krishna, S., Balas, E. A., Spencer, D. C., Griffin, J. Z., & Boren, S. A. (1997). Clinical trials of interactive computerized patient education: Implications for family practice. *Journal of Family Practice, 45*, 25–33.

Kroenke, K., Spitzer, R. L., & Williams, J. B. (2001). The PHQ-9: Validity of a brief depression severity measure. *Journal of General Internal Medicine, 16*, 606–613.

Lober, W. B., Zierler, B., Herbaugh, A., Shinstrom, S. E., Stolyar, A., Kim, E. H., et al. (2006). Barriers to the use of a personal health record by an elderly population. *American Medical Informatics Association Annual Symposium Proceedings*, 514–518.

Lorig, K., Ritter, P. L., Villa, F., & Piette, J. D. (2008). Spanish diabetes self-management with and without automated telephone reinforcement: Two randomized trials. *Diabetes Care, 31*, 408–414.

Mahoney, D. F., Tarlow, B. J., & Jones, R. N. (2003). Effects of an automated telephone support system on caregiver burden and anxiety: Findings from the REACH for TLC intervention study. *Gerontologist, 43*, 556–567.

McAlister, F. A., Stewart, S., Ferrua, S., & McMurray, J. J. (2004). Multidisciplinary strategies for the management of heart failure patients at high risk for admission: A systematic review of randomized trials. *Journal of the American College of Cardiology, 44*, 810–819.

Midanik, L. T., & Greenfield, T. K. (2008). Interactive voice response versus computer-assisted telephone interviewing (CATI) surveys and sensitive questions: The 2005 National Alcohol Survey. *Journal of Studies on Alcohol and Drugs, 69*, 580–588.

Midanik, L. T., & Greenfield, T. K. (2010). Reports of alcohol-related problems and alcohol dependence for demographic subgroups using interactive voice response versus telephone surveys: The 2005 U.S. National Alcohol Survey. *Drug and Alcohol Review, 29*, 392–398.

Millard, R. W., & Carver, J. R. (1999). Cross-sectional comparison of live and interactive voice recognition administration of the SF-12 health status survey. *American Journal of Managed Care, 5*, 153–159.

Mundt, J. C., Katzelnick, D. J., Kennedy, S. H., Eisfeld, B. S., Bouffard, B. B., & Greist, J. H. (2006). Validation of an IVRS version of the MADRS. *Journal of Psychiatric Research, 40*, 243–246.

Mundt, J. C., Kinoshita, L. M., Hsu, S., Yesavage, J. A., & Greist, J. H. (2007). Telephonic Remote Evaluation of Neuropsychological Deficits (TREND): Longitudinal monitoring of elderly community-dwelling volunteers using touch-tone telephones. *Alzheimer Disease and Associated Disorders, 21,* 218–224.

Nguyen, H. Q., Gill, D. P., Wolpin, S., Steele, B. G., & Benditt, J. O. (2009). Pilot study of a cell phone-based exercise persistence intervention post-rehabilitation for COPD. *International Journal of Chronic Obstructive Pulmonary Disease, 4,* 301–313.

Noelker, L. S., & Whitlatch, C. J. (2005). Informal caregiving. In C. J. Evanshwick (Ed.), *The continuum of long-term care* (3rd ed., pp. 29–47). Clifton Park, NY: Thomson Delmar Learning.

Ofman, J. J., Badamgarav, E., Henning, J. M., Knight, K., Gano, A. D., Jr., Levan, R. K., et al. (2004). Does disease management improve clinical and economic outcomes in patients with chronic diseases? A systematic review. *American Journal of Medicine, 117,* 182–192.

Pan American Health Organization. (2007). *Health in the Americas.* Retrieved July 1, 2011, from: http://www.paho.org/hia/archivosvol2/paisesing/honduras%20english.pdf.

Perrine, M. W., Mundt, J. C., Searles, J. S., & Lester, L. S. (1995). Validation of daily self-reported alcohol consumption using interactive voice response (IVR) technology. *Journal of Studies on Alcohol, 56,* 487–490.

Phillips, C. O., Wright, S. M., Kern, D. E., Singa, R. M., Shepperd, S., & Rubin, H. R. (2004). Comprehensive discharge planning with postdischarge support for older patients with congestive heart failure: A meta-analysis. *Journal of the American Medical Association, 291,* 1358–1367.

Piette, J. D. (1999). Patient education via automated calls: A study of English and Spanish speakers with diabetes. *American Journal of Preventive Medicine, 17,* 138–141.

Piette, J. D. (2000a). Interactive voice response systems in the diagnosis and management of chronic disease. *American Journal of Managed Care, 6,* 817–827.

Piette, J. D. (2000b). Satisfaction with automated telephone disease management calls and its relationship to their use. *Diabetes Educator, 26,* 1003–1010.

Piette, J. D. (2007). Interactive behavior change technology to support diabetes self-management: Where do we stand? *Diabetes Care, 30,* 2425–2432.

Piette, J. D., Gregor, M. A., Share, D., Heisler, M., Bernstein, S. J., Koelling, T., et al. (2008). Improving heart failure self-management support by actively engaging out-of-home caregivers: Results of a feasibility study. *Congestive Heart Failure, 14,* 12–18.

Piette, J. D., Lange, I., Issel, M., Campos, S., Bustamante, C., Sapag, J., et al. (2006). Use of telephone care in a cardiovascular disease management programme for type 2 diabetes patients in Santiago, Chile. *Chronic Illness, 2,* 87–96.

Piette, J. D., & Mah, C. A. (1997). The feasibility of automated voice messaging as an adjunct to diabetes outpatient care. *Diabetes Care, 20,* 15–21.

Piette, J. D., McPhee, S. J., Weinberger, M., Mah, C. A., & Kraemer, F. B. (1999). Use of automated telephone disease management calls in an ethnically diverse sample of low-income patients with diabetes. *Diabetes Care, 22,* 1302–1309.

Piette, J. D., Mendoza-Avelares, M., Ganser, M., Mohamed, M., Marinec, N., & Krishnan, S. (2011). A preliminary study of a cloud-computing model for chronic illness self-care support in an underdeveloped country. *American Journal of Preventive Medicine, 40,* 629–632.

Piette, J. D., Mendoza-Avelares, M. O., Milton, E. C., Lange, I., & Fajardo, R. (2010). Access to mobile communication technology and willingness to participate in automated telemedicine calls among chronically ill patients in Honduras. *Telemedicine Journal and e-Health, 16,* 1030–1041.

Piette, J. D., Rosland, A. M., Silveira, M., Kabeto, M., & Langa, K. M. (2010). The case for involving adult children outside of the household in the self-management support of older adults with chronic illnesses. *Chronic Illness, 6,* 34–45.

Piette, J. D., Weinberger, M., Kraemer, F. B., & McPhee, S. J. (2001). Impact of automated calls with nurse follow-up on diabetes treatment outcomes in a Department of Veterans Affairs Health Care System: A randomized controlled trial. *Diabetes Care, 24,* 202–208.

Piette, J. D., Weinberger, M., & McPhee, S. J. (2000). The effect of automated calls with telephone nurse follow-up on patient-centered outcomes of diabetes care: A randomized, controlled trial. *Medical Care, 38,* 218–230.

Piette, J. D., Weinberger, M., McPhee, S. J., Mah, C. A., Kraemer, F. B., & Crapo, L. M. (2000). Do automated calls with nurse follow-up improve self-care and glycemic control among vulnerable patients with diabetes? *American Journal of Medicine, 108,* 20–27.

Polinski, J. M., Patrick, A., Truppo, C., Breiner, L., Chen, Y. T., Egan, C., et al. (2006). Interactive voice response telephone calls to enhance bone mineral density testing. *American Journal of Managed Care, 12,* 321–325.

Reid, R. D., Pipe, A. L., Quinlan, B., & Oda, J. (2007). Interactive voice response telephony to promote smoking cessation in patients with heart disease: A pilot study. *Patient Education and Counseling, 66,* 319–326.

Sano, M., Egelko, S., Ferris, S., Kaye, J., Hayes, T. L., Mundt, J. C., et al. (2010). Pilot study to show the feasibility of a multicenter trial of home-based assessment of people over 75 years old. *Alzheimer Disease and Associated Disorders, 24,* 256–263.

Sarkar, U., Handley, M. A., Gupta, R., Tang, A., Murphy, E., Seligman, H. K., et al. (2008). Use of an interactive, telephone-based self-management support program to identify adverse events among ambulatory diabetes patients. *Journal of General Internal Medicine, 23,* 459–465.

Sarkar, U., Piette, J. D., Gonzales, R., Lessler, D., Chew, L. D., Reilly, B., et al. (2008). Preferences for self-management support: Findings from a survey of diabetes patients in safety-net health systems. *Patient Education and Counseling, 70,* 102–110.

Schillinger, D., Hammer, H., Wang, F., Palacios, J., McLean, I., Tang, A., et al. (2008). Seeing in 3-D: Examining the reach of diabetes self-management support strategies in a public health care system. *Health Education & Behavior, 35,* 664–682.

Schroder, K. E., & Johnson, C. J. (2009). Interactive voice response technology to measure HIV-related behavior. *Current HIV/AIDS Reports, 6,* 210–216.

Schroder, K. E., Johnson, C. J., & Wiebe, J. S. (2007). Interactive Voice Response Technology applied to sexual behavior self-reports: A comparison of three methods. *AIDS and Behavior, 11,* 313–323.

Shaw, W. S., & Verma, S. K. (2007). Data equivalence of an interactive voice response system for home assessment of back pain and function. *Pain Research & Management, 12,* 23–30.

Sherrard, H., Struthers, C., Kearns, S. A., Wells, G., Chen, L., & Mesana, T. (2009). Using technology to create a medication safety net for cardiac surgery patients: A nurse-led randomized control trial. *Canadian Journal of Cardiovascular Nursing, 19,* 9–15.

Simon, S. R., Trinacty, C. M., Soumerai, S. B., Piette, J. D., Meigs, J. B., Shi, P., et al. (2010). Improving diabetes care among patients overdue for recommended testing: A randomized controlled trial of automated telephone outreach. *Diabetes Care, 33,* 1452–1453.

Tanke, E. D., & Leirer, V. O. (1994). Automated telephone reminders in tuberculosis care. *Medical Care, 32,* 380–389.

Tanke, E. D., Martinez, C. M., & Leirer, V. O. (1997). Use of automated reminders for tuberculin skin test return. *American Journal of Preventive Medicine, 13,* 189–192.

Toll, B. A., Cooney, N. L., McKee, S. A., & O'Malley, S. S. (2005). Do daily interactive voice response reports of smoking behavior correspond with retrospective reports? *Psychology of Addictive Behaviors, 19,* 291–295.

Tucker, J. A., Foushee, H. R., Black, B. C., & Roth, D. L. (2007). Agreement between prospective interactive voice response self-monitoring and structured retrospective reports of drinking and contextual variables during natural resolution attempts. *Journal of Studies on Alcohol and Drugs, 68,* 538–542.

Turvey, C. L., Willyard, D., Hickman, D. H., Klein, D. M., & Kukoyi, O. (2007). Telehealth screen for depression in a chronic illness care management program. *Telemedicine Journal and e-Health, 13,* 51–56.

Ward, R. A., Sherman, S. R., & LaGory, M. (1984). Informal networks and knowledge of services for older persons. *Journals of Gerontology, 39,* 216–223.

Weissman, J. S., Ayanian, J. Z., Chasan-Taber, S., Sherwood, M. J., Roth, C., & Epstein, A. M. (1999). Hospital readmissions and quality of care. *Medical Care, 37,* 490–501.

Young, M., Sparrow, D., Gottlieb, D., Selim, A., & Friedman, R. (2001). A telephone-linked computer system for COPD care. *Chest, 119,* 1565–1575.

Practice Implications
and Future Directions

12

USING SOCIAL MEDIA TO ENHANCE HEALTH COMMUNICATION CAMPAIGNS

Ann M. Taubenheim, Terry Long, Jennifer Wayman, Sarah Temple, Sally McDonough, and Ashley Duncan

For a list of #HeartTruth heart disease risk factors visit hearttruth.gov and please RT (retweet) to all the women you know!

In fewer than 140 characters on Twitter, the National Heart, Lung, and Blood Institute's *The Heart Truth* campaign helps to educate and empower women to take action against their number one killer: heart disease. Social support and strong social networks make important contributions to our health (Albrecht & Goldsmith, 2003). They provide emotional and practical resources, and they make us feel cared for, loved, esteemed, and valued. Consequently, social marketers have long relied on these networks as channels to raise awareness of public health issues, facilitate behavior change, and ultimately help people live healthier, safer lives (Hughes, 2010).

Today's social networks have grown beyond neighborhoods, communities, and local organizations and are now thriving online through social media applications such as Facebook and Twitter. These digital platforms are being used to support a wide variety of health issues, from aiding suicide prevention to communicating the risks of heart disease, and they are facilitating dialogue among members of the public health community, as well. By integrating social media tactics into broader social marketing efforts, marketers are extending messaging and reach far beyond traditional expectations (Hughes, 2010).

Social marketing—a term in use since the early 1970s—is a discipline that applies consumer marketing principles to the promotion of ideas, issues, and practices to create awareness and change attitudes and behaviors regarding social and health issues. In other words, social marketers sell ideas, beliefs, and behaviors, rather than goods and services. *Social media* has been defined as a way of using the Internet to instantly collaborate, share information, and have a conversation about ideas or causes we care about (Wilcox & Kanter, 2007).

Using Web-based and mobile technologies, social media can take many different forms, including Internet forums, message boards, texting via mobile devices, blogs, social network websites such as Facebook and MySpace, wikis, podcasts, pictures, and video. Social media are less about the actual technology and more about the way the technology enables individuals to interact online (Hughes, 2010). Marketing that makes use of social media has become an increasingly important part of the integrated marketing approaches used by businesses and nonprofit organizations alike, and it has been referred to as *social media marketing* (Weinreich, 2006). Social media marketing can help to build brand awareness, increase visibility, connect more personally with customers, and achieve marketing communication goals through the use of online social networks and other Web applications. These approaches usually aim to create content that attracts attention and encourages users to share it with their own social networks, thereby increasing the reach of the message and, presumably, its credibility, since it comes from a trusted source: someone in one's own social sphere.

Using Social Media in a Public Health and Social Marketing Environment

The past three years in particular have marked a turning point in the way Americans obtain public health information via the Internet. Today one-third of adults access health-related social media (e.g., a blog about heart disease in women), and nearly 80% of physicians who use the Internet make use of social media channels to create, consume, or share medical content (Fox & Jones, 2009; Levy & Daniels, 2008; Tu & Cohen, 2008). Internet users who look for public health information online are more likely than non–health information seekers to create or work on their own blog, read someone else's blog, use a social networking site, and use status update services (Fox & Jones, 2009). Thus, being an "e-patient," an individual who looks for information about public health topics online, has become a leading indicator of other forms of social media engagement (Hughes, 2010).

This rapid evolution of digital information sharing presents a significant opportunity for the public and social marketers alike. With the broadening of traditional social networks across the Web, millions of consumers now have access to reliable public health information and interventions in real time, and social marketers have new tools for vastly expanding their reach to public audiences (Hughes, 2010).

How can social marketers take full advantage of the new opportunities presented by an expanding digital world? As with communications advances in the past, today's digital transformation generally is not replacing older media; rather, it is adding to them and expanding communications options. In planning communications efforts, today's practitioners do not have to choose one channel over the other. The opportunity exists to look across all media forms, select those that best fit the audience and issue, and integrate them into a well-planned whole.

Traditional media such as radio, television, and print may still play a strong role. And social media, with their tremendous potential for connecting people around health and social issues, have given social marketers additional options to deliver targeted messaging to a greater range of audiences than ever before.

Although digital media present social marketers with major new opportunities, they also come with substantial new responsibilities for good communications planning, formative research, program execution, and evaluation. In general, the same basic principles that guide best practices in overall health communications can be highly useful in planning and implementing a social media element of a communications initiative. These include the following key steps, which have been adapted from "Using Social Media Platforms to Amplify Public Health Messages" (Hughes, 2010).

Establish Digital Goals, Objectives, and Strategies

It may seem self-evident, but taking time to set goals and objectives for digital media that reflect the broader goals of the initiative or organization will help prevent the urge to jump on the new media bandwagon just because it's "the next big thing." Developing a digital strategy will provide a "roadmap" to show how the goals will be accomplished, and the strategy should be informed by a combination of experience, audience analysis, and formative research. As overall communications plans are developed, specific digital opportunities that are relevant and on-strategy can be integrated.

Segment and Prioritize Audiences

Audience segmentation for a digital social marketing campaign or project, like segmentation for other efforts, involves analyzing intended audiences and identifying distinct subgroups with similar needs, attitudes, or behaviors—but with a catch. For a digital plan to succeed, it is critical to know how and where audiences get their online information about the issue in question, their preferred social media networks, how they use these networks, how often, and for what purpose.

Optimize Content by "Listening" and Engaging in Bidirectional Conversation

Social marketing best practices call for research into what the message should say and where, when, and how the target audience will best receive and process it. In planning digital communications efforts, social media marketers can capture this information by "listening" to issue-specific conversations online. This means paying attention to how and where an audience is engaging online about the campaign issue, for example, through a blog or social network. Attending to online conversations can reveal how a topic is being discussed, highlight any misperceptions about it, and provide opportunities for further engagement with the audience. Soliciting feedback, another useful tactic, can proactively obtain opinions from target audiences through online surveys or discussion groups.

Evaluate Digitally

Evaluating the social media component of a communications initiative should be a key part of the overall evaluation of the initiative's effects and impact. As with evaluation of traditional communications, social media evaluation begins with setting a benchmark and ends with measuring outcomes against that benchmark. These benchmarks can be established in various ways, including, for example, looking at what "competitors" are doing online and how target audiences are discussing the issue in social media networks. Among many other possibilities, evaluation measures can include the number of followers on Twitter, unique monthly visitors to a blog post, the percentage of conversations around the message or issue, and the number of people who share a message with friends.

As various forms of social media have grown and flourished, and an increasing number of Americans have become engaged in them for health purposes, public health practitioners have begun to incorporate social media marketing as part of their communications repertoire. A growing literature is documenting practitioners' experience and results in reaching their audiences through Facebook, Twitter, YouTube, and other digital formats. For example, the North Carolina Department of Environmental and Natural Resources (DENR) adopted a variety of new media tools in the RE3.org campaign to encourage recycling among young adults ages 18–34. Along with print and broadcast media, the use of digital and social media such as websites, blogs, and social networking sites helped the campaign successfully expand its reach and double the traffic to the campaign's website (Hamilton, Dennings, & Abroms, 2008).

In 2006, MTV and the Kaiser Family Foundation employed user-generated content to foster a more personal connection with youth about HIV. The initiative engaged the target audience (youth ages 15–25) to become vloggers (video bloggers) and develop content about the impact of HIV on their generation. Nearly 100 young people submitted more than 200 hours of video footage. The selected videos were aired four times on MTV in a show called *ThinkHIV: This Is Me* and received more than three million viewings, informing youth about HIV prevention and testing and showcasing how the disease has affected their peers (Hoff, Mishel, & Rowe, 2008).

Targeting a younger demographic, the VERB Campaign used several digital/social media tools as part of its communications strategy to motivate tweens (children ages 9–13) to be more physically active. A successful example was the VERB Yellowball initiative, which started as a television commercial portraying children playing with a sun ball taken from the sky. Expanding to a broader initiative based on the Yellowball theme, 500,000 Yellowballs were distributed throughout the United States. Tweens were encouraged to play with a ball and pass it along to another tween. Through VERBnow.com and the Yellowball mini-site, tweens could track their ball, blog about their playing experience, and create a Yellowball video. During the campaign, more than 17,000 Yellowball blogs were posted and 170,000 videos created (Huhman, 2008).

In New Zealand, the government incorporated interactive Web-based and text messaging services to provide additional support for people trying to quit smoking. The website allowed members to blog about their quit journey and receive support from others. Through Txt2Quit, smokers and quitters could receive automated text messages with tips on quitting and text "crave" and "slip up" to receive immediate messages with tips on how to deal with these situations. The new website and texting services successfully attracted new members, 458 for the Web community and 317 for Txt2Quit on average per month (Li, 2009).

To engage young adults in protecting their heart health, the National Institutes of Health's National Heart, Lung, and Blood Institute (NHLBI) has funded The Early Adult Reduction of Weight through Lifestyle Intervention (EARLY) Trials. This clinical research initiative is testing innovative behavioral approaches for weight control in 18- to 35-year-old adults at high risk for weight gain. In reaching this audience, researchers plan to test the efficacy of using technology-driven methods such as mobile phones, social networks, webinars, podcasts, and Web-based college curricula.

Social Media and *The Heart Truth*

In using social media applications to expand the reach of its existing marketing and promotion tactics to reach women, *The Heart Truth* campaign serves as an evolving example of how new digital opportunities and tools can well serve a social marketing effort. In 2000, only 34% of women knew that heart disease was their leading cause of death (Mosca, Ferris, Fabunmi, & Robertson, 2004). Yet, at that time, one in three deaths in women was due to heart disease, and even today the condition kills more women than all forms of cancer combined. Consumer research showed that women perceived heart disease as a condition that overwhelmingly affects men, and they often failed to take their own risk seriously or personally (National Heart, Lung, and Blood Institute, 2002).

Recognizing the seriousness of the problem, the NHLBI convened a Strategy Development Workshop in March 2001 to gain advice from women's health leaders and other experts on an action plan to help reduce heart disease risk in women. The group unanimously recommended that the NHLBI undertake a national campaign to raise women's awareness about their risk of heart disease and how to lower it. Later that year, the NHLBI awarded a contract to Ogilvy Public Relations Worldwide to help plan and implement such a campaign. After about a year of consumer research and analysis, materials development and testing, and partnership building, the NHLBI launched *The Heart Truth* in September

2002. The twofold objective of the campaign was to (1) increase awareness among women that heart disease is their leading cause of death and (2) encourage women to talk to their doctors, find out their personal risk of heart disease, and take action to lower it.

In guiding the creation and execution of the campaign, the team followed the traditional social marketing process involving four main steps: planning and strategy development (which includes formative research); creation and testing of concepts, messages, and materials; program implementation; and assessing effectiveness/making refinements. The campaign drew on relevant behavior and social change theories and models that support the development of effective strategies for influencing attitudes and behaviors, including theories focused on determinants of behavior and stages of individual behavior change.

Designed as a social marketing initiative, the campaign also integrated a strong branding strategy that led to the creation of what became a powerful new brand for women's heart disease—The Red Dress. To emphasize that heart disease is not just a "man's disease," the red dress symbol was paired with the tag line, "Heart Disease Doesn't Care What You Wear—It's the #1 Killer of Women." The campaign's brand-driven social marketing mix of national and local programming included execution of national partnerships, high-visibility national "signature" programs, and community-level interventions, with substantial success. By 2006, more than half of women in the United States were aware that heart disease is the number one killer of women (Mosca et al., 2006). Yet to continue to move the needle of awareness upward and motivate women to adopt heart healthy behaviors, the team knew it was imperative to reach women through the newest communication channels: social media.

Nearly 56% of adult women say they use the Internet to stay in touch with people, and social media are driving and occupying their time online. Women spent an average of 16.3% of their online time on social networks in April 2010; men spent only 11.7% of their online time with social networking. Women also spent more time seeking health content online: 22.8% of women visited a health information site in April 2010; only 17.4% of men did so (Abraham, Mörn, & Vollman, 2010).

The NHLBI set out to augment existing campaign marketing and promotion strategies by creating and testing selected online communication approaches for reaching *The Heart Truth* core target audience: women ages 40–60. This is a time when women's risk for heart disease rises dramatically, and it is also the age group "most responsible for growth in social networking site usage" (Abraham et al., 2010).

The aims were to (1) connect women and foster an online community environment by designing and promoting a relevant online platform; (2) motivate women to take action to control their risk factors for heart disease through specially designed online tools; and (3) promote partnerships that amplify the campaign's messages through content integration, online engagement, and targeted outreach. The campaign's marketing efforts using social media platforms such as

Facebook, Flickr, and YouTube began with a pilot project in 2007 and increased as the campaign matured and the online world evolved. The campaign team measured results each year and adjusted and expanded tactics accordingly, focusing efforts on using social media strategies to increase the campaign's online presence in conversations about women's heart health awareness and action. The team also expanded copromotion between social media platforms (for example, providing visibility for the Twitter feed about the campaign on *The Heart Truth* Facebook page) to boost consumer conversation and engagement during and beyond February, which is American Heart Month.

The social media outreach tactics described in the next section have provided the campaign with targeted platforms to dialogue with women about heart disease. The tactics have contributed a combined impact of many millions of additional audience impressions at a relatively low cost. Results are reported through 2010, with selected updates for January/February 2011 based on available data. Overall online audience impressions for January/February 2011 totaled more than 800 million.

Social Media Tactics in *The Heart Truth*

Outreach to Bloggers and Other Social Media Influencers

In 2010, the team reached out to more than 200 influencers within social media (including blogs, social networks, and message boards) and invited them to participate in *The Heart Truth*. By carefully identifying influential, active social media contributors in categories relevant to the core audience (including health/fitness, parenting/moms, ages 55+, and fashion/style) and providing in-depth, relevant information and materials, the campaign secured accurate and positive coverage of its February "signature" activities: National Wear Red Day and the Red Dress Collection Fashion Show. In 2010, the blogger outreach program resulted in over 65 million unique monthly views from the 66 bloggers posting about *The Heart Truth* campaign and/or the Red Dress Collection Fashion Show. In February 2011 alone, blog coverage reached nearly 950,000 visitors.

Twitter

In February 2010, *The Heart Truth* launched a Twitter handle (@TheHeartTruth), which provided the campaign with a two-way channel for campaign messages and created a consistent dialogue between the campaign and those who follow @TheHeartTruth. Since the launch of the campaign Twitter page, the number of followers (those who chose to receive tweets from the campaign) has grown from 0 in February 2010 to more than 3,000 in February 2011. Countless others have seen or visited the campaign Twitter page as well or received a "retweet" (RT; a message from *The Heart Truth* that was redistributed by one the campaign's followers).

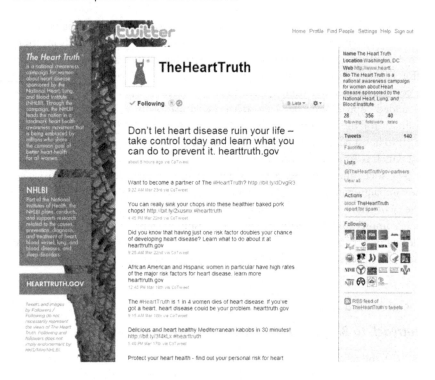

Figure 12.1 *The Heart Truth* Twitter screen capture

The campaign team initially launched the Twitter platform by offering free Twitter training to *The Heart Truth* community partners to encourage them to spread heart health messages through this platform during American Heart Month and year round. The team also promoted the handle and a universal "#HeartTruth" hashtag through other campaign platforms such as the Web page and Facebook page to encourage supporters to participate in the conversation. For the Red Dress Collection Fashion Show on February 9, 2011, the #Heart Truth hashtag was used 734 times, garnering more than 14 million audience impressions (number of people estimated to have seen a message). Celebrities participating in the fashion show tweeted about raising awareness of women and heart disease, reaching a total of more than six million followers.

To celebrate National Wear Red Day and maximize online conversation around this observance, the NHLBI hosted the first ever National Wear Red Day *Heart Truth* Twitter Party in February 2010. The goal of the event was to raise awareness about American Heart Month and the risks of heart disease and increase the number of Twitter page followers. Promotion included community partner outreach, social media outreach, *The Heart Truth* electronic magazine, and the Facebook page as well as outreach to 100 prominent women bloggers at the "Blissdom" conference and the "Clever 1000," a group of influential women working with the Clever Girls Collective. The party hosted more than 50 active participants (posting more than once) and generated more than 450 substantive Twitter posts within the one hour event. The NHLBI also provided its educational materials to participants. A similar Twitter Party held in February 2011 drew 257 active participants and resulted in nearly 1,500 tweets.

Facebook

The Heart Truth Facebook fan page, which launched in 2008, created a social forum where the campaign directly connects with consumers and provides a quick and cost-effective way to deliver campaign updates and heart health information to "fans" of the campaign. By February 2011, the page grew to include 3,546 fans (up from 800 in 2009). In addition to a substantial increase in fan membership, engagement grew with Facebook members commenting on links and photos uploaded to the page by the team. Key to the development of the Facebook fan page was the creation of compelling content that encouraged fans to interact with the material by commenting, "liking," posting, or writing on the fan page wall.

This forum not only reinforced a sense of community within *The Heart Truth* group but also helped spread the campaign messages throughout American Heart Month. In 2011, the Facebook page was enhanced to increase engagement and conversation around the issue of women and heart disease. The page was used to promote a National Wear Red Day activity in which people were asked to send in photos of themselves and/or their group wearing red, along with stories about actions they are taking for heart health. The campaign Twitter feed also was syndicated on a dedicated tab on Facebook so that fans could view the campaign-related Twitter conversation and subscribe to follow the campaign on Twitter. In addition, a new "Get Involved" tab was created to highlight ways to participate in the campaign, including how to download and use the campaign badges, how to create a "wear red" image to replace your Facebook profile photo on National Wear Red Day, and generally how to follow *The Heart Truth* on social media channels.

In addition to the campaign fan page, the team created a specific group page for *Heart Truth* Champions, health advocates and educators trained to share health information and educational materials about women and heart disease in their local communities. *The Heart Truth* team created the page in late 2009 in an effort to connect Champions. Members of the group page grew from 30 in 2010 to more than 60 members by February 2011. Group members are active, committed women who use the page to stay in touch with the campaign and consistently refresh their plans for heart health activities. The page includes links to the NHLBI, *The Heart Truth,* and the U.S. Department of Health and Human Services' Office on Women's Health websites in addition to other resources that may be of use to the Champions in promoting the campaign and women's heart health in their communities.

Bit.ly

To enable the sharing of links through multiple online channels such as Twitter and Facebook, Ogilvy created a bit.ly account. This service was used to shorten website URLs and links to resources and to track the number of clicks each link received from Twitter posts. The tactic was introduced following the launch of the overall social media campaign and therefore only partial data were collected. This tracking showed that *The Heart Truth* Web page received more than 261 click-throughs from Twitter posts alone using the following URL: bit.ly/hearttruth.

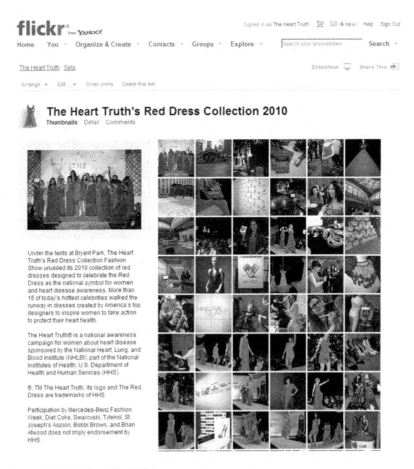

Figure 12.2 *The Heart Truth* Flickr screen capture

Flickr

In 2008, the campaign began to use Flickr, the photo- and video-hosting website. To continue promotion via Flickr, the team updated the site information for American Heart Month 2010 and 2011. The team maximized potential views by cross-promoting the designated Flickr tags, including HeartTruth, National Wear Red Day, and RedDress through outreach to social media influencers. In 2010, Flickr users uploaded more than 300 photos to the site using the prescribed tags, garnering over 3,300 views. In February 2011, there were 457 photos and nearly 14,000 views.

YouTube

More than 144 videos were posted organically by users not affiliated with the campaign to YouTube and other video sharing sites. These videos covered *The Heart Truth* campaign and Red Dress Collection 2010 Fashion Show, generating more than 43,000 views. Top videos included coverage of Red Dress Collection 2010 spokesmodel Heidi Klum (part of sponsor Diet Coke's program) on *The Ellen DeGeneres Show* and celebrity participation in the Red Dress Collection Fashion Show.

Widgets and Badges

National Wear Red Day countdown widget. First launched in 2008, the campaign's National Wear Red Day countdown widget was the federal government's first consumer-focused widget (an interactive virtual tool that provides a service). It was made available at no cost for anyone to download to their website, Facebook page, or blog. The application streamed images from *The Heart Truth* Flickr gallery and helped supporters countdown to National Wear Red Day. The tool was promoted through influencer outreach, blog postings, message boards, and social networks.

Healthy Action Community Badges. The team created the campaign's first healthy action badges in 2009. The badges—virtual tools that users can download— were designed to promote and encourage online visitors to focus on risk factors for heart disease. The team published the six badges (five in English and one in Spanish) to *The Heart Truth* Web page and Facebook page, which were promoted through social media outreach to bloggers and online influencers conducted in advance of American Heart Month. Combined badge views grew from 19,304 in 2009 to 117,031 in 2010 (a 506% increase). Combined downloading and installation of the badges on users' websites and online profiles grew from 25 in 2009 to 186 in 2010 (a 44% increase).

The Heart Truth Campaign Effects

To measure campaign results, the NHLBI sought to stretch evaluation resources by collecting some data in house and using outside sources when possible. In

I pledge to be active in 2010

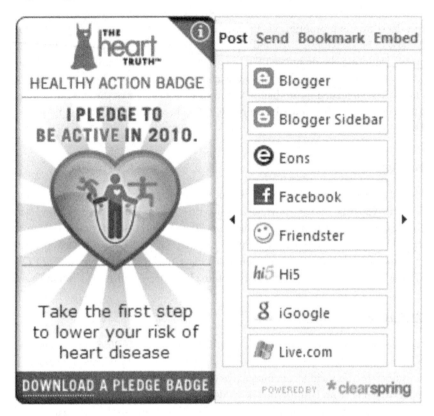

Figure 12.3 *The Heart Truth* Healthy Action Badge screen capture

general, campaign resources were used to collect data on process measures such as audience impressions (the number of people estimated to have seen a message), partner contributions, and social media and other media coverage. In measuring campaign impact—which can be more expensive—the team used national surveys and studies conducted by the American Heart Association to assess progress in raising women's awareness and motivating behavior change. In addition, the campaign's corporate and media partners provided process information such as the extent of brand promotions on product packaging and also funded audience surveys to measure impact. This combination of in-house and outside resources helped provide a cost-effective picture of progress in women's heart health.

The Heart Truth has been a catalyst in launching a substantial national awareness movement, influencing the women's health community, major corporations, local and regional community groups, and the media to work toward a common goal of greater awareness and better heart health for women. Some of the positive changes that have been observed in this area are summarized below. We cannot rule out the possible influence of extraneous variables and secular trends on these figures. However, we believe that the campaign has greatly contributed to these positive trends, especially given the leadership and work of the NHLBI and *The Heart Truth* team and the contributions of many other organizations and individuals working toward the same goal. Evidence suggests that women have become increasingly aware of *The Heart Truth* campaign over time. Awareness of the red dress symbol more than doubled between 2005 and 2008, rising from 25% to 61% (Long, Taubenheim, Wayman, Temple, & Ruoff, 2008). Awareness among women that heart disease is their leading cause of death has increased substantially. In 2000, only 34% of women knew that heart disease is the number one killer of women. This figure rose to 46% in 2003 and 54% in 2009 (Mosca, Mochari-Greenberger, Dolor, Newby, & Robb, 2010).

Rising awareness about risk does more than just inform women—it makes informed women more likely to take action. Women who are aware of the threat of heart disease are 35% more likely to be physically active and 47% more likely to report weight loss than women who are less aware (Mosca et al., 2006). Not only are more women becoming aware of the risk that heart disease poses for them but also more are talking to their doctors about it. Forty-eight percent of women report discussing heart disease with their doctors, up from 30% in 1997 (Mosca et al., 2006).

In addition to increases in awareness and associated preventive action, there has also been progress in reducing heart disease deaths in women. In 2003, of the women who died in America, one in three died of heart disease. This has shifted to one in four women (Heron et al., 2009). Although the decline in mortality is mostly associated with factors such as improved treatment, *The Heart Truth* and other campaigns have likely played a role in the increase in awareness and preventive actions that women are taking to reduce their risk (Long et al., 2008).

Discussion

The use of well-targeted social media has been playing an increasingly important role in *The Heart Truth* campaign's overall marketing and promotion strategies to reach its core audience of women. Online visibility for the campaign and its messages has grown each year since 2007 when social media tactics were introduced into the campaign's repertoire. It is expected that the yield will continue to grow over time. As the campaign's use of social media has expanded and adapted to innovations in the social media world, the team has been tracking trends and has set its own benchmarks for social media success in the context of the overall campaign. As noted previously, the campaign uses a variety of evaluation processes and resources, including results of national surveys conducted by outside organizations.

Because the campaign's resources are finite, as *The Heart Truth* moves forward, the information available about the relative contribution of social media to the overall impact may not be as robust as desired. However, the team believes that social media will continue to provide an effective means of further extending the reach of the campaign. The bottom-line advantage of the campaign's use of social media has been summarized as follows:

> For a federal government initiative without an advertising budget, the use of social media was a relatively low-budget means of raising the visibility of the campaign by substantially increasing the number of audience impressions, thereby potentially exposing many more millions of women to *The Heart Truth*. Furthermore the "viral" impact of spreading the campaign message across many websites, blogs, and social networking sites meant that far more people were reached than would have been possible through "traditional" channels alone. (Taubenheim et al., 2008, pp. 64–65)

The strong implication is that similar social media efforts, well planned and well targeted, would be a useful and effective addition to other health communications campaigns. However, in considering the useful aspects of social media—including relatively low implementation cost, ease of delivering targeted messages to targeted audiences, and ability to generate involvement and receive feedback—it is also important to keep an eye on the limitations. For example, not everyone has the means or the interest to connect online; many audiences, including the elderly and disadvantaged populations, do not fully participate in public health information online. Social media, for all their immediacy and attractiveness, are not the only answer. Public health practitioners must use good communications planning skills to identify ways to reach and engage those who are not actively seeking Web-based health information. In addition, practitioners have a responsibility to continue to learn about online approaches, use them to the best advantage in social marketing efforts, and analyze and report the results.

Conclusions and Future Directions

Social marketing is rooted in the belief that greater audience engagement translates into more powerful solutions and interventions. Social networks help facilitate engagement, and, with the advent of social media networks online, people's participation in social marketing interventions is now greater than ever. Public health programs have leveraged this growth and are successfully adopting social media platforms to influence and change people's behaviors for the better.

The expanding use of social media in *The Heart Truth* and other social marketing and health communications initiatives opens the door to much-needed additional research on its use and impact. For example, it will be important to develop additional metrics to help evaluate the impact of the social media channels being used as key elements in a social marketing campaign. Social media metrics—measures of the extent to which audiences are exposed to a particular message, develop an opinion, and/or take action regarding the issue—might include, for example, a campaign's "share of voice" about its issue and even self-reported behavior change as audience members "tweet" about changes in their health status or actions. Better process evaluation in general is needed to tease out the impact of social media in the context of a broader campaign such as *The Heart Truth* and develop a better understanding of which particular social media platforms are most effective for which audiences.

The Heart Truth represents an example of a social marketing initiative that planned for, implemented, and assessed social media approaches in the context of a larger campaign. Since its launch, *The Heart Truth* has sparked a national movement to reach women across America about their risk of heart disease. To do so, the campaign reached out to and involved the women's health community, major corporations, local and regional community groups, and traditional as well as social media. The driving force of *The Heart Truth* is its powerful brand, the Red Dress, which has contributed substantially to the campaign's success. By integrating social media approaches into the campaign in a thoughtful, well-planned manner, *The Heart Truth* has been able to extend the reach of its brand and message and make progress toward its stated objectives: to *inspire* women to become more aware about heart disease risk, *engage* them in finding out their personal risk, and *empower* them in communities nationwide to take action to reduce their risk. More information is available on the campaign's website: www.hearttruth.gov.

References

Abraham, L. B., Mörn, M. P., & Vollman, A. (2010). Women on the Web: How women are shaping the Internet. *comScore*. Retrieved June 27, 2011, from: http://www.com score.com/Press_Events/Presentations_Whitepapers/2010/Women_on_the_ Web_How_Women_are_Shaping_the_Internet.

Albrecht, T. L., & Goldsmith, D. J. (2003). Social support, social networks, and health. In T. L. Thompson, A. M. Dorsey, K. I. Miller, & R. Parrott (Eds.), *Handbook of health communication* (pp. 263–284). Mahwah, NJ: Lawrence Erlbaum Associates.

Fox, S., & Jones, S. (2009). The social life of health information. *Pew Internet & American Life Project*. Retrieved June 27, 2011, from: http://www.pewinternet.org/Reports/2009/ 8-The-Social-Life-of-Health-Information.aspx.

Hamilton, L., Dennings, K., & Abroms, L. C. (2008). RE3.org: A case study of using new media to promote recycling in North Carolina. *Cases in Public Health Communication & Marketing, 2,* 178–189.

Heron, M., Hoyert, D. L., Murphey, S. L., Xu, J., Kochaneck, K. D., & Tejada-Vera, B. (2009). Deaths: Final data for 2006. *National Vital Statistics Reports, 57,* 1–135. Retrieved June 27, 2011, from: http://www.cdc.gov/nchs/data/nvsr/nvsr57/nvsr57_14.pdf.

Hoff, T., Mishel, M., & Rowe, I. (2008). Using new media to make HIV personal: A partnership of MTV and the Kaiser Family Foundation. *Cases in Public Health Communication & Marketing, 2,* 190–197.

Hughes, A. (2010). Using social media platforms to amplify public health messages: An examination of principles and best practices. *Ogilvy Washington & The Center for Social*

Impact Communication at Georgetown University. Retrieved June 27, 2011, from: http://smexchange.ogilvypr.com/wp-content/uploads/2010/11/OW_SM_WhitePaper.pdf.

Huhman, M. E. (2008). New media and the VERB campaign: Tools to motivate tweens to be physically active. *Cases in Public Health Communication & Marketing, 2,* 126–139.

Levy, M., & Daniels, D. (2008). U.S. online specialists executive survey, 2008. *Forrester Research.* Retrieved June 27, 2011, from: http://www.forrester.com/rb/Research/us_online_specialists_executive_survey,_2008/q/id/53183/t/2.

Li, J. (2009). Mobile phones and the Internet as quitting smoking aids. *Cases in Public Health Communication & Marketing, 3,* 205–218.

Long, T., Taubenheim, A. M., Wayman, J., Temple, S., & Ruoff, B. A. (2008). The Heart Truth: Using the power of branding and social marketing to increase awareness of heart disease in women. *Social Marketing Quarterly, 14,* 3–29.

Mosca, L., Ferris, A., Fabunmi, R., & Robertson, R. (2004). Tracking women's awareness of heart disease: An American Heart Association national study. *Circulation, 109,* 573–579.

Mosca, L., Mochari, H., Christian, A., Berra, K., Taubert, K., Mills, T., et al. (2006). National study of women's awareness, preventive action, and barriers to cardiovascular health. *Circulation, 113,* 524–534.

Mosca, L., Mochari-Greenberger, H., Dolor, R. J., Newby, L. K., & Robb, K. J. (2010). Twelve-year follow-up of American women's awareness of cardiovascular disease risk and barriers to heart health. *Circulation: Cardiovascular Quality and Outcomes, 3,* 120–127.

National Heart, Lung, and Blood Institute (2002). *Report: Focus groups with mid-life women regarding women's cardiovascular health.* Unpublished manuscript, Bethesda, MD.

Taubenheim, A. M., Long, T., Smith, E. C., Jeffers, D., Wayman, J., & Temple, S. (2008). Using social media and Internet marketing to reach women with The Heart Truth. *Social Marketing Quarterly, 14,* 58–67.

Tu, H. T., & Cohen, G. R. (2008). Striking jump in consumers seeking health care information: Tracking report no. 20. *Center for Studying Health System Change.* Retrieved June 27, 2011, from: http://www.hschange.org/CONTENT/1006/.

Weinreich, N. (2006, September 6). *Social marketing vs. "social marketing" smackdown* [Web log post]. Retrieved March 22, 2011, from: http://www.socialmarketing.com/blog/2006/09/social-marketing-vs-social-marketing.html.

Wilcox, D., & Kanter, B. (2007). *Demystifying Web 2.0 for VolCom groups: Blogs, RSS, tagging, wikis, and beyond* [PowerPoint slides]. Retrieved June 27, 2011, from: http://beth.typepad.com/beths_blog/2007/01/demystifying_so.html.

13

DISSEMINATION AND IMPLEMENTATION OF eHEALTH INTERVENTIONS

Borsika A. Rabin and Russell E. Glasgow

A report from the Institute of Medicine (IOM, 2001b) states that "a basic assumption underlying intervention research is that tested interventions found to be effective are disseminated to and implemented in clinics, communities, schools, and worksites" (p. 294). Furthermore, it has been suggested that the health impact of an intervention depends not only on its effectiveness but also on the extent to which it reaches its target audience and is implemented and sustained within the target settings (Oldenburg, Sallis, Ffrench, & Owen, 1999).

While few would question that the ultimate goal of health research is to improve population health and well-being, only a small proportion of effective interventions are widely utilized in real-world settings and reach the ultimate target population (Dobbins, Cockerill, Barnsley, & Ciliska, 2001; IOM, 2001b). Dissemination and implementation (D&I) research focuses on narrowing the gap between existing efficacious interventions and their wide application. It is defined as the systematic study of processes and factors associated with the spread, uptake, and utilization of an intervention by the target audience and the integration of the intervention within the target setting (Rabin, Brownson, Haire-Joshu, Kreuter, & Weaver, 2008).

In eHealth, as with almost all areas of health and health care (McGlynn et al., 2003), there is a huge gap between the efficacy research database and what is implemented in practice. In doing the literature searches described in this chapter, we found that only a small proportion of the potentially eligible studies were conducted under translational or real world conditions. There are complex and interacting reasons for this situation (Glasgow & Emmons, 2007), but among other factors, the current scientific climate clearly reinforces discovery research more than D&I.

It cannot be assumed that an intervention tested under one set of conditions will necessarily work under a completely different set of conditions. Indeed, why would one expect results collected under optimal conditions (e.g., highly motivated, noncomplex patients receiving an intervention from experts who have perfect fidelity and are paid to do research) to apply to a totally different set of conditions (e.g., typical staff treating highly complex patients, both of whom have numerous competing demands) (Glasgow, Lichtenstein, & Marcus, 2003; Green & Glasgow, 2006)?

Indeed, one of the key points about D&I research that differentiates it from earlier stage research is a greater emphasis on external validity, or the extent to which a finding generalizes (or does not) across different conditions, populations, settings, outcomes, and time. In prior reviews of a variety of behavioral interventions across a variety of settings and for a wide range of conditions, we have consistently concluded that issues of external validity have been reported far less frequently than issues of internal validity (Glasgow, Klesges, Dzewaltowski, Bull, & Estabrooks, 2004).

This chapter explores some of these issues and reviews eHealth research that has been conducted under "T2 to T4" conditions (for definitions, see Table 13.1) (Kessler & Glasgow, 2011; Khoury et al., 2007) or more real world conditions, where an initially successful (efficacy-based) intervention has been applied more broadly. For this chapter, we have operationalized later stage (T2+) research broadly and have included studies that tested the adaptation and replication of previously tested interventions (i.e., adaptation to new modality, audience, setting, geographical areas) and studies that focused on the scale up of tested interventions (i.e., D&I to a larger audience or number of settings).

Three prior reviews of eHealth interventions (EHIs) address dissemination issues. Strecher (2007) concluded that adoption, implementation, and maintenance of EHIs by target settings and users will only happen if the programs in question have demonstrated and documented high reach, high efficacy, and low cost. He also emphasized the potential of EHIs for superior cost-effectiveness compared to

Table 13.1 Definition for types of translational research

Type	Definition	Types of research
T1	From basic biological discovery to candidate health applications	Efficacy studies
T2	From health application to evidence-based practice guidelines	Effectiveness studies Evidence synthesis
T3	From practice guidelines to health practice	Dissemination research Implementation research
T4	From practice to population health impact	Outcomes research Scaling up

traditional counterparts. Bennett and Glasgow (2009) highlighted the factors that contribute to the high dissemination potential of EHIs. These factors included low cost, scalability, adaptability, and effectiveness. Bennett and Glasgow's recommendations to realize the potential of EHIs concerned better characterization of reach of these interventions, standardized reporting usage metrics, and the integration of Web 2.0 approaches to enhance effectiveness. Tate, Finkelstein, Khavjou, and Gustafson (2009) conducted a review of cost-effectiveness studies of Internet interventions between 1995 and 2008. They observed the lack of cost data included in these studies and specifically pointed out the need for more cost-effectiveness research as the field moves to a greater focus on effectiveness studies and beyond.

Purpose

In this chapter we review the current status of the eHealth field for health promotion and disease management in terms of D&I, and on the basis of this summary, we make recommendations for future directions for this field. The following specific research questions are addressed: (1) What is the distribution of studies published on EHIs in health promotion and disease management across the research-to-practice continuum (T1 [efficacy studies] versus T2+ [adaptation studies and D&I studies]); (2) How frequently are extant external validity dimensions reported in EHIs of T2+ in health promotion and disease management; (3) What are the most important D&I-relevant characteristics of EHIs of T2+ in health promotion and disease management; and (4) Are there consistent predictors of successful D&I in EHIs of T2+ in health promotion and disease management?

Methods

We conducted a systematic literature review to identify studies of EHIs in health promotion and disease management and described these studies from a D&I perspective. We systematically searched electronic databases (i.e., Medline, OVID HealthSTAR, PsychINFO, and Cochrane Central Register for Controlled Trials) using a combination of terms related to eHealth (e.g., *e-health, interactive health communication, Web-based, Internet-based, computer-based, online, cell phone, interactive voice recognition [IVR], video game,* etc.) and the terms *health promotion, health behavior change, disease prevention, disease management,* and *self-management.* Electronic searches were limited to English-language articles published between 1980 and July 2010.

We selected the studies in two steps. First, citations from the literature search were screened using general inclusion criteria by the lead author. To ensure the completeness of the study list, we also examined reference lists of published studies on EHIs (identified through the electronic search) and reviewed and completed the final study list with relevant missing articles. We included a study if it evaluated an EHI as the main intervention component and was primarily directed toward patients and/or their caregivers rather than health care providers. T1 (or efficacy) studies had to use a controlled design using randomized or nonrandomized comparison condition(s) and had to include at least one broadly defined behavioral-oriented outcome (e.g., change in knowledge, self-efficacy, intention to change, behavior) or biological outcome (e.g., BMI, HbA1c). We excluded studies of telemedicine interventions and those expressly designed as feasibility, preliminary, or pilot studies. We included all T2+ (adaptation/replication or D&I) studies regardless of their study design or measured outcomes. A random subset of citations ($n = 100$) was reviewed by both authors to determine inter-rater reliability. The strength of the agreement between reviewers for the inclusion of articles was good (Kappa: 0.62 [95% CI: 0.461 to 0.779]).

As a second step, full articles for studies identified for inclusion were retrieved and reviewed by the lead author using the same inclusion criteria described above. Studies judged to be relevant on the basis of the full text review were included in the review as primary articles. Because the primary purpose of this review was to identify and describe D&I-relevant content reported in T2+ EHIs (rather than focus on specific outcomes), quality assessment of studies was not performed and effect sizes were not calculated. We classified included studies on the research-to-practice continuum as T1 (efficacy studies) or T2+ (adaptation studies and D&I studies). The distribution of studies across the research-to-practice continuum was determined as the percent of included studies classified as T2+.

To further analyze studies of T2+, we developed and pilot tested an abstraction protocol to code study characteristics. The lead author abstracted the following general characteristics from each study: stage on care continuum (i.e., health promotion versus disease management), target behavior(s)/risk factor(s)/disease(s) (e.g., physical activity, diet, smoking, diabetes, asthma), target population (e.g., adolescents, patients with diabetes, individuals with HIV, general population), setting (e.g., worksite, health care system, school, community), region/country, study design (randomized controlled trial, group randomized trial, quasi-experimental design), group assignment (brief description of conditions), eHealth modality (e.g., computer-generated tailored print, computer-generated tailored Web, Web-based, IVR, kiosk), theory and framework for intervention and adaptation/D&I, adaptation or D&I strategy (e.g., direct mail), and T2+ classification (e.g., adaptation to new audience, adaptation to new modality, D&I).

We also abstracted external validity dimensions using a modified version of the previously tested "Coding Sheet for Publications Reporting on RE-AIM elements" (Kaiser Permanente, n.d.). The RE-AIM framework emphasizes the multiple layers (i.e., reach, adoption, implementation, maintenance) influencing the population-level impact and D&I potential of an intervention and highlights the importance of defining efficacy or effectiveness broadly by considering various types of outcomes (behavior, quality of life, adverse outcome, cost-effectiveness) and measuring outcomes at different levels (individual and organizational/community levels) when evaluating interventions. The definition for each dimension is provided in Table 13.2. A more detailed discussion of the RE-AIM framework and its applications is provided elsewhere (Gaglio & Glasgow, in press; Glasgow &

Table 13.2 Definition for each RE-AIM dimension

RE-AIM dimension	Definition
Reach	The absolute number, proportion, and representativeness of individuals who are willing to participate in a given initiative, intervention, or program.
Effectiveness	The impact of an intervention on important outcomes, including potential negative effects, quality of life, and economic outcomes.
Adoption	The absolute number, proportion, and representativeness of settings and intervention agents (people who deliver the program) who are willing to initiate a program.
Implementation	At the setting level, implementation refers to the intervention agents' fidelity to the various elements of an intervention's protocol, including consistency of delivery as intended and the time and cost of the intervention. At the individual level, implementation refers to clients' use of the intervention strategies.
Maintenance	The extent to which a program or policy becomes institutionalized or part of the routine organizational practices and policies. Within the RE-AIM framework, maintenance also applies at the individual level. At the individual level, maintenance has been defined as the long-term effects of a program on outcomes after six or more months after the most recent intervention contact.

Linnan, 2008; Klesges, Dzewaltowski, & Glasgow, 2008). Additional abstracted D&I-relevant content included issues concerning health disparities (e.g., racial/ethnic disparities, SES, health literacy and numeracy) and reported use of participatory approaches (i.e., yes/no). Results are presented as the percentage of articles that reported on the respective criteria and are also presented by modality.

Results

A total of 2,266 citations were identified through electronic database search ($N = 1,926$), examination of review articles ($N = 329$) and reference lists ($N = 7$), and expert recommendations ($N = 4$). After reviewing the citations and full text articles, we selected 467 articles for inclusion as primary articles. Figure 13.1 summarizes the distribution of articles across the different steps of the review process along with reasons for exclusion.

Distribution of Studies across the Research-to-Practice Continuum

Of the 467 primary articles, 429 (about 92%) described T1 (efficacy) studies in either health promotion ($N = 293$) or disease management ($N = 136$), and 38 articles (about 8%) described 33 T2+ (adaptation and D&I) studies (five studies were

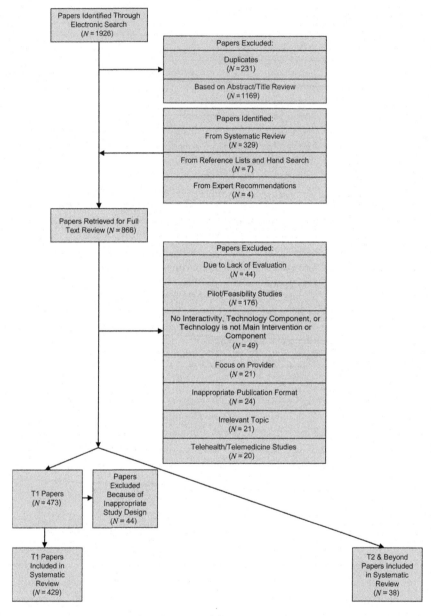

Figure 13.1 Distribution of articles across different steps of the review process

described in two articles). The majority of these T2+ studies could be classified as studies of adaptation or expansion, and focused on adaptation of an effective intervention to a new modality ($N = 16$), a new target audience ($N = 5$), a new setting or geographical area ($N = 4$), a new topic ($N = 3$), or the augmentation of a tested intervention with an additional component (N = 3). Only four articles described D&I efforts with the purpose of scale up of a tested intervention. It is also worth noting that a total of 27 efficacious interventions served as a basis for the 33 studies of T2+ (i.e., a number of included T2+ studies emerged from the adaptation/expansion or D&I of the same tested intervention [i.e., CHESS, Student Bodies, and the Chronic Disease Self-Management Program]). The rest of this chapter will focus on these 33 T2+ studies (reported in 38 articles).

General Characteristics for EHIs of T2+

General characteristics for EHIs of T2+ for health promotion and disease management are summarized in Table 13.3. The majority (N = 27) of the EHIs of T2+ focused on health promotion; only six studies of disease management were identified. The most commonly reported health promotion topics were related to healthy eating/caloric restriction and physical activity (N = 12). There were also a number of articles on smoking cessation (N = 7). The studies on disease management included topics of chronic disease management including asthma and diabetes control and management of psychosocial needs around breast cancer. None of the studies explicitly addressed patients with multiple conditions. However, two studies focused on general skill development for the management of chronic conditions. The largest percentage of the T2+ studies were community-based (N = 13) and focused on at-risk general populations (e.g., sedentary, overweight, or smoking adults) (N = 15).

The second and third most frequently reported settings were health care (N = 9) and school (N = 8) settings. The most frequent eHealth modalities were Web-based or computer-generated tailored Web (N = 21) followed by computer-generated tailored print (N = 7). Additional modalities included IVR, kiosk, computer-tailored phone, and CD-ROM. Only one study reported using multiple modalities (combination of computer-tailored print and handheld computer) and, in contrast to the recent flurry of activity around mobile health (see Abroms, Padmanabhan, & Evans and Fjeldsoe, Miller, & Marshall, this volume), none included text messaging or cell phone interventions.

External Validity Dimensions in EHIs of T2+

The different dimensions of external validity are defined in Table 13.2, and the frequency of reporting on external validity dimensions and other D&I relevant characteristics of included studies is summarized by modality in Table 13.4.

Some aspect of *reach and representativeness* was reported by all of the T2+ studies. While all of the studies reported on recruitment strategies, individual-level inclusion/exclusion criteria, and sample size, very few studies provided an explicit rationale for working with a certain target group. Reporting on participation rate

Table 13.3 General characteristics for EHIs of T2+ for health promotion and disease management

Study name[1]	Topic	HP/DM	Setting	Target population	Region/country	Modality	Study design	T2 and beyond
Becoña E, Vázquez FL.	Smoking cessation	HP	Community-based	At-risk general population (smokers)	Galicia (NW Spain)	CT-Print	RCT	Adaptation to new modality
Sunny Days, Healthy Ways (SDHW)	Sun safety	HP	Public elementary schools Licensed child-care facilities	Administrators	AZ, NV, NM, UT (USA)	Web-based	2x2 factorial post-test only	Dissemination
Active Living Every Day Internet version (ALED-I)	Physical activity	HP	Community-based	At-risk general population (sedentary)	Rural WY (USA)	Web-based	RCT	Adaptation to new modality
Curry S et al.	Smoking cessation	HP	Health care (HMO)	At-risk general population (smokers)	WA (USA)	CT-Print	RCT	Adaptation to new target audience
Active-o-meter	Physical activity	HP	School	Adolescents (12–17 yrs)	Six European countries	CT-Web	GRT	Adaptation to new target audience
De Bourdeaudhuij et al.	Diet	HP	Workplace	General population	Flanders (Belgium)	CT-Web	GRT	Dissemination
Dijkstra A et al.	Smoking cessation	HP	Community-based	At-risk general population (smokers)	The Netherlands	CT-Print	RCT	Adaptation to new target audience
HealthMedia's Balance	Weight management	HP	Health care (HMO)	At-risk population (overweight and overweight with chronic condition)	OH, CO, WA, ID (USA)	CT-Web	RCT	Expansion with additional components

Intervention	Topic	Type	Setting	Population	Location	Modality	Design	Adaptation
CHESS – Breast cancer	Breast cancer	DM	Health care (five sites)	Patients with breast cancer	Madison, WI Chicago, IL Indianapolis, IN	Web-based	RCT	Adaptation to new topic
Health Risk Appraisal for Older Persons (HRA-O)	Health risk appraisal	HP	Group practices (GP)	Patients 65 or older	London (UK)	CT-Print	GRT	Adaptation to new geographic area and modality
Student Bodies—German	Eating disorder prevention	HP	University	University students	Trier and Gottingen (Germany)	Web-based	RCT	Adaptation to new geographic area
CHESS Smoking Cessation and Relapse Prevention (CHESS SCRP)	Smoking cessation	HP	Community-based	At risk population (smokers)	Milwaukee and Madison, WI (USA)	Web-based	RCT	Adaptation to new topic
Project LIGHT—computerized version	HIV prevention	HP	School (alternative education school)	At-risk population (delinquent youths)	CA (USA)	Web-based	RCT	Adaptation to new modality
Internet-based Chronic Disease Self-Management Program (Internet-based CIDSMP)	Skill development for chronic disease management	DM	Community-based	Patients with long-term chronic conditions	USA	Web-based	RCT	Adaptation to new modality
Internet-based Arthritis Self-Management Program (Internet-based ASMP)	Pain reduction and function improvement for arthritis management	DM	Community-based	Patients with osteoarthritis, or rheumatoid arthritis, or fibromyalgia	USA	Web-based	RCT	Adaptation to new modality
Expert Patients Programme Online (EPP Online)	Skill development for chronic disease management	DM	Community-based	Patients with long-term chronic conditions	UK	Web-based	Pre-post	Adaptation to new geographical area

(Continued)

Table 13.3 (*Continued*)

Study name	Topic	HP/DM	Setting	Target population	Region/country	Modality	Study design	T2 and beyond
Marcus B, Lewis B et al.	Physical activity	HP	Community-based	At-risk population (sedentary)	Providence and Pittsburgh (USA)	CT-Web	RCT	Adaptation to new modality
Project STRIDE	Physical activity	HP	Community-based	At-risk population (sedentary)	USA	CT-Phone	RCT	Adaptation to new modality
Active Living website	Physical activity	HP	Workplace	General population	Australia	CT-Web	RCT	Adaptation to new modality
Focusing Implementation to Bring Effective Reminders (FIBER)	Colorectal cancer screening	HP	Health care setting (HMO)	At-risk population (due for CRC screening)	WA, OR (USA)	IVR	RCT	Adaptation to new modality
Muñoz RF et al.	Smoking cessation	HP	Community-based	At-risk population (smokers)	Not Specified	Web-based	Pre-post RCT	Adaptation to new modality
CHESS Stomp Out Smokes (CHESS SOS)	Smoking cessation	HP	Community-based + medical clinics	At-risk population (adolescent smokers)	Rochester, MN Madison, WI Hartford, CT	Web-based	RCT	Adaptation to new topic
High 5, Low Fat (H5LF)	Diet	HP	Parents as Teachers National Training Center	Families	Nationwide (USA)	CD-ROM	Cross-sectional	Adaptation to new modality Dissemination
Piette JD et al.	Diabetes management	DM	General medicine clinics Diabetes clinic (VA)	Patients with diabetes	N Cal (USA)	IVR	RCT	Adaptation to new target audience
PACE+ classroom version	Multiple health behavior (Physical activity and Diet)	HP	Middle school	Adolescents	San Diego, CA (USA)	CT-Print	RCT	Adaptation to new setting
Prochaska JO et al.	Smoking cessation	HP	Managed care setting	At-risk population (smokers)	Not Specified	CT-Print Hand-held computer	RCT	Expansion with additional component

Name	Topic		Setting	Population	Location	Modality	Design	Purpose
U-CAN-POOP-TOO	Pediatric encopresis	DM	Health care	Families of children with encopresis	VA, TN (USA)	Web-based	RCT	Adaptation to new modality
Spittaels et al.	Physical activity	HP	Community-based	General population (Parents and staff of primary and secondary schools)	Belgium	CT-Web	GRT	Adaptation to new modality
Computer-tailored nutrition education tool (CTT)	Diet	HP	Community-based	General population (14 years and older)	Maastricht, Netherlands	CT-Print	Post only	Dissemination
Electronic Check-Up to Go (E-CHUG)	Alcohol/heavy drinking	HP	University	Students (1st year university students)	Southern Region, United States	Web-based	RCT	Adaptation to new modality
Nutrition for a Lifetime System (NLS-1 and NLS-2)	Diet	HP	Supermarket	General population	Not Specified	Kiosk	RCT	Adaptation to new modality
Student Bodies	Eating disorder prevention	HP	University	At risk population (female students with elevated body image concerns)	West Coast, U.S.	Web-based	RCT	Adaptation to new target audience
Student Bodies—extended	Eating disorder prevention	HP	University	At-risk population (female students with elevated body image concerns)	West Coast, U.S.	Web-based	RCT	Expansion with additional component

[1] A list of complete citations for those studies included in the table can be accessed by contacting the authors of the chapter

HP—Health promotion; DM—Disease management; CT-Print—Computer-generated tailored print; CT-Web—Computer-generated tailored Web; CT-Phone—Computer-tailored phone

($N = 24$) and the characteristics of participants ($N = 29$) was less consistent. Only two studies reported on characteristics of nonparticipants, and four studies did not provide any information on the characteristics of individual participants. Nine studies provided reasons for nonparticipation but did not describe characteristics of nonparticipants.

Multiple measures were included in all T2+ studies. However, the measures reported were not very broad and were usually restricted to a few variables measuring the same construct (e.g., physical activity measured by multiple variables). Three of the studies did not report on *effectiveness* measures (i.e., their focus was on process measures) and none of the studies documented unanticipated effects (i.e., adverse events). Only four studies included measures of quality of life as an outcome. A smaller number of studies included reports on sub-analyses to determine possible differential effects and to draw conclusions about impact on subgroups (e.g., gender, at-risk status).

Measures of *adoption* were seldom reported, despite their importance in understanding the context for intervention results. In particular, only two studies reported on the participation rate among settings, and nine studies reported on the characteristics among adopting settings (e.g., clinics, worksites, schools). No studies reported on characteristics of settings that refused to participate.

A majority of studies ($N = 23$) reported at least one measure of *implementation*. The most commonly reported information was level of use of the EHI (i.e., engagement measured by number of logins, activities completed, time spent on different pages, number of sessions attended, reported use of intervention), but these measures were largely idiosyncratic. Very few studies reported on the impact of intervention intensity on outcome measures, and only two studies reported information regarding the cost of the intervention. One of the two studies, Piette, Weinberger, Kraemer, and McPhee (2001), described the evaluation of an IVR program for diabetes management with nurse follow-up and provided a detailed discussion on intervention costs per patient annually. This study also provided estimates on the savings that the national implementation of the program within the VA system could generate.

Maintenance was commonly reported at the individual level but seldom, if ever, at the setting level. While all the studies reported follow-up time, long-term follow-up (at least 12 months) was reported for less than half of the studies (45%). The follow-up time ranged between three weeks and 25 months, with a median follow-up time of nine months. It was striking that there were no reports of sustainability at the setting/organizational/contextual level or reports of how an intervention was adapted or modified once the evaluation study period was over. A positive finding was that 85% of studies reported on attrition rate, and the majority of those reported on differential attrition across conditions and compared characteristics of dropouts to those who remained in the study. The median attrition rate at 12-month follow-up for studies that reported long-term follow-up outcomes was 19.95%, with a range of 3% (in a study testing an intervention

Table 13.4 Percentage of EHIs of T2+ reporting external validity dimensions and other D&I relevant characteristics (overall and by modality)

Construct	Overall (N=33)	CT-Print (N=6)	CT-Web (N=6)	CT-Phone (N=1)	Web-based (N=15)	Kiosk (N=1)	IVR (N=2)	CD-ROM (N=1)	Multiple (N=1)
Reach and representativeness (individual level)									
Target population identification	100%	100%	100%	100%	100%	100%	100%	100%	100%
Individual inclusion/exclusion criteria	100%	100%	100%	100%	100%	100%	100%	100%	100%
Sample size	100%	100%	100%	100%	100%	100%	100%	100%	100%
Participation rate	73%	67%	83%	100%	60%	100%	100%	100%	100%
Characteristics of participants	88%	83%	83%	100%	87%	100%	100%	100%	100%
Characteristics of nonparticipants	6%	0%	33%	0%	0%	0%	0%	0%	0%
Effectiveness (outcomes of intervention)									
Multiple measures	100%	100%	100%	100%	100%	100%	100%	100%	100%
Measure of effectiveness	91%	84%	84%	100%	93%	100%	100%	100%	100%
Differential outcome by subgroups	27%	67%	50%	0%	13%	0%	0%	0%	0%
Quality of life measure	12%	0%	0%	0%	27%	0%	0%	0%	0%
Adverse consequences	0%	0%	0%	0%	0%	0%	0%	0%	0%
Adoption (setting level)									
Target setting identification	55%	50%	83%	0%	47%	100%	50%	100%	0%
Setting inclusion/exclusion criteria	15%	50%	0%	0%	7%	0%	0%	100%	0%
Number of settings	73%	67%	83%	0%	67%	100%	100%	100%	100%
Participation rate for settings	6%	17%	0%	0%	7%	0%	0%	0%	0%
Characteristics of adopting settings	27%	33%	33%	0%	13%	100%	50%	100%	0%
Characteristics of nonadopting settings	0%	0%	0%	0%	0%	0%	0%	0%	0%

(Continued)

Table 13.4 (*Continued*)

Construct	Overall (N=33)	CT-Print (N=6)	CT-Web (N=6)	CT-Phone (N=1)	Web-based (N=15)	Kiosk (N=1)	IVR (N=2)	CD-ROM (N=1)	Multiple (N=1)
Implementation									
Extent protocol implemented as intended	58%	67%	67%	0%	67%	0%	50%	0%	0%
Expertise or training of delivery agents	27%	33%	0%	0%	33%	0%	50%	100%	0%
Intervention intensity	36%	17%	17%	0%	90%	0%	50%	0%	0%
Differential implementation by staff	9%	0%	33%	0%	7%	0%	0%	0%	0%
Program adaptation/fidelity	9%	17%	17%	0%	7%	0%	0%	0%	0%
Cost measures	6%	0%	0%	0%	7%	0%	50%	0%	0%
Maintenance and institutionalization									
Follow-up time	100%	100%	100%	100%	100%	100%	100%	100%	100%
Long-term effects measured (at least 12 month)	45%	67%	33%	100%	33%	0%	50%	100%	100%
Attrition rate reported	85%	67%	100%	100%	87%	100%	100%	0%	100%
Differential attrition by condition tested	67%	67%	83%	100%	60%	0%	100%	0%	100%
Characteristics of drop-outs	30%	33%	50%	0%	27%	0%	0%	0%	100%
Other D&I-relevant characteristics									
Theory used for intervention	52%	33%	67%	100%	53%	100%	0%	0%	100%
Theory used for adaptation/D&I	15%	17%	17%	0%	7%	0%	0%	100%	100%
Health disparities	24%	17%	0%	0%	33%	0%	50%	100%	0%
Participatory approach	9%	17%	0%	0%	7%	0%	0%	100%	0%
Human contact	48%	33%	33%	0%	60%	0%	50%	100%	100%

CT-Print—Computer-generated tailored print; CT-Web—Computer-generated tailored Web; CT-Phone: Computer-tailored phone involving personalized feedback and telephone counseling in an HMO setting) to as high as 65% (in a study evaluating a smoking cessation website with participation from the general public).

Other D&I-Relevant Characteristics for eHealth Studies of T2+

Study design. The most frequent design used was the randomized controlled trial (RCT) ($N = 25$), although there is likely publication bias on this factor in which studies with highly controlled RCT designs are more likely to get published than their counterparts with more contextualized and less controlled designs (Kessler & Glasgow, 2011). Four studies reported on innovative designs such as the group randomized trial (GRT) or fractional factorial design. The most common types of comparison conditions reported were no treatment or wait list ($N = 10$) or minimal treatment/component control ($N = 3$). A common comparative effectiveness design was to compare the basic form of the intervention to its augmented (i.e., expanded with additional components) format ($N = 9$). A number of studies compared different interventions or modalities such as in-person versus Internet delivery of the same intervention ($N = 6$). Three studies used no comparison groups.

D&I strategies. Few studies ($N = 4$) reported on explicit use of theories or frameworks to inform the adaptation/expansion and D&I efforts. The theories and frameworks mentioned were the diffusion of innovations theory (Rogers, 2003), the RE-AIM framework (Glasgow, Vogt, & Boles, 1999), and the transtheoretical model (Prochaska, 1992). As discussed earlier, the majority of T2+ studies described the adaptation or expansion of a tested intervention, and very few reported on dissemination activities. Among the ones that did, few reported on creative D&I strategies. An exception was De Bourdeaudhuij and colleagues (2007), who used local health promotion services and existing mediating organizations to identify potential worksites and guide the dissemination of their tested computer-tailored fat intake reduction intervention.

Health disparities. Due to the diversity of target populations across studies, it is difficult to make conclusions about who is more likely to participate in and/ or benefit from EHIs. Only eight T2+ studies mentioned explicitly taking into account at least one driver of health disparities (e.g., racial/ethnic, low socioeconomic status, gender) when designing their intervention or recruiting for their study. None of the studies discussed issues of health literacy and numeracy, and only a few addressed the digital divide. In a study addressing the digital divide, Gustafson and colleagues (2008) provided a computer and Internet subscription along with extensive personal training on use of computers and the Internet to study participants. Additional support in the form of a manual, follow-up training, and a toll-free helpline was also available. However, these resources were revoked after the termination of the study, and thus the sustainability of this approach is questionable.

Participatory approach. Few studies reported on using an approach that actively engaged either the potential target audience or organizational adopters (e.g., clinicians, teachers, etc.). However, developers of all three CHESS programs included in this chapter (Gustafson et al., 2001; Japuntich et al., 2006; Patten et al., 2006) used clinician and patient panels and an iterative process to identify content for the respective programs. The Expert Patient Programme Online used a reference group of key stakeholders to advise how to access possible target networks and used peers to moderate online program activities (Lorig et al., 2008). Finally, the High 5, Low Fat program was developed and disseminated with a close partnership between the Parents as Teachers National Training Center and the research team (Nanney et al., 2007).

Human contact. About half of the interventions were designed to have no need for human contact with participants (e.g., mailed tailored report or CD-ROM, fully automated website or IVR, automated email and call reminders). For the interventions that included human contact with participants, the frequency, type, amount, and timing of contact and training needs of contact staff differed widely but often included reminder calls or follow-up visits with decreasing frequency over time. Very few studies evaluated the added value of human contact from trained staff members (e.g., research assistant) or health care professionals (e.g., nurse).

Fidelity and adaptation. Very few studies provided information on the adaptation of programs to local context or on any variation in implementation by staff or setting. For the evaluation of the Activ-O-Meter computer-tailored physical activity intervention, De Bourdeaudhuij and colleagues (2010) reported variations in implementation strategies across six participating countries due to the scarcity of local resources and varying level of endorsement by adopting teachers. Included T2+ studies did not commonly report on how or the extent to which the intervention evolved over time.

Discussion

One of the most disappointing findings of this review was that only 8% of the EHIs could be classified as T2+. For example, we identified 71 primary articles on physical activity and 53 articles on smoking in the T1 group but only eight physical activity and seven smoking articles on T2+. Furthermore, the majority of the articles of T2+ described adaptation or expansion of tested interventions and many fewer articles (less than 1%) described scale up or dissemination. One possible explanation for this is that funding for T2+ research has been much more limited than for T1 research. Especially in cases in which T2+ studies use designs different from RCTs, such studies can be harder to get funded and published (Kessler & Glasgow, 2011; Szilagyi, 2009).

Only one study included both managed care and community health care settings (Gustafson et al., 2001). Few eHealth researchers have partnered with implementation settings to form research-practice partnerships (International Health

Informatics, n.d.). The work of Strecher and colleagues (2008) in partnering with HMOs and worksites is an example of this type of relationship. Including diverse settings, as recommended by proponents of practical and pragmatic trials (Glasgow, Magid, Beck, Ritzwoller, & Estabrooks, 2005; Thorpe et al., 2009; Tunis, Stryer, & Clancy, 2003), would increase the generalizability of study findings (i.e., practical clinical trials).

Only 6% of studies reported on the percentage of settings that participated after being approached, and none reported on their representativeness. This lack of reporting on setting and contextual factors (Glasgow, Bull, Piette, & Steiner, 2004; Klesges et al., 2008) reflects the more general trend of health research to value and report internal validity issues over external validity. EHIs will need to give enhanced value to external validity and contextual concerns if they are to succeed at T2–T4 research and going to scale (Green & Glasgow, 2006). We found no reports of T2+ studies using Web 2.0, social media, or mobile health interventions, but we expect this to change substantially in future years. We encourage reports on the use of multiple EHIs and interventions that are platform independent (i.e., can be delivered by multiple devices [Glasgow, Bull et al., 2004]), as technologies will undoubtedly continue to evolve, especially convergence devices such as the iPad.

Our review revealed acute needs for greater reporting on the *representativeness* of patients, providers, and settings studied and for broader reporting on outcomes and factors related to outcomes. Such outcomes should include contextual analysis and qualitative/mixed methods reporting on setting, timing, economic, political, policy, and historical factors related to implementation and outcomes.

We also encourage more standardized reporting on both outcomes and eHealth technology-related factors as advocated by Harrington and Noar (in press) and Tate et al. (2009). Without such "data harmonization" (e.g., Grid-Enabled Measures Database [GEM] [National Cancer Institute, 2010]), it is difficult to compare results across studies. Brief, well-normed measures of quality of life (e.g., Patient Reported Outcomes Measurement Information System [PROMIS] [National Institutes of Health, n.d.]) are available and we encourage reporting on unanticipated outcomes, both positive and negative. Such patient-centered measures complement biological outcomes, can help us understand the participant's perspective, and can enhance evaluation of how well the intervention will perform under real world conditions (Glasgow, Magid et al., 2005; Society of Behavioral Medicine, 2010; Tunis et al., 2003). They also provide a common metric across studies of different chronic conditions, and some authors have argued that quality adjusted life years is the ultimate health outcome (Kaplan, 1993).

Cost and cost-effectiveness of EHIs (only 6% of T2+ studies reported on this) are two of the least often reported and most needed outcomes. This is often the first—and sometimes only—question asked by potential adopting organizations, and if it is not answered satisfactorily, it is often the end of the conversation. Cost analyses can favor EHIs, especially if initial development costs are already invested, because scalability or delivering interventions efficiently to large numbers of participants is frequently a strength of EHIs versus face-to-face interventions. We recommend that EHIs include transparent cost data that include costs for development, recruitment, training and supervision, site maintenance, and intervention implementation, as described by Gold, Siegel, Russell, and Weinstein (1996), Ritzwoller, Sukhanova, Gaglio, and Glasgow (2009), and Ritzwoller and colleagues (2005). Sensitivity analyses should be included to investigate the impact of factors such as scale and different recruitment, intervention, and assessment procedures.

Maintenance was reported moderately often at the individual level (45% of T2+ studies reported at least 12 month results), although it is subject to the attrition issues described above. We recommend use of imputation procedures and models in situations having greater than 10% attrition. Studies such as that of Couper, Peytchev, Strecher, Rothert, and Anderson (2007) that investigate the characteristics and outcomes of participants who do not participate in follow-up assessments are also important. Such intensive follow-up procedures can be informative and surprising. For example, those participants not participating in follow-up assessments in a weight loss study appear to have lost as much weight as those who did (Couper et al., 2007).

Maintenance at the setting level, or sustainability, was never reported in the T2+ studies of this review. More research on the extent to which EHIs are maintained, adapted, or discontinued following an initial evaluation, and the reasons for such actions, are essential to evaluate public health impact. The measurement of sustainability when applied to EHIs, however, is complex because they often change dynamically. This complexity reflects evolving evidence, societal trends, user feedback, and rapid technology developments especially given the advent of social media and Web 2.0 applications.

General Issues

The current status of the literature on T2+ EHIs reflects the status of the field of health behavior change more generally (Glanz, Rimer, & Viswanath, 2008; Glasgow et al., 2004b). Progress has been made, and we conclude, similar to other reviews of the general eHealth literature (Ahern, Kreslake, & Phalen, 2006; Bennett & Glasgow, 2009; Harrington & Noar, in press; Strecher, 2007; Tate et al., 2009), that tailored health behavior change interventions appear efficacious (and in our case, effective). They have broad dissemination potential given a number of factors, including accessibility, societal trends, and scalability. However, much more research is needed. These benefits need to be measured and documented, rather than simply hoped for.

Particular areas in need of research include the impact of EHIs on health disparities, not only racial and ethnic disparities, which are of critical importance, but also disparities in terms of reach and effectiveness; implementation; initial and long-term outcomes related to factors such as age, gender, health, and computer literacy (especially the evolving field of health numeracy); rural-urban residence; employment; types of computer connections; and so forth. Common to all of these areas is establishing a denominator database of the settings, staff, and participants approached for participation and using this information as a basis for reporting representativeness. Guidance for this reporting is provided in Glasgow and colleagues (2010). Computational tools, including "reach and adoption calculators," are available at http://www.re-aim.org/.

Retaining participant engagement in EHIs remains an important challenge. More work needs to be done on conceptualization and measures of engagement (Danaher & Seeley, 2009), as well as interventions to enhance engagement. It is not clear for most EHIs if there is a robust linear relationship between engagement and outcomes or if there is a typical "threshold level" of involvement necessary for benefit. A key issue for eHealth research is the type, timing, and amount of human contact (and modality) that is most cost-effective for producing specified outcomes (Gaglio & Glasgow, in press).

A final general issue was how challenging it was to infer the extent to which participatory approaches were used. We estimated that 9% of the T2+ studies used some type of participatory approach, but this often required a fairly high level of inference. We expected that community-based participatory research principles (Minkler & Wallerstein, 2003) with stakeholder groups would be commonly applied, but this was not reported frequently. It is never too early to begin planning for dissemination, and the involvement of both patients/end users and individuals who will be responsible for adopting and/or sustaining EHIs increases the likelihood of large-scale application and sustainability (Glasgow, 2007).

Methods Issues

The majority of T2+ studies used either a patient randomized design (76%) or a group randomized design (12%). We were disappointed to see that there were not more creative, dynamic, and adaptive evaluation designs. The eHealth medium lends itself to dynamic, adaptive, and iterative type designs (Collins, Murphy, & Strecher, 2007) and possibly multiple baseline, sequential intervention, quality improvement, and replication design strategies more than traditional RCTs (Glasgow, Toobert, Barrera, & Strycker, 2005; Kessler & Glasgow, 2011). As mentioned earlier, this may be a consequence of the types of science that get funded and published (Kessler & Glasgow, 2011). However, there is a disconnect between the potential of EHIs and the designs employed to date. In particular, we emphasize the need for research that is stronger on relevance and external validity (Bennett & Glasgow, 2009; Glasgow, 2008; Green & Glasgow, 2006; Rothwell, 2005).

Iterative interventions and research designs to evaluate such interventions are especially relevant given the advent of social media and participatory research, which are open-ended and evolving. Unfortunately, few review groups or Institutional Review Boards are well positioned to evaluate such programs and proposals

(Kessler & Glasgow, 2011). We hypothesize that the extent to which an EHI provides fresh material, is responsive to user feedback, and links to current events and context should be strong predictors of keeping users engaged and of long-term success.

Two final methods issues are interrelated: the use of comparative effectiveness research (CER) designs and the level of human contact in EHIs. CER research is likely to dominate much of the near future funding agenda (Clancy & Collins, 2010; Institute of Medicine, 2009), and EHIs should be strong candidates for CER. Details on CER definitions and characteristics are available elsewhere (Glasgow & Steiner, in press; Institute of Medicine, 2009), but the key characteristics involve pragmatic evaluations that test feasible interventions under real world settings and that employ real world alternative interventions (often current state-of-the-field or standard interventions) as comparison conditions as opposed to no treatment or placebo controls (Glasgow, Magid et al., 2005; Tunis et al., 2003; Zwarenstein et al., 2008). We refer readers to recent work by the CONSORT Work Group on Pragmatic Trials and the Pragmatic Explanatory Continuum Indicator Scale (PRECIS) tool and work by Harrington and Noar in press to enhance transparent reporting (Thorpe et al., 2009).

One of the most important questions for EHIs is the type, amount, and timing of human contact needed to enhance intervention outcomes. Most but not all reports that have evaluated the impact of added contact have found such contact via in-person meetings, emails, or other avenues to enhance outcomes (Glasgow et al., 2011; Tate et al., 2009; Tate, Jackvony, & Wing, 2003). Investigations of the conditions under which contact enhances outcomes and the cost-effectiveness of increased amount of human contact evaluated from a realist review perspective (Pawson, Greenhalgh, Harvey, & Walshe, 2005) are especially needed to advance our knowledge and improve the practicality of EHIs.

Conclusion

Our overall conclusion about the literature on implementation and dissemination of EHIs is decidedly mixed and variable across areas. There are important eHealth areas upon which to build. The majority of T2+ studies were relatively strong on internal validity, with over half reporting follow-up assessments of 12 months or longer and most addressing differential attrition across conditions. Further, studies addressed a variety of health conditions and eHealth platforms/modalities.

More research is needed, however, and the type of research needed is not "more of the same." Only 8% of eHealth research met criteria for T2+. This is of concern, especially given calls over the past decade for research that is more relevant to real world problems (Glasgow et al., 1999; Green & Glasgow, 2006; Rothwell, 2005; Tunis et al., 2003). It is alarming that less than 1% of the studies addressed scale up or dissemination, given the frequent claims regarding the generalizability and scalability of EHIs (Bennett & Glasgow, 2009; Bonander & Gates, 2010;

Strecher, 2007). We believe that research conducted on the issues identified in this review will provide more responsive and rapid answers to the question: "Which type of EHIs, administered under what conditions are most cost-effective for producing which outcomes for which types of patients?" (Bennett & Glasgow, 2009; Pawson et al., 2005).

Furthermore, this research will inform the field and help EHIs achieve their potential in terms of enhancing care that is patient-centered, broadly available, equitable, efficient, safe, and effective (Institute of Medicine, 2001a). There have been modest structural changes in this direction, as evidenced by the establishment of a standing NIH study section for dissemination and implementation research and the increasing attendance and number of submissions to the annual NIH Dissemination and Implementation Conference. We hope that publications such as this will help to enhance the visibility of this evolving science, its funding, and understanding of its importance for eHealth and other fields.

Acknowledgments

The authors are thankful to Ms. Laura E. Muhs and Ms. Edina Rozsa for their assistance with the preparation of this chapter. Funding for the preparation of this chapter was provided through the National Cancer Institute CRN Cancer Communication Research Center (1P20 CA137219). The content and opinions expressed in this article do not necessarily reflect those of the National Cancer Institute.

References

Ahern, D. K., Kreslake, J. M., & Phalen, J. M. (2006). What is eHealth: Perspectives on the evolution of eHealth research. *Journal of Medical Internet Research, 8,* e4.

Bennett, G. G., & Glasgow, R. E. (2009). The delivery of public health interventions via the Internet: Actualizing their potential. *Annual Review of Public Health, 30,* 273–292.

Bonander, J., & Gates, S. (2010). Public health in an era of personal health records: Opportunities for innovation and new partnerships. *Journal of Medical Internet Research, 12,* e33.

Clancy, C., & Collins, F. S. (2010). Patient-Centered Outcomes Research Institute: The intersection of science and health care. *Science Translational Medicine, 2,* 37cm18.

Collins, L., Murphy, S. A., & Strecher, V. (2007). The Multiphase Optimization Strategy (MOST) and the Sequential Multiple Assignment Randomized Trial (SMART): New methods for more potent eHealth interventions. *American Journal of Preventive Medicine, 32,* S112–S118.

Couper, M. P., Peytchev, A., Strecher, V. J., Rothert, K., & Anderson, J. (2007). Following up nonrespondents to an online weight management intervention: Randomized trial comparing mail versus telephone. *Journal of Medical Internet Research, 9,* e16.

Danaher, B. G., & Seeley, J. R. (2009). Methodological issues in research on Web-based behavioral interventions. *Annals of Behavioral Medicine, 38,* 28–39.

De Bourdeaudhuij, I., Maes, L., De Henauw, S., De Vriendt, T., Moreno, L. A., Kersting, M., et al. (2010). Evaluation of a computer-tailored physical activity intervention in adolescents in six European countries: The Activ-O-Meter in the HELENA intervention study. *Journal of Adolescent Health, 46,* 458–466.

De Bourdeaudhuij, I., Stevens, V., Vandelanotte, C., & Brug, J. (2007). Evaluation of an interactive computer-tailored nutrition intervention in a real-life setting. *Annals of Behavioral Medicine, 33,* 39–48.

Dobbins, M., Cockerill, R., Barnsley, J., & Ciliska, D. (2001). Factors of the innovation, organization, environment, and individual that predict the influence five systematic reviews had on public health decisions. *International Journal of Technology Assessment in Health Care, 17,* 467–478.

Gaglio, B., & Glasgow, R. E. (in press). Evaluation approaches for dissemination and implementation research. In R. C. Brownson, G. Colditz, & E. Proctor (Eds.), *Dissemination and implementation research in health: Translating science to practice.* New York: Oxford University Press.

Glanz, K., Rimer, B. K., & Viswanath, K. (Eds.) (2008). *Health behavior and health education: Theory, research, and practice* (4th ed.). San Francisco: Jossey-Bass.

Glasgow, R. E. (2007). eHealth evaluation and dissemination research. *American Journal of Preventive Medicine, 32,* S119–S126.

Glasgow, R. E. (2008). What types of evidence are most needed to advance behavioral medicine? *Annals of Behavioral Medicine, 35,* 19–25.

Glasgow, R. E., Bull, S. S., Piette, J. D., & Steiner, J. F. (2004a). Interactive behavior change technology: A partial solution to the competing demands of primary care. *American Journal of Preventive Medicine, 27,* 80–87.

Glasgow, R. E., Dickinson, P., Fisher, L., Christiansen, S., Toobert, D. J., & Bender, B. G. (2011). *Patient-centered assessment, communication, and outcomes in the primary care medical home: Use of RE-AIM to develop a multi-media facilitation tool.* Manuscript submitted for publication.

Glasgow, R. E., & Emmons, K. M. (2007). How can we increase translation of research into practice? Types of evidence needed. *Annual Review of Public Health, 28,* 413–433.

Glasgow, R. E., Klesges, L. M., Dzewaltowski, D. A., Bull, S. S., & Estabrooks, P. (2004b). The future of health behavior change research: What is needed to improve translation of research into health promotion practice? *Annals of Behavioral Medicine, 27,* 3–12.

Glasgow, R. E., Lichtenstein, E., & Marcus, A. C. (2003). Why don't we see more translation of health promotion research to practice? Rethinking the efficacy-to-effectiveness transition. *American Journal of Public Health, 93,* 1261–1267.

Glasgow, R. E., & Linnan, L. A. (2008). Evaluation of theory-based interventions. In K. Glanz, B. K. Rimer, & K. Viswanath (Eds.), *Health behavior and health education: Theory, research, and practice* (4th ed., pp. 487–503). San Francisco: Jossey-Bass.

Glasgow, R. E., Magid, D. J., Beck, A., Ritzwoller, D., & Estabrooks, P. A. (2005). Practical clinical trials for translating research to practice: Design and measurement recommendations. *Medical Care, 43,* 551–557.

Glasgow, R. E., & Steiner, J. F. (in press). Comparative effectiveness research to accelerate translation: Recommendations for "CERT-T." In R. C. Brownson, G. Colditz, & E. Proctor (Eds.), *Dissemination and implementation research in health: Translating science to practice.* New York: Oxford University Press.

Glasgow, R. E., Strycker, L. A., Kurz, D., Faber, A., Bell, H., Dickman, J. M., et al. (2010). Recruitment for an Internet-based diabetes self-management program: Scientific and ethical implications. *Annals of Behavioral Medicine, 40,* 40–48.

Glasgow, R. E., Toobert, D. J., Barrera, M., Jr., & Strycker, L. A. (2005). The Chronic Illness Resources Survey: Cross-validation and sensitivity to intervention. *Health Education Research, 20,* 402–409.

Glasgow, R. E., Vogt, T. M., & Boles, S. M. (1999). Evaluating the public health impact of health promotion interventions: The RE-AIM framework. *American Journal of Public Health, 89,* 1322–1327.

Gold, M. R., Siegel, J. E., Russell, L. B., & Weinstein, M. C. (1996). *Cost-effectiveness in health and medicine.* Oxford, United Kingdom: Oxford University Press.

Green, L. W., & Glasgow, R. E. (2006). Evaluating the relevance, generalization, and applicability of research: Issues in external validation and translation methodology. *Evaluation & the Health Professions, 29,* 126–153.

Gustafson, D. H., Hawkins, R., McTavish, F., Pingree, S., Chen, W. C., Volrathongchai, K., et al. (2008). Internet-based interactive support for cancer patients: Are integrated systems better? *Journal of Communication, 58*(2), 238–257.

Gustafson, D. H., Hawkins, R., Pingree, S., McTavish, F., Arora, N. K., Mendenhall, J., et al. (2001). Effect of computer support on younger women with breast cancer. *Journal of General Internal Medicine, 16,* 435–445.

Harrington, N. G., & Noar, S. M. (in press). Reporting standards for studies of tailored interventions. *Health Education Research.*

Institute of Medicine. (2001a, March). *Crossing the quality chasm: A new health system for the 21st century* [Report brief]. Washington, DC: Committee on Quality of Health Care in America. Retrieved July 6, 2011, from: www.nap.edu/html/quality_chasm/reportbrief.pdf.

Institute of Medicine. (2001b). *Health and behavior. The interplay of biological, behavioral, and societal influences.* Washington, DC: National Academies Press.

Institute of Medicine. (2009, June). *Initial national priorities for comparative effectiveness research* [Report brief]. Washington, DC: Committee on Comparative Effectiveness Research Prioritization. Retrieved July 6, 2011 from: http://www.iom.edu/~/media/Files/Report%20Files/2009/ComparativeEffectivenessResearchPriorities/CER%20report%20brief%2008-13-09.pdf.

International Health Informatics. (n.d.). *2010 Association for Computing Machinery International Health Informatics Symposium website.* Retrieved July 8, 2011, from: http://ihi2010.sighi.org/.

Japuntich, S. J., Zehner, M. E., Smith, S. S., Jorenby, D. E., Valdez, J. A., Fiore, M. C., et al. (2006). Smoking cessation via the Internet: A randomized clinical trial of an Internet intervention as adjuvant treatment in a smoking cessation intervention. *Nicotine & Tobacco Research, 8,* S59–S67.

Kaiser Permanente (n.d.). *Coding sheet for publications reporting on RE-AIM elements.* Retrieved July 8, 2011, from: http://www.re-aim.org/tools/figures-and-tables/coding-sheet-for-publications.aspx.

Kaplan, R. M. (1993). *The Hippocratic predicament: Affordability, access, and accountability in American health care.* San Diego: Academic Press.

Kessler, R., & Glasgow, R. E. (2011). A proposal to speed translation of healthcare research into practice: Dramatic change is needed. *American Journal of Preventive Medicine, 40,* 637–644.

Khoury, M. J., Gwinn, M., Yoon, P. W., Dowling, N., Moore, C. A., & Bradley, L. (2007). The continuum of translation research in genomic medicine: How can we accelerate the appropriate integration of human genome discoveries into health care and disease prevention. *Genetics in Medicine, 9,* 665–674.

Klesges, L. M., Dzewaltowski, D. A., & Glasgow, R. E. (2008). Review of external validity reporting in childhood obesity prevention research. *American Journal of Preventive Medicine, 34,* 216–223.

Lorig, K. R., Ritter, P. L., Dost, A., Plant, K., Laurent, D. D., & McNeil, I. (2008). The Expert Patients Programme Online, a 1-year study of an Internet-based self-management programme for people with long-term conditions. *Chronic Illness, 4,* 247–256.

McGlynn, E. A., Asch, S. M., Adams, J., Keesey, J., Hicks, J., DeCristofaro, A., et al. (2003). The quality of health care delivered to adults in the United States. *New England Journal of Medicine, 348,* 2635–2645.

Minkler, M., & Wallerstein, N. (Eds.). (2003). *Community-based participatory research for health.* San Francisco: Jossey-Bass.

Nanney, M. S., Haire-Joshu, D., Brownson, R. C., Kostelc, J., Stephen, M., & Elliott, M. (2007). Awareness and adoption of a nationally disseminated dietary curriculum. *American Journal of Health Behavior, 31,* 64–73.

National Cancer Institute. (2010, November 1). *Grid-enabled measures (GEM) database beta.* Retrieved July 8, 2011, from: https://www.gem-beta.org.

National Institutes of Health. (n.d.). *PROMIS: Dynamic tools to measure health outcomes from the patient perspective.* Retrieved July 8, 2011, from: http://www.nihpromis.org/default. aspx.

Oldenburg, B. F., Sallis, J. F., Ffrench, M. L., & Owen, N. (1999). Health promotion research and the diffusion and institutionalization of interventions. *Health Education Research, 14,* 121–130.

Patten, C. A., Croghan, I. T., Meis, T. M., Decker, P. A., Pingree, S., Colligan, R. C., et al. (2006). Randomized clinical trial of an Internet-based versus brief office intervention for adolescent smoking cessation. *Patient Education and Counseling, 64,* 249–258.

Pawson, R., Greenhalgh, T., Harvey, G., & Walshe, K. (2005). Realist review—A new method of systematic review designed for complex policy interventions. *Journal of Health Services Research & Policy, 10,* S21–S34.

Piette, J. D., Weinberger, M., Kraemer, F. B., & McPhee, S. J. (2001). Impact of automated calls with nurse follow-up on diabetes treatment outcomes in a Department of Veterans Affairs health care system: A randomized controlled trial. *Diabetes Care, 24,* 202–208.

Prochaska, J. O. (1992). A transtheoretical model of behavior change: Learning from mistakes with majority populations. In D. M. Becker, D. R. Hill, & J. S. Jackson (Eds.), *Health behavior research in minority populations: Access, design, and implementation* (pp. 105–111). Bethesda, MD: National Institutes of Health.

Rabin, B. A., Brownson, R. C., Haire-Joshu, D., Kreuter, M. W., & Weaver, N. L. (2008). A glossary for dissemination and implementation research in health. *Journal of Public Health Management and Practice, 14,* 117–123.

Ritzwoller, D. P., Goodman, M. J., Maciosek, M. V., Elston Lafata, J., Meenan, R., Hornbrook, M. C., et al. (2005). Creating standard cost measures across integrated health care delivery systems. *Journal of the National Cancer Institute Monographs, 35,* 80–87.

Ritzwoller, D. P., Sukhanova, A., Gaglio, B., & Glasgow, R. E. (2009). Costing behavioral interventions: A practical guide to enhance translation. *Annals of Behavioral Medicine, 37,* 218–227.

Rogers, E. M. (2003). *Diffusion of innovations* (5th ed.). New York: Free Press.

Rothwell, P. M. (2005). External validity of randomised controlled trials: "To whom do the results of this trial apply?" *Lancet, 365,* 82–93.

Society of Behavioral Medicine. (2010, November). *The public health need for patient-reported measures and health behaviors in electronic health records: A policy statement of the Society of Behavioral Medicine* [Report brief]. Milwaukee, WI: Society of Behavioral Medicine Public Policy Statements. Retrieved July 7, 2011, from: http://www.sbm.org/UserFiles/file/ patient-reported_measures.pdf.

Strecher, V. J. (2007). Internet methods for delivering behavioral and health-related interventions (eHealth). *Annual Review of Clinical Psychology, 3,* 53–76.

Strecher, V. J., McClure, J. B., Alexander, G. L., Chakraborty, B., Nair, V. N., Konkel, J. M., et al. (2008). Web-based smoking-cessation programs: Results of a randomized trial. *American Journal of Preventive Medicine, 34,* 373–381.

Szilagyi, P. G. (2009). Translational research and pediatrics. *Academic Pediatrics, 9,* 71–80.

Tate, D. F., Finkelstein, E. A., Khavjou, O., & Gustafson, A. (2009). Cost effectiveness of Internet interventions: Review and recommendations. *Annals of Behavioral Medicine, 38,* 40–45.

Tate, D. F., Jackvony, E. H., & Wing, R. R. (2003). Effects of Internet behavioral counseling on weight loss in adults at risk for type 2 diabetes: A randomized trial. *Journal of the American Medical Association, 289,* 1833–1836.

Thorpe, K. E., Zwarenstein, M., Oxman, A. D., Treweek, S., Furberg, C. D., Altman, D. G., et al. (2009). A pragmatic-explanatory continuum indicator summary (PRECIS): A tool to help trial designers. *Canadian Medical Association Journal, 180,* E47–E57.

Tunis, S. R., Stryer, D. B., & Clancy, C. M. (2003). Practical clinical trials: Increasing the value of clinical research for decision making in clinical and health policy. *Journal of the American Medical Association, 290,* 1624–1632.

Zwarenstein, M., Treweek, S., Gagnier, J. J., Altman, D. G., Tunis, S., Haynes, B., et al. (2008). Improving the reporting of pragmatic trials: An extension of the CONSORT statement. *British Medical Journal, 337,* a2390.

14

HEALTH INFORMATION
TECHNOLOGY POLICY ISSUES

Relevance and Implications for eHealth Applications

Cynthia Baur

> My medical history may not mean much to others, but it is an important part of my life and I would like others to treat it with the respect it deserves—a patient's commentary on electronic health information exchange.
> *(MacDonald, 2001, p. 287)*

> I'm an e-patient: empowered, engaged, equipped, enabled—e-patient Dave's blog posting at a conference on shared decision-making.
> *(DeBronkart, 2010)*

In the late 1990s, the Science Panel on Interactive Communication and Health issued its report with a proposed policy framework to maximize societal benefit of the use of health information technologies (health IT) (Science Panel on Interactive Communication and Health, 1999). The members' recommendations reflected the reality of the marketplace and the technological and policy environment of their times as well as their projections for the future. The Internet was a relatively new phenomenon, and the unequal distribution of technological resources in society was a primary concern. In 1998, only 22% of households had any type of Internet access (U.S. Department of Commerce, 1999).

Yet the panel recognized the potential power of combining people and technology to communicate about and manage minor and major health concerns. The panel projected that interactive health communication (or eHealth) technologies would demonstrate great value and diffuse rapidly as people understood the potential for technologies to promote and improve individual and community health. Panel members also outlined key policy issues. These issues included privacy and confidentiality protections, quality standards and evaluation criteria, provider liability, public and private responsibilities for investment, payment and reimbursement for services, access to technologies, and data exchange rules. Panel members stated that if policy makers paid appropriate attention to these issues, then eHealth could be used to the great benefit of individuals and communities.

A decade and a half later, the same enthusiasm about IT for health improvement still exists (President's Council of Advisors on Science and Technology, 2010). The spotlight is now on electronic health records (EHRs), personal health records (PHRs), and electronic health information exchange. Although many of the information technologies in use have matured and new technologies have emerged, many of the policy issues identified by the Science Panel are still being decided. Policy making has both advanced and is in flux in the wake of recent, significant federal legislation. Two pieces of legislation—the Patient Protection and Affordable Care Act (ACA) and the Health Information Technology for Economic and Clinical Health (HITECH) Act—elevate the importance of health care and health IT issues, particularly EHRs, on the national policy agenda. These pieces of legislation provide a framework for policy discussion and debates that did not exist when the Science Panel made its recommendations.

Although many eHealth applications might not have been covered by federal and state laws or regulations in the past, the emerging interoperability of systems and electronic data exchange will affect eHealth applications. Researchers, developers, and evaluators of eHealth applications need to be aware of—if not actively addressing—policy issues such as data exchange standards and privacy and security protections. Even without laws or regulations, ethical considerations may be relevant to design features, dissemination strategies, and evaluation methods (Baur, 2008; Goodman & Cava, 2008).

If the pace of technology change has been rapid, the inclusion of individuals, communities, and consumer-oriented eHealth technologies in the care process has been slower (Ferguson with the e-Patients Scholars Working Group, 2007). Despite the Science Panel's recommendations, subsequent reports on consumer eHealth, and multiple reports from the Institute of Medicine, people are far from full partners in the care process (Berwick, 2009; Institute of Medicine, 2001, 2003, 2009; U.S. Department of Health and Human Services, 2006). Although people can use social media to reach hundreds of "friends" to tell them about a diagnosis seconds after getting the news, the majority of patients cannot use electronic communication with their own doctors, let alone access digital tools that meet their needs and interface with their EHRs (National Cancer Institute, 2007). E-patient Dave, quoted at the beginning of the chapter, is the anomaly, not the rule.

The HITECH legislation created a new policy lever—"meaningful use"—that could change the terms for consumer engagement and eHealth. Clinical services that use certified EHRs and want to receive government payments will have to meet the standard of "meaningful use," or the use of health IT in ways that meet broad health care improvement goals (Buntin, Jain, & Blumenthal, 2010). As federal policy about meaningful use evolves, some groups have taken the position that directly engaging patients and measuring and reporting their experiences are essential steps to achieve the overall goals of safer, more effective, and less costly health care services (Ralston, Coleman, Reid, Handley & Larson, 2010).

Even while policy is evolving, consumers already are creating their own "meaningful use" as they "mash up" data from multiple sources and compare other peoples' experiences with their own. Health information seekers can use a search engine to locate information, social media to connect with other people with the same experiences, and downloadable applications that allow them to customize and manage information for their specific needs. In academic and policy terms, consumers are engaged in "personal information management," which is the "collection of tasks that people perform in order to acquire, organize, maintain, retrieve and use *information items . . . to complete tasks* and *fulfill their various roles*" (Agarwal & Khuntia, 2009, p. 5).

This chapter uses the Science Panel's policy framework and the recent federal legislation as starting points for summarizing policy issues most relevant to consumer eHealth. This chapter takes a slice of the much larger health IT field and focuses on the policy aspects of eHealth of greatest relevance to health communication. These aspects include (1) meaningful use for consumers and patients; (2) privacy, security, and control of health information; (3) access to technology; (4) quality and integrity of applications and services; and (5) the cost and payment for applications and services. eHealth researchers and practitioners should at least be aware of, if not actively contributing to, health IT policy making. If eHealth applications are going to live in the "real world," not just the lab, then they will need to be designed and tested with accessibility, privacy, security, interoperability, and quality standards and policies in mind.

Federal Legislation as the New Health IT Policy Framework

Regardless of their ultimate effects on health care delivery and outcomes, the HITECH and ACA laws mark the beginning of a new era for policy making in health care and health IT. Table 14.1 lists the federal government agency names and acronyms with primary responsibility for health IT policy making. The HITECH provisions create an infrastructure and focal point for policy making and funding for digital health that heretofore did not exist in the federal government. HITECH established the Office of the National Coordinator for Health Information Technology (ONC) in the U.S. Department of Health and Human Services. ONC is the principal federal entity to coordinate health IT and the electronic exchange of health information.[1] Both the HITECH Act and ACA fundamentally reorient the foundations of public and private health care. The ONC leadership team observes, "Although HITECH may be viewed narrowly as legislation to stimulate the adoption of health information technology (IT), it is better understood as an essential foundation for our broader efforts to restructure health care delivery" (Buntin, Jain, & Blumenthal, 2010, p. 1214). The HITECH Act and ACA share several

Table 14.1 Federal government agencies with primary health IT policy responsibilities

Name of agency	Acronym	Responsibility for health IT policy
Office of the National Coordinator for Health IT	ONC	Federal coordination for all health IT and electronic health information exchange
Office for Civil Rights	OCR	Federal regulatory agency for privacy and security protections
Food and Drug Administration	FDA	Software as a medical device, labeling, health claims
Centers for Medicare and Medicaid Services	CMS	Meaningful use and incentive payments
Federal Trade Commission	FTC	Labeling, health claims, online privacy, advertising and marketing

goals, including improving the quality, reducing the cost, and increasing access to health care services. Electronic data storage and exchange are essential elements of the work necessary to accomplish these goals (Buntin et al., 2010).

Although it has a leadership and coordination role, ONC is not the only federal agency or office with policy and regulatory authority for health IT issues. Specific responsibilities related to the privacy and security of protected health information are assigned to the HHS Office for Civil Rights (OCR). OCR is the federal regulatory agency for privacy and security protections for personal health information. The Privacy Rule of the Health Insurance Portability and Accountability Act (HIPAA) covers who can look at and exchange health information and the rights of patients to access or restrict access of health information. The Privacy Rule applies to "covered entities," which are primarily health care providers, facilities, and insurers. HIPAA applies to all health information managed by covered entities, not just information electronically stored and exchanged. The HIPAA Security Rule provides multiple standards for health information protection.

In addition to ONC and OCR, there are other governmental actors who help define the standards and policies that pertain to the functionality, inter-connectedness, and conditions of use of health IT applications. For example, the HHS Food and Drug Administration (FDA) regulates medical devices. The Federal Food, Drug and Cosmetic Act covers health IT software as a medical device, although the agency has not enforced regulatory requirements (Shuren, 2010). A small number of safety issues, such as accessing incorrect patient information or overwriting patient data, making errors in data entry, and encountering software incompatibilities, have been reported to the FDA. The director of the FDA unit in charge of medical devices testified "because these reports are purely voluntary, they may represent only the tip of the iceberg in terms of the HIT-related problems that exist" (Shuren, 2010, p. 2). The quality of health IT system implementation and the integrity of the source data and algorithms may be issues that have not been fully recognized or addressed (Sittig & Classen, 2010). Maintaining information integrity is both a safety and ethical concern (Baur & Deering, 2006). In addition to the FDA's role for HIT software, the National Institute of Standards and Technology (NIST) has a role in developing standards for many dimensions of health IT and runs health IT testing programs.

The FDA and the Federal Trade Commission (FTC) both have some responsibility for labeling and claims made about health devices and products (Federal Trade Commission, n.d.). As part of its consumer protection mandate, the FTC monitors online privacy, advertising, and marketing practices. The FTC has proposed a privacy framework that would make privacy protection part of regular business practices. The agency calls the approach "privacy by design" (Federal Trade Commission, 2010). The U.S. Commerce Department reinforced the idea that federal oversight of data privacy is essential to the successful evolution of digital technologies. The department has issued its own framework for commercial data privacy (Department of Commerce Internet Policy Task Force, 2010).

Private sector organizations and state governments also are part of the policy-making process. For example, URAC, an independent accreditation and measurement organization, has had a health website and health content vendor accreditation program for a number of years (URAC, n.d.). Organizations that have health content on their website can have the sites reviewed to evaluate editorial, linking, and advertising policies and practices. For information on state laws, Georgetown University's Center on Medical Record Rights and Privacy links to state laws regarding privacy and medical records.

From a consumer, researcher, and developer perspective, locating responsibility for health IT oversight can be daunting among the "alphabet soup" of agencies and organizations that have some authority in the consumer eHealth space. The current situation requires users and developers to have a large amount of bureaucratic and legal savvy to determine if an eHealth product is under the jurisdiction of a particular agency or subject to a set of regulations or standards. Yet making such a determination is a necessary step if a user has questions or concerns about an eHealth application, in particular if federal or state laws for the protection of personal health information apply, or if a developer is trying to comply with the law. The notions of consumer empowerment and engagement are seriously challenged when consumers must navigate such a complex set of organizations and practices to know, understand, and protect their rights, many of which are still undefined.

Of the many health IT public policy issues that federal and state agencies are considering, five are most relevant for consumer eHealth: (1) meaningful use; (2) privacy, security, and control of health information; (3) access to health information; (4) quality and integrity of applications and health information; and (5) the cost and payment for eHealth services. For the purposes of this chapter, "health information" includes person-level data as well as more general, aggregated health information such as that found on a public website about a health condition. Although there are multiple regulatory and legal nuances to each of the topic areas, this overview highlights those issues that relate most directly to health communication and the applications covered in this edited volume. Each of these five issues has the potential to affect researchers' and practitioners' decisions about the design and testing of eHealth applications that will connect to other technology and health care systems.

Meaningful Use

Policy makers are writing the full definition of meaningful use in three phases over five years, concluding in 2015. The HITECH legislation introduced the concept of "meaningful use" and identified three main elements: using a certified EHR in a "meaningful" manner, electronically exchanging health information to improve care, and submitting clinical quality and other measures to the federal Centers for Medicare and Medicaid Services (CMS) (Centers for Medicare and Medicaid Services, 2010). CMS issued the phase one criteria in 2010.

In this first phase, patients will be able to do basic tasks, such as request copies of their electronic medical records, but ONC proposes that "empowering consumers and patients" is part of the promise of meaningful use that will be realized in later phases (Daniel, 2010; Maxson et al., 2010). Much of the empowerment and engagement is premised on consumers' and patients' access to information—their own clinical data and information potentially integrated or at least available through other sources, such as online rating systems and provider directories. The underlying notion is to provide patients access to what has traditionally been the property of health care facilities and providers—patient data stored in paper records. Although most patients do not ask their providers for copies of personal health information or medical records in electronic format, about 60% of patients say it is important they can get secure access if they want to see their records (Markle Connecting for Health, 2010a).

At the same time that policy makers are working on the access and engagement rules for EHRs, "e-patients" are articulating a view of meaningful use that envisions a power sharing relationship between patients and the medical community. "E-patients" are people who often have life-threatening or chronic illnesses and use the Internet for medical research, communication, and advocacy for patients as full partners in the care process (Ferguson with the e-Patients Scholars Working Group, 2007). Their basic position can be summarized as "nothing about me without me" (Delbanco et al., 2001). Former CMS director Dr. Donald Berwick has called for the health care system to embrace "patient-centeredness," which is driven by patients' needs and wants (Berwick, 2009). Some of the Beacon communities—those ONC-funded communities with already high rates of health IT—have patient empowerment components (Maxson et al., 2010). How far these projects will go toward demonstrating a full clinical-patient partnership based on secure and open information exchange and patients' needs and wants is unknown.

Privacy, Security, and Control of Health Information

Because privacy and security protections continually rate as the most important health IT issues for consumers, privacy and security topics often occupy a large part of the policy agenda (Diamond, Goldstein, Lansky, & Verhulst, 2008; Goldstein & Rein, 2010; Markle Connecting for Health, 2010b). According to a white paper commissioned by ONC, "the issue of whether, to what extent, and how individuals should have the ability to exercise control over their health information represents one of the foremost policy challenges related to the electronic exchange of health information" (Goldstein & Rein, 2010, p. ES-1). The earliest proposals for a nationwide health information network recognized that ensuring privacy and the secure electronic exchange of personal health information was necessary for public acceptance of digital health care (National Committee on Vital and Health Statistics, 1998, 2001). According to Dr. David Blumenthal, former national Health IT coordinator, and Georgina Verdugo, director of the HHS Office for Civil Rights, "one of the Department's (HHS) guiding principles is that the benefits of health IT can only be fully realized if patients and providers are confident that electronic health information is kept private and secure" (Blumethal & Verdugo, 2010).

Although the current policy focus is on electronic health information that is exchanged, privacy and security protections can relate to eHealth applications that are stand-alone, such as online educational or behavioral modification tools that consumers or patients use for a specific health issue. The extensive profiles of users' habits and preferences built to drive tailoring algorithms, for example, create data repositories that require security mechanisms and policies. Stand-alone applications have not been covered by the HIPAA Privacy Rule to date, although they could be subject to state laws (Goldstein & Rein, 2010). Noncovered entities for the purposes of HIPAA may offer their own privacy policies, although the FTC has noted these policies are often long, confusing, and difficult to find (Federal Trade Commission, 2010). The FTC suggests steps companies can take to make it easier for consumers to understand privacy practices and to control the flow and use of their personal information.

Stand-alone applications, however, are not the future of health IT. The premise of the HITECH Act is that the greatest value to health care quality, safety, and cost will come from health information exchanged among clinicians, facilities, and patients (Blumenthal, 2010). The HITECH legislation includes provisions to review and update privacy and security policies and standards in line with the goal of advancing electronic health information exchange. OCR has proposed extending HIPAA to business associates, and notification requirements and penalties for unauthorized information release have increased (Blumenthal & Verdugo, 2010).

If eHealth applications are to be interoperable with or successfully integrated into health care services, they will need to be consistent with the existing and emerging privacy practices and security mechanisms of EHRs and PHRs.

In addition to privacy policies, consumer control of personal health information is another model for assuring privacy and allowing information exchange (Goldstein & Rein, 2010). The President's Council of Advisors on Science and Technology (2010) has proposed allowing consumers to "tag" their data in small chunks so that they can create different exchange rules, depending on the type of data. In general, though, consumers are not familiar with or attentive to the ways companies use technology and innovation for sophisticated tracking and marketing of personal information (Department of Commerce Internet Policy Task Force, 2010; Federal Trade Commission, 2010).

Multiple national surveys find the public "considers privacy safeguards important to all health information technology efforts" (Markle Connecting for Health, 2010b, slide 2). Patients and doctors report they want notifications when an unauthorized information release occurs, and they want to have audit trails, choices about information uses, and options to make corrections when errors are found (Markle Connecting for Health, 2010b). Similarly, a large focus group study of consumer attitudes about health IT design, including privacy and security issues, found that "privacy and security were the main concerns of a large majority of the participants" (Schneider, Kerwin, Robins, & Dean, 2009). Even though study participants said they should have a role in deciding how their information is accessed and used, they also said they were confused about how to influence decisions about health IT and thought experts should play the leading role in health IT design decisions (Schneider et al., 2009).

The matter of information control and exchange has in part been framed as a matter of trust—primarily trust of patients in health IT systems as a safer, more effective means for doctors, nurses, hospitals, clinicians, and the rest of the massive health care infrastructure to provide high-quality care (Blumenthal & Verdugo, 2010; Goldstein & Rein, 2010). Policies and practices for information control are also a matter of professional ethics (Baur & Deering, 2006; Wynia, 2010). Harm to the provider-patient relationship that may follow an unauthorized information release or mistakes in data entry in a patient record should be considered. Health IT systems and business relations are not currently part of patients' everyday experiences with health care; doctors, nurses, hospitals, and clinics are. Patients expect their providers to act ethically and in the patients' best interests. As Dr. Matthew Wynia, a noted medical ethicist observes, patients already trust their doctors (and nurses). The question is, are doctors and other actors in the clinical system acting in trustworthy and ethical ways when they handle patients' health information? Are they using appropriate precautions and limiting the amount of information shared (Wynia, 2010)? The FTC analysis of online information practices indicates most consumers place unwarranted trust in online information and service providers, in part because consumers do not know much about how personal information is collected, stored, and shared, nor do they know what the options are, if any, to protect their privacy online (Department of Commerce Internet Policy Force, 2010; Federal Trade Commission, 2010). Even if eHealth applications are not yet covered by law or regulation, developers have an ethical obligation to safeguard personal health information stored in eHealth applications and be transparent in their information practices.

Access to Health Information

The consumer appeal and relative affordability of new technologies are changing the ways people access health information and services. Mobile devices, such as smartphones and lightweight, portable computers, make it possible for some people to access health information wherever and whenever they choose (see Abroms, Padmanabhan, & Evans, and Fjeldsoe, Miller, & Marshall, this volume). In the late 1990s, the policy questions related to access were the following: Who has access to the Internet? What demographic differences, such as income or race and ethnicity, affect who has access? Is technology creating a social divide that should be addressed through policy mechanisms? The Internet was too new to generate much data about what people did online, and there was a lot of speculation about what people could do or would want to do. A decade and a half later, questions of access still are relevant (U.S. Department of Commerce, 2010). Questions about use—who uses technology for which purposes—have taken on greater importance (Fox, 2006, 2011).

Trend data on technology access and use suggest that the marketplace has not fully eliminated disparities as a topic of interest for policy making or the health communication and public health fields (Baur, 2008). Differences in technology access and use persist by educational attainment, income levels, age groups, and urban or rural community type (Pew Internet and American Life Project, 2010; U.S. Department of Commerce, 2010). As survey research from the Pew Internet and American Life Project shows, "Those in higher-income households are different from other Americans in their tech ownership and use" (Jansen, 2010, p. 2). According to the Pew Project, higher-income people are more likely to have multiple ways to connect to the Internet and use the Internet for finance and news (Jansen, 2010). Even though there is a gap in cell phone ownership between the highest and lowest income levels (95% ownership at the highest and 75% at the lowest income levels), it is the smallest difference among the categories of broadband at home, Internet use, and cell phone ownership (Jansen, 2010).

The data about cell phones and mobile access to the Internet complicate the picture of disparities. The Pew Internet and American Life Project survey results also show that adult African Americans and English-speaking Latinos have higher rates of cell phone ownership and use more features than whites (Smith, 2010). Cell phone owners take pictures and send or receive text messages more frequently than any other activities (Smith, 2010). Cell phone ownership is ubiquitous (90%)

among people ages 18–29 (Smith, 2010). Although racial and ethnic disparities in technology access may persist for older adults, the data suggest that disparities may diminish among groups of younger adults because of similarities across racial and ethnic lines in product tastes, affordability, and social norms in technology use.

Given the shift to mobile devices and their acceptance among minority populations, two sets of policy issues are relevant. The first set pertains to universal access. The existing policy goal of universal access to EHRs relies on universal access to the infrastructure and devices compatible with EHR applications. Although mobile technologies appear to be popular points of access, will EHRs, PHRs, and other applications be compatible with mobile devices and provide sufficient security features to protect personal information? The data on Internet and cell phone use suggest population segments already have preferences and habits that will influence their interest in and adoption of eHealth applications.

The second set of issues pertains to populations' reactions to accessing health applications and personal health data on mobile devices. Will the habits they developed using communication and entertainment functions transfer to the health domain? The high rates of diabetes, heart disease, asthma, and other chronic conditions in minority populations indicate there could be a significant market for chronic disease management applications that work on mobile devices and target minority users, if the applications fit their existing patterns and habits or are sufficiently engaging to attract and maintain their attention.

The applications must also be sensitive to the health literacy barriers in these populations (Baur, 2008). Fifty-eight percent of adult African Americans and 66% of English-speaking Hispanic adults have basic or below basic health literacy skills (Kutner, Greenberg, Jin, & Paulsen, 2006). Even if African American and Hispanic users are comfortable with the technology, some still may be challenged in understanding and applying the information in the applications. They may also be challenged by the off-putting language and complexity of choice in data use consent forms (Goldstein & Rein, 2010). If minority users or other high-risk populations are not interested in online and/or mobile health applications and content, then what public or private incentives might be necessary to stimulate the use of effective eHealth applications, especially EHRs? In addition to the content, there may be differences in the types of concerns that different populations have about the privacy and security of personal health information and the mechanisms required or desired to exercise control over the sharing of the information.

Quality and Integrity of Online Health Applications and Information

Health application and information quality is a public policy issue of relevance to eHealth developers and researchers. The popularity of online health information sources, consumers' reliance on this information for decision making, and the negative social consequences when inaccurate or misleading information is easily available has generated concern in the medical and health education communities since the mid-to-late 1990s (Seidman, Steinwachs, & Rubin, 2003; Silberg, Lundberg, & Musacchio, 1997). At the same time, governmental evaluation of information quality or sponsorship of such evaluation raises questions about censorship, appropriateness of standards, and sufficiency of evidence (Baur & Deering, 2001).

The need to assure the quality of health applications and information is relevant in at least two contexts: public or semi-public resources, such as a website or social media application, and semi-private or private resources, such as a provider portal open to patients through registration, clinical EHR, or consumer-controlled PHR. Closed or stand-alone applications, such as disease management or social support tools, would fit the second category because these applications are usually not accessible online or allow only limited access through registration. These tools, which can be part of larger systems, require high levels of quality from a safety perspective but also safe implementation and safe use by clinicians and patients in health care contexts. If the algorithms and databases driving these tools have inaccurate data or calculations, then the outputs that end users rely on will be greatly compromised.

A literature on online information quality has developed over the last 15 years (Eysenbach, Powell, Kuss, & Sa, 2002; Silberg et al., 1997). Numerous organizations have proposed health information quality standards, including URAC, the first organization to offer accreditation of health websites (URAC, n.d.). Online health information remains an important enough issue that *Healthy People 2020,* the nation's prevention agenda, continues to track and report data on health website quality metrics for the second decade (U.S. Department of Health and Human Services, n.d.). Healthy People data from 2006 indicate developers provided a privacy policy as the most common quality assurance measure; least common was disclosing content development practices and providing regular reviews and content updates (CDC Wonder, n.d.). Given consumers' concerns about privacy discussed earlier in this chapter, the availability of privacy policies is noteworthy but in practical terms, not as significant as it could be, given the policies' complexity and jargon. The virtual absence of transparent and reliable content development practices is troubling when only 25% of online health information seekers report they always or most of the time check the source and date of the information they find (Fox, 2006). These data suggest consumers are unlikely to confirm the accuracy of the algorithms and database content driving applications and services.

Consumer-generated content challenges the traditional notions of information quality and online privacy. Social networking sites such as StrengthOfUs.org or PatientsLikeMe.com draw members with the promise of connecting them to people like themselves and allowing them to share and exchange information about their situations (ACOR, n.d.). In this context, expert opinion often carries less weight than hearing from others with the same concerns and conditions. The payoff for users is that sharing information can bring quick feedback and support from others (Meier, Lyons, Frydman, Forlenza, & Rimer, 2007). Consumer-generated content demonstrates consumers want to decide for themselves what information they will and will not share and what information is relevant. This content and these decisions fall outside existing policy frameworks for information quality and reliability and represent many of the features of the "wild west" some observers noted when health information first became freely available online (Silberg et al., 1997). Consumers' lack of interest in independent verification suggests eHealth developers bear major responsibility to ensure content accuracy and overall application quality and integrity, including content available through links or other referral mechanisms.

Cost and Payment for Consumer eHealth Services

The business models for consumer and patient eHealth applications are evolving, and the need for public policy to address cost and payment is unclear. In the late 1990s, the Science Panel envisioned public investment in eHealth might be necessary to "make the market" and address the needs of underserved populations. By 2010, IT industry leaders, such as Microsoft, have entered the PHR market, and health "apps" are available for purchase and download from popular online stores. How quickly consumers and patients choose to purchase applications and how many receive access through another means, such as health insurance or an employer, will likely influence the need for policy to address gaps in access or diversity of applications.

A panel of PHR industry leaders outlined three business models for PHRs, and these models likely have applicability for other eHealth applications (Office of the National Coordinator for Health IT, 2010). One model is PHRs available to members of health care organizations, such as Kaiser Permanente or Group Health Cooperative, or health insurers such as Aetna. Kaiser and Group Health provide PHRs and related patient eHealth applications as part of the regular member costs. A second model focuses on employers as the PHR sponsor. Aetna and independent PHR vendors such as Dossia and Microsoft HealthVault market their applications to employers and health plans that purchase the applications for employees or beneficiaries. A third model is grant-funded work. A fourth model, one not identified by the panel, is the free-standing PHR that consumers and patients purchase on their own. This model might provide some safeguards and peace of mind in terms of denying employers and insurers access, but also might be limited in connectivity to other applications and patients' EHRs.

Similar to PHRs, telemedicine services have struggled to cover costs and generate reimbursements for services since their inception (see Bashshur, Reardon, & Shannon, 2000, for definitions and an historical review of telemedicine). In many ways, telemedicine and consumer eHealth share common limitations from an economic perspective. Telemedicine provided benefits primarily to the patient, not the clinician or health care facility. Patients who tried telemedicine services were often geographically isolated from health care services and welcomed telemedicine as a means to avoid lengthy and costly travel to distant specialists and facilities. On the other hand, the clinicians and facilities were expected to invest in expensive equipment without the promise of extra reimbursement. Consumer eHealth provides similar benefits to consumers and patients and similar costs to clinicians and facilities. If relatively healthy consumers can purchase and download an "app" from an online store to track their weight, exercise habits, and tobacco use, or manage their diabetes, then they may have fewer reasons to visit the doctor or use the digital tools provided by the clinic or health plan. Yet, as a result of the HITECH Act, clinicians and facilities are investing in EHRs to modernize their own business operations and meet federal requirements, even if their patients look elsewhere for online support. eHealth developers may need to decide if they want to compete or cooperate with clinicians, mainstream technology companies, and EHR and PHR systems for patient "eyeballs" and loyalty.

Implications of Health IT Policy Developments for eHealth

The eHealth applications covered in this volume are part of the evolving health IT policy landscape. Even if HIPAA does not fully apply to eHealth applications yet, the amount of personal health information that people must provide to use most eHealth applications places it in the thick of debates about privacy and security protections. The relevance of privacy and security issues will only increase for eHealth developers and researchers as eHealth applications interconnect with or become fully integrated with EHRs and PHRs. Issues of access, information, and application quality and cost also will increase in relevance as developers and researchers decide if and how they will distribute eHealth applications to populations with limited financial resources and health literacy.

Because eHealth has at least partial roots in the academic discipline of communication, researchers in communication and related fields such as psychology and consumer marketing are well-positioned to challenge notions of technological and marketplace determinism that often drives policy debates and decisions. Computer codes, data standards, and complex policies and interfaces should not be used to separate people from their personal health information and create barriers to informed decision making and necessary care. Researchers can offer options for authentic consumer and patient engagement based on models of trusting and reciprocal exchanges rather than technocratic approaches that separate people from data and existing relationships with clinicians. eHealth can be an exemplar to enhance transparency and dialogue in health services if developers and researchers engage in the significant policy work happening at the federal and state levels. eHealth can help create more e-patient Daves than worried patients who view eHealth as one more hurdle to getting the health services they need and want.

More than a decade ago, the Science Panel looked into the future and anticipated many of the issues that would confront today's policy experts, application developers, clinicians, researchers, consumers, and patients. Recent federal legislation has created the infrastructure and provided resources to address many of these longstanding policy issues. Marketplace pressures may drive technology to overtake the policy apparatus. eHealth developers, researchers, and evaluators should offer their findings and expertise in this process to help shape policies that will multiply the truly empowered e-patient Daves of the present and future.[2]

Notes

1. Readers should refer to the U.S. Department of Health and Human Services's (HHS) Office of the National Coordinator for Health Information Technology (ONC) website for up to date information on evolving legal, technical, and financial policies and standards and initiatives for electronic health records and health information exchange (www.healthit.hhs.gov).
2. The findings and conclusions in this chapter are those of the author and do not necessarily represent the views of the Centers for Disease Control and Prevention/the Agency for Toxic Substances and Disease Registry.

References

ACOR. (n.d.) *About ACOR*. Retrieved January 28, 2011, from: http://www.acor.org/about/about.html.

Agarwal, R., & Khuntia, J. (2009). *Personal health information and the design of consumer health information technology: Background report*. (AHRQ Publication No. 09–0075-EF). Rockville, MD: Agency for Healthcare Research and Quality.

Bashshur, R. L., Reardon, T. G., & Shannon, G. W. (2000). Telemedicine: A new health care delivery system. *Annual Review of Public Health, 21,* 613–637.

Baur, C. (2008). An analysis of factors underlying e-Health disparities. *Cambridge Quarterly of Healthcare Ethics, 17,* 417–428.

Baur, C., & Deering, M. J. (2001). Commentary on "Review of Internet Health Information Quality Initiatives." *Journal of Medical Internet Research, 3,* e29. Retrieved February 1, 2011, from: http://www.jmir.org/2001/4/e29/.

Baur, C., & Deering, M. J. (2006). E-Health for consumers, patients and caregivers. In L. B. Harman (Ed.), *Ethical challenges in the management of health information* (pp. 381–401). Sudbury, MA: Jones and Bartlett Publishers.

Berwick, D. M. (2009). What "patient-centered" should mean: Confessions of an extremist [Electronic version]. *Health Affairs, 28,* w555–565. Retrieved January 30, 2011, from: http://content.healthaffairs.org/content/28/4/w555.abstract.

Blumenthal, D. (2010, July 13). Advancing the future of health care with Electronic Health Records. *HealthITBuzz*. Retrieved February 2, 2011, from: http://healthit.hhs.gov/blog/onc/index.php/2010/07/13/advancing-the-future-of-health-care-with-electronic-health-records-2/.

Blumenthal, D., & Verdugo, G. (2010, July 8). *Building trust in health information exchange: Statement on privacy and security*. Retrieved February 2, 2011, from: http://healthit.hhs.gov/portal/server.pt?CommunityID=2994&spaceID=11&parentname=CommunityEditor&control=SetCommunity&parentid=9&in_hi_userid=11673&PageID=0&space=CommunityPage.

Buntin, M. B., Jain, S. H., & Blumenthal, D. (2010). Health information technology: Laying the Infrastructure for National Health Reform. *Health Affairs, 29*, 1214–1219.

CDC Wonder. (n.d.). *Data 2010, the Healthy People 2010 Database, Objective 11–4.* Retrieved February 2, 2011, from: http://wonder.cdc.gov/scripts/broker.exe.

Centers for Medicare and Medicaid Services. (2010). *Frequently asked questions: What is meaningful use and how does it apply to Medicare and Medicaid Electronic Health Record Incentive Programs?* Retrieved February 2, 2011, from: http://questions.cms.hhs.gov/app/answers/detail/a_id/10084/session/L3NpZC9iZnp5TXhnaw%3D%3D.

Daniel, J. (2010, November 19). Strategy for empowering consumers, round two—continuing the discussion. *HealthITBuzz*. Retrieved February 2, 2011, from: http://healthit.hhs.gov/blog/onc/index.php/2010/11/19/strategy-for-empowering-consumers-round-two-%e2%80%93-continuing-the-discussion/.

DeBronkart, D. (2010, December 23). Back to the future: Tom Ferguson's "epatients" emerge in shared decision-making. *BMJ Group Blogs.* Retrieved February 2, 2011, from: http://blogs.bmj.com/bmj/2010/12/23/%E2%80%9Ce-patient-dave%E2%80%9D-debronkart-back-to-the-future-tom-ferguson%E2%80%99s-%E2%80%9Ce-patients%E2%80%9D-emerge-in-shared-decision-making/.

Delbanco, T., Berwick, D. M., Boufford, J. I., Edgman-Levitan, S., Ollenschlager, G., Plamping, D., et al. (2001). Healthcare in a land called PeoplePower: Nothing about me without me. *Health Expectations, 4,* 144–150.

Department of Commerce Internet Policy Task Force. (2010). *Commercial data privacy and innovation in the Internet economy: A dynamic policy framework.* Washington, DC: U.S. Department of Commerce. Retrieved February 2, 2011, from: www.ntia.doc.gov/reports/2010/IPTF_Privacy_GreenPaper_12162010.pdf.

Diamond, C., Goldstein, M., Lansky, D., & Verhulst, S. (2008). An architecture for privacy in a networked health information environment. *Cambridge Quarterly of Healthcare Ethics, 17,* 429–440.

Eysenbach, G., Powell, J., Kuss, O., & Sa, E. R. (2002). Empirical studies assessing the quality of health information for consumers on the World Wide Web: A systematic review [Electronic version]. *Journal of the American Medical Association, 287,* 2691–2726.

Federal Trade Commission. (2010). *Protecting consumer privacy in an era of rapid change.* Retrieved February 2, 2011, from: www.ftc.gov/os/2010/12/101201privacyreport.pdf.

Federal Trade Commission. (n.d.). *Health page.* Retrieved February 2, 2011, from: http://www.ftc.gov/bcp/menus/consumer/health.shtm.

Ferguson, T. with the e-Patient Scholars Working Group. (2007). *White Paper: e-patients: How they can help us help healthcare.* Retrieved February 2, 2011, from http://e-patients.net/e-Patients_White_Paper.pdf.

Fox, S. (2006). *Online health search 2006.* Retrieved February 2, 2011, from: http://pewinternet.org/Reports/2006/Online-Health-Search-2006.aspx.

Fox, S. (2011). *Health Topics 80% of Internet users look for health information online.* Retrieved February 1, 2011, from: http://www.pewinternet.org/~/media//Files/Reports/2011/PIP_HealthTopics.pdf.

Goldstein, M. M., & Rein, A. L. (2010). *Consumer consent options for electronic health information exchange: Policy considerations and analysis.* Retrieved February 2, 2011, from: http://healthit.hhs.gov/portal/server.pt?open=512&objID=1147&parentname=CommunityPage&parentid=32&mode=2&in_hi_userid=11113&cached=true.

Goodman, K. W., & Cava, A. (2008). Bioethics, business ethics, and science: Bioinformatics and the future of healthcare. *Cambridge Quarterly of Healthcare Ethics, 17,* 361–372.

Institute of Medicine. (2001). *Crossing the quality chasm: A new health system for the 21st Century.* Washington, DC: National Academies Press.

Institute of Medicine. (2003). *Priority areas for national action: Transforming health care quality.* Washington, DC: National Academies Press.

Institute of Medicine. (2009). *Toward health equity and patient-centeredness: Integrating health literacy, disparities reduction, and quality improvement: Workshop summary.* Washington, DC: National Academies Press.

Jansen, J. (2010). *Use of the Internet in higher-income households.* Retrieved January 28, 2011, from: http://www.pewinternet.org/Reports/2010/Better-off-households.aspx.

Kutner, M., Greenberg, E., Jin, Y., & Paulsen, C. (2006). *The health literacy of America's adults: Results from the 2003 National Assessment of Adult Literacy.* Washington, DC: National Center for Education Statistics.

MacDonald, R. (2001). Commentary: A patient's viewpoint [Electronic version]. *British Medical Journal, 322,* 287.

Markle Connecting for Health. (2010a). *Markle survey on health in a networked life 2010 snapshot: The public and doctors agree with "Blue Button" idea.* Retrieved February 2, 2011, from: http://www.markle.org/downloadable_assets/20101007_bluebutton_summary.pdf.

Markle Connecting for Health. (2010b). *Markle survey on health in a networked life 2010 snapshot: The public and doctors express importance of specific privacy policies.* Retrieved February 2, 2011, from: http://www.markle.org/downloadable_assets/20101203_phr_roundtable.pdf.

Maxson, E. R., Jain, S. H., McKethan, A. N., Brammer, C., Buntin, M. B., Cronin, K., et al. (2010). Beacon communities aim to use health information technology to transform the delivery of care. *Health Affairs, 29,* 1671–1677.

Meier, A., Lyons, E. J., Frydman, G., Forlenza, M., & Rimer, B. K. (2007). How cancer survivors provide support on cancer-related Internet mailing lists. *Journal of Medical Internet Research, 9,* e12. Retrieved January 28, 2011, from: http://www.jmir.org/2007/2/e12/.

National Cancer Institute. (2007). *Health Information National Trends Survey (HINTS) 2007 Question HC18c.* Retrieved February 2, 2011, from: http://hints.cancer.gov/questions/question-details.jsp?qid=761&dataset=2007&method=combined.

National Committee on Vital and Health Statistics. (1998). *Assuring a health dimension for the national information infrastructure.* Washington, DC: U.S. Department of Health and Human Services. Retrieved February 2, 2011, from: http://www.ncvhs.hhs.gov/hii-nii.htm.

National Committee on Vital and Health Statistics. (2001). *NHII–Information for health: A strategy for building the national health information infrastructure.* Washington, DC: U.S. Department of Health and Human Services. Retrieved February 2, 2011, from: http://www.ncvhs.hhs.gov/nhiilayo.pdf.

Office of the National Coordinator for Health IT. (2010, December 3). *ONC Roundtable: Personal health records: Understanding the evolving landscape* [Panel 1 remarks]. Washington, DC.

Pew Internet and American Life Project. (2010, May). *Trend data–demographics of Internet users.* Retrieved February 2, 2011, from: http://www.pewinternet.org/Static-Pages/Trend-Data/Whos-Online.aspx.

President's Council of Advisors on Science and Technology. (2010). *Report to the President realizing the full potential of health information technology to improve healthcare for Americans: The path forward.* Retrieved February 2, 2011, from: http://www.whitehouse.gov/sites/default/files/microsites/ostp/pcast-health-it-report.pdf.

Ralston, J. D., Coleman, K., Reid, R. J., Handley, M. R., & Larson, E. B. (2010). Patient experience should be part of meaningful-use criteria. *Health Affairs, 29*, 607–613.

Schneider, S., Kerwin, J., Robins, C., & Dean, D. (2009). *Consumer engagement in developing electronic health information systems: Final Report.* AHRQ Publication Number 09–0081-EF. Rockville, MD: Agency for Healthcare Research and Quality. Retrieved January 28, 2011, from: http://healthit.ahrq.gov/portal/server.pt?open=512&objID=650&parentname=CommunityPage&parentid=7&mode=2&in_hi_userid=3882&cached=true.

Science Panel on Interactive Communication and Health. (1999). *Wired for health and well-being: The emergence of interactive health communication.* (HHS Office of Disease Prevention and Health Promotion Publication). Washington, DC: U.S. Government Printing Office.

Seidman, J. J., Steinwachs, D., & Rubin, H. R. (2003, November 27). Conceptual framework for a new tool for evaluating the quality of diabetes consumer-information websites. *Journal of Medical Internet Research, 5*, e29. Retrieved January 28, 2011, from: http://www.jmir.org/2003/4/e29/.

Shuren, J. (2010, February). *Testimony of Jeffrey Shuren, Director of FDA's Center for Devices and Radiological Health.* Health Information Technology Policy Committee Adoption/Certification Workgroup.

Silberg, W. M., Lundberg, G. D., & Musacchio, R. A. (1997). Assessing, controlling, and assuring the quality of medical information on the Internet: Caveat lector et viewor—Let the reader and viewer beware. *Journal of the American Medical Association, 277*, 1244–1245.

Sittig, D. F., & Classen, D. C. (2010). Safe electronic health record use requires a comprehensive monitoring and evaluation framework. *Journal of the American Medical Association, 303,* 450–451.

Smith, A. (2010). *Mobile Access 2010.* Retrieved January 28, 2011, from: http://www.pewinternet.org/Reports/2010/Mobile-Access-2010.aspx.

URAC. (n.d.) *URAC's health website and health content vendor accreditation programs.* Retrieved February 2, 2011, from: http://www.urac.org/programs/prog_accred_HWS_po.aspx.

U.S. Department of Commerce. (1999). *Falling through the Net: Defining the Digital Divide.* Retrieved May 26, 2011, from: http://www.ntia.doc.gov/ntiahome/fttn99/.

U.S. Department of Commerce. (2010). *Exploring the digital nation: Home broadband Internet adoption in the United States.* (Economics and Statistics Administration and the National Telecommunications and Information Administration Publication). Retrieved January 31, 2011, from: http://www.ntia.doc.gov/reports/2010/ESA_NTIA_US_Broadband_Adoption_Report_11082010.pdf.

U.S. Department of Health and Human Services. (2006). *Expanding the reach and impact of consumer e-health tools.* Retrieved February 2, 2011, from http://www.health.gov/communication/ehealth/ehealthTools/default.htm.

U.S. Department of Health and Human Services. (n.d.). *Healthy People 2020: Health communication and health IT objectives.* Retrieved February 2, 2011, from: http://www.healthypeople.gov/2020/topicsobjectives2020/overview.aspx?topicid=18.

Wynia, M. (Speaker). (2010, Dec. 3). *ONC Roundtable: Personal health records: Understanding the evolving landscape.* Washington, DC. Retrieved March 2, 2011, from: http://healthit.hhs.gov/portal/server.pt/community/healthit_hhs_gov__personal_health_records_%E2%80%93_phr_roundtable/3169/.

15

BUILDING AN EVIDENCE BASE FOR eHEALTH APPLICATIONS

Research Questions and Practice Implications

Nancy Grant Harrington and Seth M. Noar

> I'm sick of following my dreams. I'm just going to ask where they're going
> and hook up with them later.
>
> —*Mitch Hedberg*

Observations and Reflections on eHealth Applications

The ultimate goal of health communication interventions is to improve public health and well-being. A society free from the burdens of illness and disease may sound like a dream, but with the creative and innovative development and effective dissemination of theory- and research-based eHealth applications, we are closer to that dream than ever before. As we consider the topics and issues surrounding the eHealth applications addressed in this volume, several questions arise. What technologies are available, who is using them, and how are they using them? What are the advantages and disadvantages of particular technologies? What are the challenges in their application? What makes them unique? What is the most effective way to use technology to promote health? How do we best evaluate eHealth interventions? How do we disseminate and implement them? And, what is the ultimate impact of eHealth interventions on health behavior change and health outcomes?

The chapters in this volume address all of these questions and more. In this concluding chapter, we offer our thoughts on where we believe the field of eHealth interventions stands and the pressing issues that should be considered as research and development in the area moves forward. We begin with matters related to research and then address matters related to practice.

Research Matters

The variety of health conditions addressed by the applications covered in this volume is impressive, as is the diversity of populations targeted. From basic research being conducted in laboratories to field research that applies what has been developed in the lab to various settings, we have learned a great deal about eHealth applications and their effects. eHealth applications are clearly capable of influencing the gamut of variables along the behavior change continuum, from knowledge to attitudes to behavioral intentions to behavior. The applications may at times act through mediating variables (such as self-efficacy or social support) or have direct effects on outcomes of interest. Many studies reviewed in the applications chapters in this volume show behavioral effects; perhaps even more important, evidence across many of the chapters supports the notion that eHealth applications can influence not only behavior change but also critical health outcomes. For example, eHealth applications have demonstrated reductions in asthma symptoms, depression, and missed school and work days as well as improvements in weight loss, diabetes symptoms, and quality of life. Clearly, many eHealth applications have been successful in reaching their disease management and health promotion goals, and this is very promising for the field. But there is still a lot to learn. Table 15.1 poses some of the important, broad-based research questions in this area using the RE-AIM model (Glasgow, Lichtenstein, & Marcus, 2003) as an organizing guide.

One question is whether some applications are better at influencing certain variables than other applications and what those relationships might be. Each technology will be defined by its platform and features, including the nature and extent of interactivity. Each is also defined by a set of unique characteristics. Do these differences matter, and if so, how? Strecher (2007) distinguishes among four ways in which users can interact with Internet-based programs. These include user navigation (users search the Internet), collaborative filtering (algorithms make recommendations for patients based on what has worked with a similar patient), expert systems (automated computer counseling), and human-to-human interaction (counseling and social support via the Internet). How can these various types of interactivity be best matched based on individual characteristics and particular health issues? And in what circumstances are these strategies best deployed individually versus deployed in combination in the context of more comprehensive programs? As Strecher discusses, these questions should be the basis for much future research.

Another compelling question is the influence of eHealth applications on interpersonal relationships. A team-based game may be designed to improve a health outcome, but it also may affect relationships between team members. An avatar may be a fine way for a patient to present a health concern to her new physician, but it also could lay the foundation for a better face-to-face relationship. The CarePartners program detailed in Piette and Beard's chapter undoubtedly

Table 15.1 Some broad-based research questions on eHealth applications

RE-AIM dimensions	Research questions
Reach	Which populations are using which technologies, and how is use changing over time?
	How are technologies being used differently across individuals and populations?
	Who can be reached with particular eHealth applications? Who cannot?
	How do we best match eHealth applications to individuals and populations?
	How can study samples be recruited and retained in eHealth studies?
	How can eHealth applications extend the reach of interventions and campaigns?
Efficacy	Which types of eHealth applications are most efficacious with which individuals/populations?
	Can eHealth applications outperform standard interventions and practices?
	Which features of eHealth applications make them more or less efficacious?
	What are mediators and moderators of efficacious eHealth applications?
	How can we best evaluate eHealth applications, including social media?
	In which cases are eHealth applications best used as stand-alone interventions versus supplements to human-delivered or media-based interventions?
	What is the impact of eHealth applications on interpersonal relationships?
Adoption/ Implementation/ Maintenance	How can reach/efficacy research be best designed for ultimate dissemination?
	What are cost and other advantages of eHealth applications over other interventions?
	How can eHealth applications be developed with ease of adoption in mind?
	What are the barriers and facilitators to adoption of eHealth applications in various settings?
	How can efficacious eHealth applications be "brought to market" in the public and private sectors?
	How do current and emerging policies affect the ability to disseminate eHealth applications?
	How can consumers be incentivized to engage with eHealth applications?
	How can the use of eHealth applications be sustained over time (at both the individual and institutional levels)?

influences the relationship between the patient and the family member or friend serving as the partner. Whether these applications have a positive impact and how eHealth applications can be designed to promote that, in addition to meeting (and not compromising) the primary objective of positively influencing health behaviors and outcomes, should be of interest to researchers.

The above discussion raises a larger question of the role of eHealth applications. While some applications may be designed as stand-alone programs, others are so-called hybrid programs designed to supplement or extend more traditional health communication efforts (Bull, 2011). Different health communication contexts will call for different approaches. For example, many Internet-based interventions discussed in Buller and Floyd's chapter and in the literature (Lustria, Cortese, Noar, & Glueckauf, 2009; Ritterband, Thorndike, Cox, Kovatchev, & Gonder-Frederick, 2009) are clearly designed as stand-alone programs. In fact, many of these programs are designed as "expert systems" that essentially replace a human counselor with automated computerized counseling (Strecher, 2007). This approach was also exemplified in our chapter on tailored interventions in which the TIPSS program was described as being tested as a replacement for face-to-face counseling (Noar et al., 2011b). The approach has several advantages, the most critical being low cost to deliver when compared with the cost of human counseling.

In some contexts, replacing human counselors altogether may not make sense, but rather employing "online therapists" may be most effective (Tate & Zabinski, 2004). For example, several studies by Tate and colleagues have demonstrated the efficacy of counseling conducted via email or online for weight loss (Tate, Jackvony, & Wing, 2003, 2006; Tate, Wing, & Winett, 2001). In one study, email counseling significantly enhanced the effects of an Internet-based program (Tate et al., 2003), while in another study, online counseling better sustained weight loss effects when compared to an automated, tailored Internet-based intervention (Tate et al., 2006). Together, these studies suggest that in the weight loss area (mediated) human support may be critical to success.

Finally, in still other cases, eHealth applications can be used as supplements to more traditional health promotion efforts. For example, many of the health video games described in the chapter by Lieberman—such as the *Packy & Marlon* game—could be used to supplement regular visits with one's doctor. Also, many newer technologies being integrated into health campaigns, such as social media (described in the Taubenheim et al. chapter), are being used to extend the reach and impact of campaigns, rather than to replace particular communication channels (Abroms, Schiavo, & Lefebvre, 2008). As technology continues to become a larger part of our lives, understanding the best ways to supplement or in some cases replace face-to-face interaction with computer-mediated interaction will become increasingly important.

Another research-related question regards evaluation. We know that evaluation can be facilitated and enhanced through technology. Survey data can be collected and entered into a database simultaneously, large samples can be easily obtained through online recruiting, attrition can be reduced through follow-up with participants via their mobile phones instead of landlines, data quality can be enhanced through greater anonymity, and data beyond standard questionnaire responses can be collected through various applications (e.g., length of time the subject uses the application, performance data). However, there are also numerous challenges to eHealth evaluation, especially online, with issues related to privacy, informed consent, user identity, delivering incentives, retention, and data integrity being particularly apparent (Bull, 2011; Pequegnat et al., 2007). There are also concerns regarding evaluation lagging behind the rapid changes in the technology field (Bull, 2011; Strecher, 2007) because, by definition, careful evaluation takes time.

As was described in virtually all of the applications chapters in this volume, rigorous evaluation designs such as randomized controlled trials (RCTs) have been broadly applied in the eHealth field. This is a positive development since strong evaluation is extraordinarily important to understanding what does and does not work. As the current volume demonstrates, such trials have begun to build a significant evidence base for the effects of eHealth applications. Recent work has also discussed the relevance of CONSORT reporting requirements to eHealth applications (Baker et al., 2010). These important recommendations encourage authors to be thoughtful and clear in their reporting of RCTs testing eHealth applications and can help to build an even stronger literature in the future.

We also know, however, that depending on the stage of development of an intervention, rigorous evaluation by traditional standards may be difficult or impossible. For example, Rabin and Glasgow point out in their chapter that as we move toward more dissemination and implementation (T2+) research, issues of external validity necessarily take precedence over issues of internal validity. This recognition is critical because the eHealth field should be focused not only on what works but also on how we can translate what works into practice (Glasgow, 2007; Noar, 2011). Thus, more flexible research designs will need to be applied in T2+ studies in order to balance both rigor and practical application. Glasgow (2007) recommends that in future eHealth research, we conduct "practical clinical trials": trials that study representative patients, are conducted in multiple settings, employ alternative interventions as control groups, and report on outcomes relevant to several audiences, including policymakers. Surely, we must take care to *not* repeat the mistakes of earlier health behavior change research in which efficacy was almost the sole focus of the field, at the expense of critical dimensions relevant to translation and dissemination (Glasgow et al., 2003).

Moreover, it is important to point out that the rapidly growing platforms for eHealth, such as social media, do not readily lend themselves to neat RCTs. The very nature of social media is such that success means one's message is no longer "controlled," such as when something "goes viral." This is at odds with traditional experimental design in which all elements are under the investigator's control. What can be done in this situation? One approach would be to simulate an online environment, but in a controlled study, in order to gather some clues as to whether the approach is engaging and shows some promise. Then, the program could be applied in a real-world manner in which a more flexible design (e.g., quasi-experimental design) would be applied. While from a research design perspective the study would have lower internal validity than an RCT, from a translational perspective the study would have much greater external validity. This situation is in many ways analogous to the health communication campaigns literature, in which RCTs can seldom be applied and thus quasi-experimental designs often take their place. In that case, there are several things evaluators can do to make such designs as strong as possible (see Hornik, 2002; Noar, Palmgreen, & Zimmerman, 2009).

Another important area to address is theory. The eHealth applications included in this volume all have been or can be informed by common health behavior change theories, such as social cognitive theory (Bandura, 1986), the theory of reasoned action/planned behavior/integrated model (Fishbein & Ajzen, 2010), and the transtheoretical model (Prochaska, DiClemente, & Norcross, 1992). Some applications have been very strongly theory driven, such as tailored interventions; other areas, such as games and mobile phone applications, have had spotty application of theory. Internet-based interventions appear to fall somewhere in between these two extremes. What is clear is that while existing theory is useful for guiding research on processes such as learning and attitude and behavior change, there is a need for theory development to describe and explain the functions and effects of interactive technologies themselves (Neuhauser & Kreps, 2003). Several chapters in this volume (including Buller & Floyd, Noar & Harrington, and Abroms, Padmanabhan, & Evans) make this point, and such work will require scholars in interactivity and health communication to collaborate. As demonstrated in the chapter by Chung, interactivity is a complex construct, and understanding what its effects are (both theoretically and empirically) in eHealth applications will take careful research aimed at such a purpose. This discussion also relates to a larger point about eHealth applications: To the extent that we can understand principles of effective applications, we can transcend the technology of the moment and create knowledge that may be applicable when the next technology emerges. Research with such a focus will be helpful in building a cumulative eHealth literature base that not only tells us *what* works but also helps inform the question of *why* it works in the first place (Noar, Harrington, Van Stee, & Aldrich, 2011; Strecher, 2009).

Finally, an important research-related issue to address is the relative role of the individual and society in public health. We noted in the introductory chapter that several chronic conditions are rooted in human behavior and that 50% of annual deaths in the United States could be prevented if people changed their risk-related health behavior (e.g., smoking, diet, exercise, alcohol consumption). Such observations frame the individual as the source of the problem and suggest that it is individuals who must be reached with messages to change their problematic behavior. Indeed, the eHealth applications presented in this book target individuals: Text messages reach individuals through their mobile phones, tailored interventions reach individuals through computer kiosks, YouTube campaign videos reach individuals through the Internet. While individuals need to be responsible for their behavioral choices, we also recognize that social, environmental, economic, and other societal forces are a powerful influence on behavior (McLeroy, Bibeau, Steckler, & Glanz, 1988). A clear case in point is the movement to ban smoking in public places, whether in restaurants or shopping malls, university campuses, or entire cities. A person who wants to quit smoking—with or without the aid of an eHealth application—is positioned to have much greater success in an environment that bans the behavior than allows it.

With this observation, we believe it is time to explicitly consider how eHealth applications can be applied beyond the level of the individual. As the health behavior change field increasingly focuses on the influence of factors beyond the individual level, there are increasing calls for both theory (DiClemente, Crosby, & Kegler, 2009) and intervention (Blankenship, Friedman, Dworkin, & Mantell, 2006) at that broader level. Perhaps the approach that currently comes closest to this is the use of social media as part of community-level campaign efforts, such as that discussed in Taubenheim et al. (this volume). Another promising approach could be the application of eHealth to media advocacy. *Media advocacy* is defined as "the strategic use of mass media in combination with community organizing to advance health public policies" (Wallack & Dorfman, 2001, p. 389). It recognizes social inequities as the root cause of public health problems, and it works to change public policy through reaching the powerbrokers and decision makers. Historically, media advocacy has emphasized getting the message out through traditional news media and advertising, but today these outlets are evolving or being replaced entirely with new media. When we consider that social media fired a revolution that ended the 30-year rule of Egyptian president Hosni Mubarak, and that new media played a significant role in electing President Barack Obama (Abroms & Lefebvre, 2009), the idea of improving public health through eHealth media advocacy seems like one whose time has come.

Practice Matters

The question of what goes on in actual practice provides an opportunity to raise some concerns. One concern regards the quality of the applications and health information currently available. Abroms, Padmanabhan, and Evans (this volume) cited a study (Dolan, 2010) that estimated there were approximately 6,000 health-related apps available for smartphones. How much development and testing went into those applications? It could be a great deal; it could be next to none. The applications may prove helpful; they may have no impact; they could do harm. In most cases, we do not know.

Apps of questionable quality are not the only concern, of course. With interactivity being the hallmark of Web 2.0, we must also question the quality of user-provided information. In her chapter, Baur refers to the "wild west" nature of the information landscape, where the quality and reliability of information provided by users is unknown. The information may be accurate, of course, and the social and psychological benefits of blogging for the user can represent positive outcomes, as Chung (this volume) observes. Still, we must always be on alert for potentially negative effects. The need for a media and health literate population has never been more apparent.

On a more positive note, as research evolves and we develop a more thorough understanding of the interactions between applications, target populations, and health behaviors, one of the most exciting implications for practice is the ability of eHealth applications to address the broad array of health conditions. From prevention to treatment, from managing chronic conditions to treating addictions, from confronting physical disease to mental illness, the potential for eHealth applications to have a positive impact is clear. The promise is particularly exciting for mental health issues. These conditions continue to suffer the burden of stigma, which may compromise a person's willingness to seek treatment. eHealth applications not only can revolutionize approaches to treatment (such as using a virtual environment to treat phobias) but also can be a gateway to help for individuals who otherwise may not have access to treatment (e.g., online access to social support groups) (Wright, 2009).

Issues of access introduce the question of the digital divide: the gap in access to technology between the "haves" and the "have nots." With eHealth applications, the digital divide is much more complicated than mere access, although that does continue to be a problem in some areas. Instead, we have new divides introduced by differences in features of technologies, differences in patterns of use, and differences in interest and motivation among audience members. The variety of mobile phones available today is staggering. An application delivered via one of the many kinds of smartphones may provide a different experience for its user than the application delivered via a different phone. Such an application likely cannot be accessed at all via a phone that only allows voice and text messaging. Different groups of users will use the same technologies differently. As Abroms et al. (this volume) point out, although mobile phones are ubiquitous in the United States, they are more common among African Americans and Hispanics than whites, and African Americans and Hispanics are also heavier users than whites. As Fjeldsoe, Miller, and Marshall (this volume) observe, although persons in developing countries may have mobile phones, they rely on them for voice communication instead of texting (as is common in more developed countries). Even among affluent populations with no limits on access to technology, individual differences in interest and motivation will result in subgroups, some of whom may resemble Luddites. These differences suggest a role for tailoring within applications to meet individual needs.

Assuming digital divides can be crossed, the promise of eHealth applications will only be realized if these applications see the light of day. Indeed, a major concern in health behavior change intervention research is the issue of dissemination and implementation (see Rabin & Glasgow, this volume). This is actually a two-part question: (1) how to make the translation from research project to marketable product and (2) how to reach audiences once a product makes it to the market. Too many promising interventions sit on shelves in academic offices because of the chasm between academe and industry. This situation highlights the importance of interdisciplinary, team-based research. As Lieberman observes in her chapter, the development of a game to improve health requires a host of players: social behavioral scientists, content experts, target population experts, game designers, and game researchers. To this list we would add experts in product development, business, and marketing. Even if every intervention shown to be effective in T1 trials did end up on the market, though, as Buller and Floyd (this volume) and others have observed, the question of how to get the target audience to actually use the intervention remains. Expertise in product development and marketing can certainly help in this area.

One of the issues at the heart of the divide between research-based program development and translation on a large scale to the public is this divide between academe and industry. Although there are notable exceptions, academic researchers for the most part are not business people. We are trained to be experts in our respective fields; to design and conduct rigorous, theory-based research; and to publish our work in academic outlets. Our universities reward this type of productivity through promotion and tenure; we might even receive an award from our professional disciplines if we're fortunate. Contrast this with business and industry, an environment that requires a different skill set and mind-set, an environment with a profit motive, an environment that rewards the bottom line. In the 2 (design effectiveness: low, high) × 2 (dissemination effectiveness: low, high) factorial design of life, academe shows a main effect for design, and business shows a main effect for dissemination. What is needed is an interaction.

To be sure, there are some academics who also thrive in the business world, often by splitting their time but sometimes by crossing over entirely (but not forgetting their academic roots and training in theory-based research and development). Further, some universities are now encouraging and rewarding the entrepreneurial faculty member. The University of Kentucky, for example, has an office for commercialization and economic development (with the slogan "research means business"). The office works to develop university-industry partnerships, promote start-up companies, and commercialize university-based intellectual properties and technologies. We believe it is the exceptional individual, though, who has the time, energy, and ability to be both an academic and an entrepreneur. If this trend is to become the norm, graduate program curricula will need to be modified to include required courses in business and marketing, and the reward structure of the university will need to be restructured to value more than extramural grants and peer-reviewed publications.

Finally, we do not want to leave out the possibility of public sector dissemination. Historically, we have not done as good a job in this area as we would like, and recent efforts have attempted to improve on this situation. For instance, the Centers for Disease Control and Prevention's Diffusion of Effective Behavioral Interventions constitutes an explicit effort to improve the diffusion of evidence-based HIV prevention interventions into practice (Collins, Harshbarger, Sawyer, & Hamdallah, 2006). However, the eHealth arena brings with it new dissemination challenges, since technology infrastructure and expertise are needed to deliver such interventions. As was discussed in our chapter on tailored interventions, technical issues have contributed to the startling lack of dissemination of most individually tailored interventions.

One compelling model that has already emerged in the eHealth area, and that was discussed in the Abroms et al. chapter (this volume), is text4baby. Text4baby is a text messaging service for expectant mothers, designed with the goal to decrease infant mortality. Expectant mothers receive text messages timed to their baby's delivery date, which users input when they sign up. This program was developed and is implemented by a coalition made up of numerous founding partners, sponsors, mobile partners, U.S. government partners, and implementation partners, although a nonprofit group is the lead agency. The service is entirely free for users, including the usual cost of text messages that come to one's phone. As of February 2010, the service had delivered more than one million text messages to over 36,000 women across the country (Text4baby, 2011). Given their success to date, including the significant coalition that was amassed for this effort and the response from the target audience, text4baby represents one very important model for eHealth practice.

Conclusion

An important concluding observation is the following: We are still learning how to best utilize newer technologies such as text messaging, social media, and Internet-based interventions to promote public health. The platforms and features of applications will influence the nature of messages designed for them. How, then, should messages be adapted to meet the limitations of or take advantage of the flexibility of a particular technology? Often, when new technologies emerge, we begin using them in a traditional manner, such as when the Internet was being used simply as an information transfer technology. As Web 2.0 emerged, the potential of the Internet as much more than a simple information delivery channel was realized (Cassell, Jackson, & Cheuvront, 1998; Thackeray, Neiger, Hanson, & McKenzie, 2008). Similarly, in many areas of eHealth, we are just beginning to appreciate how to use these technologies and take advantage of their unique strengths and attributes. This journey will take time.

When we think about the rapid pace of development in technology—how much has changed in the past 10 years alone—we are inspired by the promise and possibilities of the future of eHealth applications. Of course, we need to keep in mind one truism: Just because something can be done, doesn't mean it should be done. Developing creative, innovative technology-based interventions to promote health is a fine endeavor as long as it does not replace an approach that works perfectly well. At the same time, the use of new media technology should be applied beyond interventions that target individual level health behaviors to broader approaches that capitalize on the power of societal level change. Then, when we catch up with our dreams, we may find that the burden of illness and disease has been greatly alleviated and people everywhere are enjoying the gift of good health.

References

Abroms, L. C., & Lefebvre, R. C. (2009). Obama's wired campaign: Lessons for public health communication. *Journal of Health Communication, 14,* 415–423.

Abroms, L. C., Schiavo, R., & Lefebvre, R. C. (2008). New media cases in Cases in Public Health Communication & Marketing: The promise and potential. *Cases in Public Health Communication & Marketing, 2,* 3–10.

Baker, T. B., Gustafson, D. H., Shaw, B., Hawkins, R., Pingree, S., Roberts, L., et al. (2010). Relevance of CONSORT reporting criteria for research on eHealth interventions. *Patient Education and Counseling, 81*(Suppl 1), S77–S86.

Bandura, A. (1986). *Social foundations of thought and action: A social cognitive theory.* Englewood Cliffs, NJ: Prentice-Hall.

Blankenship, K. M., Friedman, S. R., Dworkin, S., & Mantell, J. E. (2006). Structural interventions: Concepts, challenges and opportunities for research. *Journal of Urban Health, 83,* 59–72.

Bull, S. (2011). *Technology-based health promotion.* Thousand Oaks, CA: Sage.

Cassell, M. M., Jackson, C., & Cheuvront, B. (1998). Health communication on the Internet: An effective channel for health behavior change? *Journal of Health Communication, 3,* 71–79.

Collins, C., Harshbarger, C., Sawyer, R., & Hamdallah, M. (2006). The diffusion of effective behavioral interventions project: Development, implementation, and lessons learned. *AIDS Education & Prevention, 18,* 5–20.

DiClemente, R. J., Crosby, R. A., & Kegler, M. C. (2009). *Emerging theories in health promotion practice and research* (2nd ed.). San Francisco, CA: Jossey-Bass.

Dolan, B. (2010). 3 million downloads for Android health apps. *MobiHealthNews.* Retrieved August 25, 2011, from: http://mobihealthnews.com/6908/3-million-downloads-for-android-health-apps.

Fishbein, M., & Ajzen, I. (2010). *Predicting and changing behavior: The reasoned action approach.* New York, NY: Psychology Press.

Glasgow, R. E. (2007). eHealth evaluation and dissemination research. *American Journal of Preventive Medicine, 32*(5, Suppl 1), S119–S126.

Glasgow, R. E., Lichtenstein, E., & Marcus, A. C. (2003). Why don't we see more translation of health promotion research to practice? Rethinking the efficacy-to-effectiveness transition. *American Journal of Public Health, 93,* 1261–1267.

Hornik, R. C. (2002). Epilogue: Evaluation design for public health communication programs. In R. C. Hornik (Ed.), *Public health communication: Evidence for behavior change* (pp. 385–406). Mahwah, NJ: Lawrence Erlbaum Associates.

Lustria, M. L., Cortese, J., Noar, S. M., & Glueckauf, R. L. (2009). Computer-tailored health interventions delivered over the Web: Review and analysis of key components. *Patient Education & Counseling, 74,* 156–173.

McLeroy, K. R., Bibeau, D., Steckler, A., & Glanz, K. (1988). An ecological perspective on health promotion programs. *Health Education Quarterly, 15,* 351–377.

Neuhauser, L., & Kreps, G. L. (2003). Rethinking communication in the e-health area. *Journal of Health Psychology, 8,* 7–23.

Noar, S. M. (2011). Computer technology-based interventions in HIV prevention: State of the evidence and future directions for research. *AIDS Care, 23,* 525–533.

Noar, S. M., Harrington, N. G., Van Stee, S. K., & Aldrich, R. S. (2011a). Tailored health communication to change lifestyle behaviors. *American Journal of Lifestyle Medicine, 5,* 112–122.

Noar, S. M., Palmgreen, P., & Zimmerman, R. S. (2009). Reflections on evaluating health communication campaigns. *Communication Methods & Measures, 3,* 105–114.

Noar, S. M., Webb, E. M., Van Stee, S. K., Redding, C. A., Feist-Price, S., Crosby, R., et al. (2011b). Using computer technology for HIV prevention among African-Americans: Development of a tailored information program for safer sex (TIPSS). *Health Education Research, 26,* 393–406.

Pequegnat, W., Rosser, B. R. S., Bowen, A. M., Bull, S. S., DiClemente, R. J., Bockting, W. O., et al. (2007). Conducting Internet-based HIV/STD prevention survey research: Considerations in design and evaluation. *AIDS and Behavior, 11,* 505–521.

Prochaska, J. O., DiClemente, C. C., & Norcross, J. C. (1992). In search of how people change: Applications to addictive behaviors. *American Psychologist, 47,* 1102–1114.

Ritterband, L. M., Thorndike, F. P., Cox, D. J., Kovatchev, B. P., & Gonder-Frederick, L. A. (2009). A behavior change model for Internet interventions. *Annals of Behavioral Medicine, 38,* 18–27.

Strecher, V. J. (2007). Internet methods for delivering behavioral and health-related interventions (eHealth). *Annual Review of Clinical Psychology, 3,* 53–76.

Strecher, V. J. (2009). Interactive health communications for cancer prevention and control. In S. M. Miller, D. J. Bowen, R. T. Croyle, & J. H. Rowland (Eds.), *Handbook of cancer control and behavioral science: A resource for researchers, practitioners, and policymakers* (pp. 547–558). Washington, DC: American Psychological Association.

Tate, D. F., Jackvony, E. H., & Wing, R. R. (2003). Effects of Internet behavioral counseling on weight loss in adults at risk for type 2 diabetes: A randomized trial. *Journal of the American Medical Association, 289,* 1833–1836.

Tate, D. F., Jackvony, E. H., & Wing, R. R. (2006). A randomized trial comparing human e-mail counseling, computer-automated tailored counseling, and no counseling in an Internet weight loss program. *Archives of Internal Medicine, 166,* 1620–1625.

Tate, D. F., Wing, R. R., & Winett, R. A. (2001). Using Internet technology to deliver a behavioral weight loss program. *Journal of the American Medical Association, 285*(9), 1172–1177.

Tate, D. F., & Zabinski, M. F. (2004). Computer and Internet applications for psychological treatment: Update for clinicians. *Journal of Clinical Psychology, 60*(2), 209–220.

Text4baby. (2011). *Text4baby.* Retrieved September 7, 2011, from: http://www.text-4baby.org/.

Thackeray, R., Neiger, B. L., Hanson, C. L., & McKenzie, J. F. (2008). Enhancing promotional strategies within social marketing programs: Use of Web 2.0 social media. *Health Promotion Practice, 9,* 338–343.

Wallack, L. M., & Dorfman, L. (2001). Putting policy into health communication: The role of media advocacy. In R. E. Rice & C. K. Atkin (Eds.), *Public communication campaigns* (3rd ed., pp. 389–401). Thousand Oaks, CA: Sage Publications.

Wright, K. B. (2009). Increasing computer-mediated social support. In J. C. Parker & E. Thorson (Eds.), *Health communication in the new media landscape* (pp. 243–265). New York, NY: Springer Publishing Co.

CONTRIBUTORS

Victor J. Strecher, Ph.D., is a professor and director of innovation and social entrepreneurship at the University of Michigan School of Public Health. Dr. Strecher is also founder of HealthMedia Inc., an Ann Arbor–based company that develops and disseminates award-winning tailored health interventions in numerous behavioral areas. Dr. Strecher has been a leading investigator on over \$45 million in grant-funded studies in the digital health communications technologies area. He has published over 100 journal articles and chapters, and he serves on the editorial board of the *American Journal of Preventive Medicine.* Dr. Strecher was appointed in 1998 by Al Gore to serve on the Department of Health and Human Service's Science Panel on Interactive Health Communications and he currently serves on the National Cancer Institute's Board of Scientific Advisors. Dr. Strecher and the organizations he founded—the University of Michigan Center for Health Communications Research and HealthMedia, Inc.—have also won numerous national and international awards for their work.

Seth M. Noar, Ph.D., is an associate professor in the School of Journalism and Mass Communication and a member of the Lineberger Comprehensive Cancer Center at the University of North Carolina at Chapel Hill. He received his Ph.D. in psychology from the University of Rhode Island. His work addresses health behavior theories, message design and media campaigns, eHealth applications, tailored communication, and methodological topics including meta-analysis and evaluation. Dr. Noar and his colleagues have conducted extensive work examining effective health communication strategies for promoting health behavior change, in particular focusing on the development and evaluation of mass media and computer-based interventions. He has published more than 75 articles and chapters in a wide range of outlets in the social, behavioral, health, and communication sciences, and he serves on the editorial boards of several journals including *Health Communication, Journal of Applied Communication Research,* and *Journal of Communication.* Dr. Noar and colleagues conducted the first meta-analysis of computer-tailored interventions (published in *Psychological Bulletin* in 2007) and the first meta-analysis of computer technology–based HIV prevention interventions (published in *AIDS* in 2009). He was the principal investigator of a NIMH-funded study to develop a computer-tailored safer sex intervention for at-risk African Americans and a co-investigator on several NIH and CDC-funded projects. Dr. Noar also recently co-edited *Communication Perspectives on HIV/ AIDS for the 21st Century,* published by Routledge in 2008.

Nancy Grant Harrington, Ph.D., is a professor in the Department of Communication and associate dean for research in the College of Communications and Information Studies at the University of Kentucky. She also holds an academic appointment in the College of Public Health and is a faculty associate of the Multidisciplinary Center on Drug and Alcohol Research. She received her Ph.D. from the University of Kentucky. Dr. Harrington has been a principal investigator, co-investigator, or principal evaluator on several NIH-funded and CDC-funded studies totaling nearly $8.5 million. She has published more than 40 journal articles or chapters in outlets such as *Health Communication, Communication Monographs, Communication Yearbook,* and *Health Education & Behavior,* and she serves on the editorial boards of nine journals, including *Journal of Communication, Health Communication,* and *Journal of Applied Communication Research.* She was a founding member of the Coalition for Health Communication and served as its chair from 2006 to 2008; she served as chair to the Health Communication division of the National Communication Association from 2004 to 2005. She teaches undergraduate and graduate courses in persuasive message design, health communication, interpersonal communication, communication theory, and research methods. Her research focuses on persuasive message design in a health behavior change context, particularly as it relates to risk behavior prevention/health promotion and interactive health communication using computer technology.

Sheana Bull, Ph.D., M.P.H., is trained in public health and sociology and works as an associate professor with appointments in the Department of Community and Behavioral Health, Colorado School of Public Health and in the Department of Health and Behavioral Sciences, both at the University of Colorado Denver. She has been researching the use of technology for health promotion for over a decade and has developed and tested numerous technology-based interventions to facilitate prevention of sexually transmitted infections, including HIV, and to promote improvements in physical activity and nutrition. Her work includes collaborations with researchers and public health experts in Colorado, Wyoming, California, Pennsylvania, Virginia, Kentucky, and Texas, and she is involved in technology-based research for HIV prevention in Uganda, East Africa. She has published over four dozen research articles related to public health and is nationally and internationally recognized as a leader and innovator in the field of technology-based health promotion.

Deborah S. Chung, Ph.D., is an associate professor in the School of Journalism and Telecommunications at the University of Kentucky. She earned her Ph.D. from Indiana University–Bloomington. Her research focuses on the changing dynamics between communication professionals and their audiences through emergent information communication technologies (ICTs) and in particular focuses on how ICTs may empower information consumers. She has studied the concepts of interactivity, participatory communication, and convergence.

David B. Buller, Ph.D., is a senior scientist at Klein Buendel, Inc., a health communication research and media development company in Golden, Colorado. He received his Ph.D. in communication from Michigan State University. In his research, Dr. Buller tests theory-based health communication strategies for reducing chronic disease among children and adults, including over the Internet and on mobile devices. He has published over 130 books, chapters, and articles on his research.

Anna H. L. Floyd, Ph.D., is and independent consultant in health and social psychology. She was previously a postdoctoral fellow with Klein Buendel, Inc., conducting research on health behavior and behavior change. She received her Ph.D. in social and health psychology from Stony Brook University. Her current research projects focus on assessment and reduction of risk behaviors in college student populations, with a focus on addictive behaviors such as cigarette smoking.

Lynn Carol Miller, Ph.D., is a professor in the Annenberg School for Communication and Journalism and the Department of Psychology at the University of Southern California. Dr. Miller is a personality and interpersonal psychologist by training and an expert in the use of virtual interactive technologies (interactive video, intelligent agents/games) for changing risky behavior for men who have sex with men. With Stephen Read, she has developed biologically inspired social computational models of personality and emotion that are used in games and for robots. As principal investigator, she has received over $11 million in funding and has published one edited volume and over 70 peer reviewed articles and book chapters.

Paul Robert Appleby, Ph.D., is a social psychologist and research assistant professor in the Annenberg School for Communication and Journalism and the Keck School of Medicine at the University of Southern California. Dr. Appleby's research focuses on HIV and drug use prevention among youth and adults. Dr. Appleby is interested in using new technology such as interactive video and serious games for HIV and drug prevention as well as other health promotion programs.

John L. Christensen, Ph.D., received his doctoral training in social psychology at the University of Southern California. He has held a fellowship with the American Psychological Association's Minority Fellowship Program as well as research traineeships from the National Institutes of Health and the RAND Corporation. He is currently a postdoctoral fellow at the Annenberg School for Communication at the University of Pennsylvania. His research interests include decision making, emotion, message framing, and the tailoring of appeals to individual differences in future time perspective.

Carlos Godoy, Ph.D., J.D., is an assistant professor of communication and a senior research associate at the Social and Behavioral Research Laboratory's Center for Games Research at Rensselaer Polytechnic Institute. He holds an M.A. and Ph.D. in communication from the University of Southern California's Annenberg School for Communication and a J.D. from the University of California, Berkeley. His research focuses on the role that virtual environments may play in diagnosing and changing real life decision making and behavior.

Mei Si, Ph.D., is an assistant professor in the Department of Cognitive Science, Rensselaer Polytechnic Institute. Her research interests include interactive narrative, serious games, embodied conversational agents, computational modeling of emotion, multi-agent systems, and human-computer interaction. Dr. Si's work on the "Thespian" multi-agent framework for interactive narratives has been applied to authoring dozens of virtual characters in various interactive narratives, including multi-scene language and culture training scenarios and Aesop fables.

Charisse Corsbie-Massay, M.A., earned undergraduate degrees in brain and cognitive science and comparative media studies from MIT, with an emphasis on psychological development, television, and new media. She also earned an M.A. from USC's School for Cinematic Arts in critical studies while conducting research with the Keck School of Medicine to develop cognitively efficient interactive interfaces for medical students. Her doctoral research focuses on demographic representation in media and its effect on internalized norms and self-perceptions, as well as group identity and message retention.

Stephen J. Read, Ph.D., is a social psychologist and cognitive scientist who is an expert in the computational modeling of human social behavior and social reasoning, as well as in the use of interactive technologies, such as interactive video and 3-D games, for changing risky sexual behavior in men who have sex with men. His research covers work on human decision making, social perception, causal reasoning, attitudes and attitude change, and human motivation and personality. He has published two edited books and 84 articles.

Stacy Marsella, Ph.D., is a research associate professor in the Department of Computer Science at the University of Southern California (USC), associate director at the Institute for Creative Technology (ICT) and a co-director of USC's Computational Emotion Group. He received his B.A. in economics from Harvard and his Ph.D. in computer science from Rutgers University. Dr. Marsella's research is in computational models of human cognition, emotion and social behavior, as well as the use of those models in a variety of research, education and analysis applications; he has published over 150 research articles.

Alexandra N. Anderson received a B.S. in kinesiology and a B.A. in psychology and is currently an M.P.H. student in the Global Health Leadership track in the Keck School of Medicine at the University of Southern California (USC). She has been awarded a student fellowship at the Institute for Global Health and works with Hollywood, Health & Society at the Norman Lear Center at USC. Her research interests include racial and ethnic disparities in health and health behaviors, cultural sensitivity in intervention design, and using transmedia approaches to develop effective health interventions.

Jennifer Klatt, M.Sc., is a doctoral student in the Department of Social Psychology: Media and Communication at the University of Duisburg-Essen, Germany. She earned a master's degree in cognition and media science at the University of Duisburg-Essen; her thesis focused on modeling Theory of Mind in the context of HIV prevention. Her research interests include psychological effects of interactivity in games, embodied conversational agents and multi-agent systems, and emotional reactions to an embodied conversational agent that is accompanied by different styles of music.

Jesse Fox, Ph.D., is an assistant professor at Ohio State University. She received her Ph.D. from Stanford University. Her research is concerned with the effects and implications of new media technologies, including virtual worlds, video games, social networking sites, websites, blogs, and mobile applications, particularly in the domains of health and sex, gender, and sexuality. With regard to health, Dr. Fox is interested in how new technologies affect psychological and physical health outcomes; how virtual representations can be used as persuasive agents; and how avatars may be implemented in patient-provider and patient-patient interaction.

Debra A. Lieberman, Ph.D., is a communication researcher at the University of California, Santa Barbara. Her research focuses on processes of learning and behavior change with interactive media, with special interests in digital games, health media, and children's media. She directs Health Games Research, a national program funded by the Robert Wood Johnson Foundation to improve and advance the research, design, and effectiveness of health games. Before joining UC Santa Barbara, she was vice president of research at several companies that developed innovative health games and telehealth systems, and before that she was a faculty member in the Department of Telecommunications at Indiana University, Bloomington. She holds an Ed.M. in media and learning from the Harvard Graduate School of Education and a Ph.D. in communication research from Stanford University.

Lorien C. Abroms, Sc.D., is an assistant professor of prevention and community health in the Public Health Communication and Marketing Program at the School of Public Health and Health Services at The George Washington University (GWU). Her research focuses on the application of communication technologies—including emails, text messaging, and smartphone apps—for smoking cessation and other health behaviors. She has developed and is currently leading an evaluation of the Text2Quit Program, an interactive text messaging program for smoking cessation.

Nalini Padmanabhan, M.P.H., is a consultant with the Public Health Communication and Marketing Program in the School of Public Health and Health Services at The George Washington University (GWU), and a writer/editor at the National Institute of Allergy and Infectious Diseases, part of the National Institutes of Health. She received a B.A. from the University of California, Berkeley in 2007, and a master's of public health from GWU in 2009. She has conducted research on various new media and health topics, such as mobile apps for smoking cessation and the literacy demands of health blogs.

W. Douglas Evans, Ph.D., is professor of prevention and community health, and of global health, and director of the Public Health Communication and Marketing Program in the School of Public Health and Health Services at The George Washington University (GWU). He has published widely on the effectiveness of social marketing and behavior change interventions in various subject areas and global settings. His current research focuses on the use of branding strategies in public health and evaluation methods using new and mobile media. In 2008, he published the volume *Public Health Branding* and is currently finishing a second book, *Global Social Marketing Research,* both from Oxford University Press.

Brianna S. Fjeldsoe, Ph.D., is a human movement scientist and health psychologist working as a teaching fellow at the Cancer Prevention Research Centre in The University of Queensland. Her research and teaching focus on understanding and influencing health behaviors in a population health framework and on developing, implementing, and evaluating physical activity interventions delivered via text messaging for the primary prevention of chronic disease.

Yvette D. Miller, Ph.D., is a health psychologist and behavioral epidemiologist working as a research fellow in the School of Psychology at the University of Queensland. Her research focuses on population approaches to health behavior change, including the application of behavioral theories to achieve large-scale change in disease prevention and health promotion. Dr. Miller's research is largely applied and addresses the translation of behavioral interventions that have proven small-scale effectiveness to field settings to establish their potential for population health impact.

Alison L. Marshall, Ph.D., is a human movement scientist and behavioral epidemiologist and is principal research fellow with the School of Public Health and Human Health and Wellbeing domain in the Institute of Health and Biomedical

Innovation Queensland University of Technology. Her research has a strong community focus, as well as an emphasis on epidemiological methods and contemporary theoretical frameworks to develop innovative physical activity interventions to assist in chronic disease prevention and management. This includes the development, implementation, and evaluation of population-based self-help programs delivered through print, phone, and most recently via the Internet and text messaging.

John D. Piette, Ph.D., is a Department of Veterans Affairs senior research career scientist, VA Ann Arbor Healthcare System, Ann Arbor, Michigan, United States. He is the director of the program on Quality Improvement for Complex Chronic Conditions (QUICCC) and a professor of internal medicine at the University of Michigan. His research focuses on the development and evaluation of low-cost strategies for improving chronic illness care, with an emphasis on socioeconomically vulnerable patients in the United States, patients served by the U.S. Department of Veterans Affairs healthcare system, and patients with complex chronic illnesses in developing countries.

Ashley J. Beard, Ph.D., is a Department of Veterans Affairs (VA) research health science specialist, Ann Arbor VA Healthcare System, Ann Arbor, Michigan, and research investigator in the Department of Internal Medicine at the University of Michigan. Her research focuses on the quality and context of care for older adults with multiple chronic illnesses. She is particularly interested in the intersection of informal and formal systems of care and ways to maximize the utility of both to improve medication use and health outcomes.

Ann M. Taubenheim, Ph.D., MSN, is the chief of the Health Campaigns and Consumer Services Branch, Office of Communications at the National Heart, Lung, and Blood Institute (NHLBLI). She serves as the NHLBI's project director for *The Heart Truth* campaign, overseeing strategic program planning and development, implementation, and evaluation. She also serves as the project officer for the NHLBI Health Information Center and leads the Center's work in developing new technologies for responding to public inquiries and marketing and promoting the Institute's health information to patients, health professionals, and the public.

Terry Long served as the communications director of the National Heart, Lung, and Blood Institute (NHLBI) where she directed media relations, education campaigns, and product marketing for NHLBI's research and education programs. She was the senior manager of *The Heart Truth* campaign since its inception in 2002. Before joining the NHLBI, Ms. Long managed media relations, campaigns, and prevention programs for other agencies of the U.S. Department of Health and Human Services. She retired from the National Institutes of Health in 2007 and is now a consultant in social marketing and health communications.

Jennifer Wayman, M.H.S., is an executive vice president with Ogilvy Public Relations Worldwide, and director of Ogilvy's Social Marketing Practice in Washington, DC. She specializes in the strategic development, implementation, and evaluation of national social marketing and health communications campaigns, with an emphasis on women's health. Currently, Ms. Wayman serves as corporate monitor for Ogilvy's work on the National Heart, Lung, and Blood Institute's *The Heart Truth* campaign, after serving as the project director for five years.

Sarah Temple is a senior vice president and director of client affairs in Ogilvy's Social Marketing practice in Washington, DC. She specializes in strategic health communications planning, public/private partnership development, and corporate social responsibility programming. Currently, Ms. Temple is the project director for Ogilvy's work on the National Heart, Lung, and Blood Institute's *The Heart Truth* campaign and also serves as partnership director for the campaign, guiding outreach and engagement of all partners in the corporate, media, and nonprofit sectors.

Sally McDonough is the director of the Office of Communications for the National Heart, Lung, and Blood Institute (NHLBI). She leads the Institute on communications strategy and the execution of all public affairs and media activities and oversees the Institute's health information center and its public health campaigns. Before joining the NHLBI, Ms. McDonough served as special assistant to the president and director of communications and press secretary to First Lady Laura Bush and as vice president and director of cause-related programming at Ogilvy Public Relations Worldwide, where she managed a broad portfolio of accounts.

Ashley Duncan is an account supervisor with Ogilvy Public Relations Worldwide in Washington, DC, where she manages and implements comprehensive communications strategies for social marketing initiatives. On behalf of the National Heart, Lung, and Blood Institute (NHLBI), Ms. Duncan manages media relations for the Institute and its national awareness campaign for women about heart disease—*The Heart Truth*. She coordinates media outreach and onsite media activities, arranges live programming and promotional elements, and directs national media partnerships with major publications and outlets.

Borsika A. Rabin, M.P.H., Pharm.D., Ph.D., is a staff researcher at the Institute for Health Research at Kaiser Permanente Colorado. She also serves as the research coordinator for the Cancer Research Network Cancer Communication Research Center, one of five National Cancer Institute funded Centers of Excellence in Cancer Communication Research. Dr. Rabin holds a Ph.D. in public health studies and a master's in public health from Saint Louis University, St. Louis, Missouri, and a Doctor of Pharmacy degree from Semmelweis University, Budapest, Hungary. Her research focuses on the dissemination and implementation of evidence-based cancer control interventions with an increasing emphasis on interactive tools. Dr. Rabin was named a Cancer Research Network Research Scholar for 2009–2011.

Russell E. Glasgow, Ph.D., is the deputy director of dissemination and implementation science in the National Cancer Institute's Division of Cancer Control and Population Sciences. He earned his Ph.D. degree in clinical psychology from the University of Oregon, Eugene. Dr. Glasgow is a behavioral scientist specializing in the design and evaluation of practical and generalizable behavior change interventions, especially using interactive technologies, for use in health care, worksite, and community settings. In his current position, Dr. Glasgow provides leadership on numerous research projects to close the gap between research discovery and program delivery in public health, clinical practice, and health policy. He has 30 years of experience in applied research and has been the recipient of key awards and honors in his field, including the Society of Behavioral Medicine's Distinguished Scientist Award and the American Diabetes Association's Behavioral Medicine and Psychology Council Lectureship for Distinguished Contributions.

Cynthia Baur, Ph.D., is the senior adviser for Health Literacy, Office of the Associate Director for Communication, Centers for Disease Control and Prevention (CDC), U.S. Department of Health and Human Services (HHS). Before CDC, Dr. Baur was the Team Leader for Health Communication in the HHS Office of Disease Prevention and Health Promotion. During her time at HHS and CDC, Dr. Baur has led or participated in projects on health literacy, consumer e-health, dissemination of information to vulnerable populations, social marketing, innovative methods in formative research, evaluation of health communication campaigns and interventions and national health objectives in health communication and health information technology.

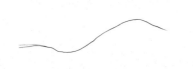

AUTHOR INDEX

SUBJECT INDEX

CPSIA information can be obtained
at www.ICGtesting.com
Printed in the USA
FSOW04n2237231215
14872FS